Elsevier's
VETERINARY ASSISTING
EXAM REVIEW

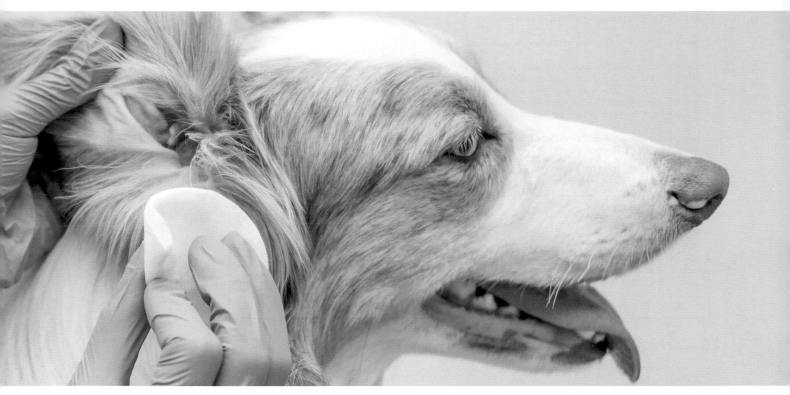

Elsevier's

VETERINARY ASSISTING
EXAM REVIEW

Margi Sirois, EdD, MS, CVT, LAT, VTES

Consultant
TVTS Educational Services
Port Richey, Florida

ELSEVIER

Elsevier
3251 Riverport Lane
St. Louis, Missouri 63043

ELSEVIER'S VETERINARY ASSISTING EXAM REVIEW ISBN: 978-0-323-69442-1

Notice

Practitioners and researchers must always rely on their own experience and knowledge in evaluating and using any information, methods, compounds or experiments described herein. Because of rapid advances in the medical sciences, in particular, independent verification of diagnoses and drug dosages should be made. To the fullest extent of the law, no responsibility is assumed by Elsevier, authors, editors or contributors for any injury and/or damage to persons or property as a matter of products liability, negligence or otherwise, or from any use or operation of any methods, products, instructions, or ideas contained in the material herein.

Library of Congress Control Number: 2020950858

Senior Content Strategist: Brandi Graham
Senior Content Development Specialist: Luke Held
Publishing Services Manager: Julie Eddy
Project Manager: Grace Onderlinde
Design Direction: Brian Salisbury

Printed in India

Last digit is the print number: 9 8 7 6 5 4 3 2 1

Preface

Veterinary assistants have become vitally important members of the veterinary health care team. An educated assistant working directly with a credentialed veterinary technician helps create a powerful team that greatly improves the ability of the veterinarian to attend to animals in their care. Veterinary assistants are also involved in many of the business aspects of veterinary practice and often work closely with management staff in the practice. As the veterinary assistant has become increasingly incorporated into the veterinary health care team, more educational programs have been created to provide the veterinary assistant with the knowledge and skill needed to perform their vital role. Additionally, numerous state and national agencies and organizations have developed examinations to allow the veterinary assistant to obtain a veterinary assistant credential. This book was designed to aid the veterinary assistant in preparing to take credentialing examinations.

Each chapter begins with learning objectives, a chapter outline, and key terms. Recommended readings provide additional sources of detailed information on the topics.

The text is designed to adhere to the model curricula for veterinary assistant training as published by the Association of Veterinary Technician Educators (AVTE) and the National Association of Veterinary Technicians in America (NAVTA). The companion test bank is organized to reflect the domains of knowledge on credentialing examinations, as well as additional information on basic foundations of veterinary assisting. Relative percentages of questions from each domain reflect the general weight indicated for each domain by the largest of the credentialing agencies.

ACKNOWLEDGMENTS

This book would not have been possible without the cooperation of the numerous agencies and organizations that shared information on their examination blueprints. I am grateful for their assistance.

Margi Sirois

Always for my family—especially Dan, Jen, and Daniel.

Contents

Foundations of Veterinary Assisting

KEY TERMS

Appendicular skeleton
Autonomic nervous
  system
Axial skeleton
Buccal
Cardiac cycle
Caudal
Central nervous system
Compound word
Cranial

Dental formula
Distal
Dorsal
Endocrine glands
General senses
Gestation
Integument
Lateral
Lymphatic system
Medial

Mesial
Occlusal
Palmar
Parturition
Peripheral
Plantar
Proximal
Recumbent
Reproductive system
Root word

Rostral
Skeletal muscle
Smooth muscle
Special senses
Tissues
Urinary system
Ventral

LEARNING OBJECTIVES

1. Describe types of cells and tissues of the body.
2. List the names of organs and structures that make up the various body systems.
3. Describe the general and special senses of the body and their functions.
4. Construct medical terms from word parts.
5. Define the meanings of common prefixes and suffixes used in medical terms.
6. Define terms used for common surgical procedures, diseases, instruments, procedures, and dentistry.
7. Describe anatomic terms for direction.
8. Define common abbreviations.

ANATOMY AND PHYSIOLOGY

Cells

- Basic structural and functional units of life
- All living things are composed of cells.
- Many different types of cells may be present, each with its own place and function

Tissues and Organs

- Groups of specialized cells
- Types of **tissues**
  - Epithelial tissue
    - Covers the interior and exterior surfaces of the body, lines body cavities, and forms glands; does not contain blood vessels

- Connective tissue: holds the different tissues together and provides support
  - Adipose connective tissue: lipid-storing cells
  - Loose connective tissue: fiber-producing cells, fibroblasts, collagen fibers, reticular fibers, and elastic fibers
  - Dense connective tissue: same components as loose connective tissue but more densely packed
  - Elastic connective tissue: tendons, ligaments
  - Blood-specialized connective tissue: cells suspended in plasma
  - Cartilage: chondrocytes and various types and amounts of fibers embedded in a thick, gelatinous, intercellular substance; hyaline cartilage, fibrous cartilage, elastic cartilage
  - Bone: osteocytes embedded in a matrix that has become mineralized through the process of ossification
    - Types: long bones, flat bones, irregular bones, sesamoid bones, pneumatic bones
- Muscle tissue: composed of myocytes
- Nervous tissue: composed of neurons; specialized cells that respond to stimuli and conduct impulses from one part of a cell to another
- Organs are composed of functional groupings of tissues.
  - Organ systems are groups of organs that are involved in a common activity.

Musculoskeletal Systems

Skeleton: bones that support and protect the soft tissues of the body (Fig. 1.1)

- **Axial skeleton:** bones of the skull, spinal column, ribs, and sternum

- Spinal column: composed of a series of individual bones—the vertebrae
  - Cervical vertebrae are in the neck region; first cervical vertebra (C1) is the atlas that forms a joint with the skull.
  - Thoracic vertebrae form joints with the **dorsal** ends of the ribs.
  - Lumbar vertebrae serve as the site of attachment for the large sling muscles that support the abdomen.
  - Sacral vertebrae are fused together to form the sacrum.
  - Coccygeal vertebrae form the tail.
  - The number of vertebrae in each region varies with species.
- Ribs: form the **lateral** walls of the thorax or chest
  - Number varies with the species; number of rib pairs is usually the same as the number of thoracic vertebrae.
  - The spaces between ribs are referred to as intercostal spaces.
- Sternum: forms the **ventral** portion of the thorax; composed of a series of bones called *sternebrae*
  - The manubrium sterni is the cranialmost sternebra, and the xiphoid process is the caudalmost.
- Skull: consists of many bones, most of which are held together by immovable joints called *sutures*
- **Appendicular skeleton:** bones of the limbs
  - Thoracic limb: forelimb; scapula, humerus, radius and ulna, carpal bones, metacarpal bones, and phalanges
  - Pelvic limb: hindlimb; pelvis, femur, patella, tibia and fibula, tarsal bones, metatarsal bones, and phalanges
- Visceral skeleton: may be present in soft tissues of the body

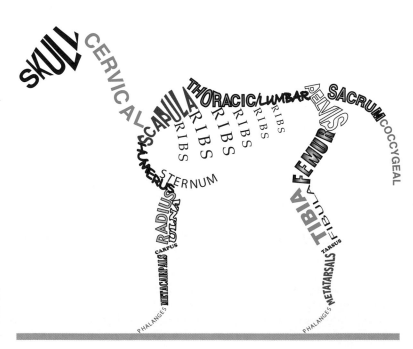

FIGURE 1.1 Word skeleton, the main bones of the axial and appendicular portions of the skeleton. (From Colville TP: *Clinical anatomy and physiology for veterinary technicians*, ed 2, St Louis, 2008, Mosby.)

- Joints: fibrous joints (immovable), cartilaginous joints (slightly movable), diarthrodial, or synovial joints (freely movable)

Muscular system: skeletal muscle, cardiac muscle, and smooth muscle

- **Skeletal muscle:** moves the skeleton; responds to impulses delivered by nerves
  - Also known as voluntary striated muscle; under conscious control; cells have a striped or striated appearance.
  - Skeletal muscles are usually attached to bones at both ends by tendons.
- Cardiac muscle: found only in the heart.
  - Also known as involuntary striated muscle; not under conscious control, and cells have a striped or striated appearance.
  - Cardiac muscle cells form an intricate branching network in the heart and have an innate contractile rhythm that does not require an external nerve supply.
- **Smooth muscle:** found mainly in internal organs
  - Cells do not show any stripes or striations; not under conscious control.
  - Two types of smooth muscle—visceral smooth muscle and multiunit smooth muscle
    - Visceral smooth muscle occurs in large sheets in the walls of the gastrointestinal tract, uterus, and urinary bladder.
    - Multiunit smooth muscle is found where fine, involuntary movements are needed, such as in the iris and ciliary body of the eye and walls of blood vessels.

Integument

- **Integument:** outer covering of the body; consists of the skin, hair, claws or hooves, and horns. In nonmammalian species it also includes such structures as feathers and scales.
- Functions as a protective organ and contains a large number of sensory receptors
  - Helps in regulating body temperature through its ability to adjust blood flow to the skin, adjust the position of hairs, and secrete sweat
  - Produces vitamin D and secretes and excretes a number of substances through various types of skin glands
  - Skin: largest body organ; consists of two main layers, the superficial epithelial layer (epidermis) and the deep connective tissue layer (dermis)
    - The epidermis is composed of keratinized, stratified squamous epithelium.
      - The surface layer of the epidermis dries out and is converted to a tough horny substance called keratin, which also makes up the bulk of hair, claws, hooves, and horns (antlers).
    - Dermis layer of skin is composed of collagen, elastic, and reticular fibers and contains various

sensitive nerve endings, blood vessels, hair follicles, sebaceous glands (oil glands), sudoriferous glands, and arrector pili muscles.
- Hair: covers most of the body surface of most animals; composed of densely compacted keratinized cells produced in glandlike structures called hair follicles
  - At the base of some hair roots, a tiny muscle is attached: the arrector pili muscle.
  - When it contracts, it pulls the hair into a more upright position. This produces what is called goosebumps or raised hackles.
- Claws and hooves are horny structures that cover the **distal** ends of the digits.
  - Composed of parallel bundles of keratinized cells organized into an outer wall and a bottom sole

Respiratory and Cardiovascular Systems
Circulatory (Cardiovascular) System

- Functions to transport substances throughout the body, such as cells, antibodies, nutrients, oxygen, carbon dioxide, metabolic wastes, and hormones
- Two main divisions are the blood vascular system (systemic and pulmonary circulation) and **lymphatic system.**
  - Blood vascular system: closed system of blood vessels through which blood is propelled by the heart to the body tissues and back to the heart
    - Three types of blood vessels—arteries, capillaries, and veins
    - Arteries carry blood away from the heart to the capillaries.
    - The aorta (the largest and main artery) originates from the left ventricle of the heart and carries oxygenated blood to various body tissues.
    - Capillaries are composed of a single layer of endothelium and permit substances to move freely between the extracellular fluid (fluid surrounding cells) and blood.
    - Nutrients, waste products, gases, hormones, and other substances are exchanged at the capillaries.
    - From the capillaries the CO_2-laden, waste-filled blood passes first into small venules and then into veins for the return trip to the heart.
    - The veins take the blood back to the heart and to the **cranial** and **caudal** venae cavae, which open into the right atrium of the heart.
    - Many veins contain tiny one-way valves along their length that help propel blood back to the heart, assisted by movement of muscles in the area.
    - The pulmonary artery carries CO_2-rich blood from the right ventricle of the heart to the lungs for purification (oxygenation).
    - The pulmonary veins bring oxygenated blood from the lungs to the left atrium of the heart.
    - The heart has four chambers, two atria (right and left atrium), and two ventricles (right and left ventricles).

- **Cardiac cycle** refers to the series of events happening during one heartbeat.
  - Includes the relaxation of the heart chambers (diastole) to receive the blood and contraction of the heart chambers (systole) to pump the blood into body tissues and lungs
- Blood
  - Blood is a specialized connective tissue composed of fluid and cellular portions.
  - The fluid portion is plasma, and the cellular portion is composed of red blood cells, white blood cells, and platelets (Fig. 1.2).
  - Plasma is composed of 91% water, 7% protein molecules, and 2% other substances and electrolytes.
  - Red blood cells (RBCs), also called *erythrocytes*, are the most numerous of the blood cells, typically numbering in the millions per microliter of blood.
    - In mammalian species RBCs do not normally contain a nucleus and are shaped like biconcave discs.
    - The protein hemoglobin, which gives erythrocytes their red color, also gives them the ability to carry large amounts of O_2 to the body's cells.

- White blood cells (WBCs), also called leukocytes, typically number in the tens of thousands per microliter of blood.
  - They are divided into granulocytes (neutrophils, eosinophils, and basophils) and agranulocytes (lymphocytes and monocytes).
- Lymphatic system: vascular system that returns excess tissue fluid to the blood vascular system
  - Filters the tissue fluid, examines it for foreign invaders, and manufactures defensive cells and antibodies to help keep the body healthy
  - Lymph capillaries begin peripherally as blind-ended vessels that pick up excess tissue fluid, called lymph, and move it toward the thorax.
  - Lymph vessels contain small one-way valves, similar to the valves in veins.
  - Combined with body movements, these one-way valves help propel the lymph to the thorax, where it is deposited back into the bloodstream.
  - Lymph nodes: found along the network of lymph vessels are small lumps of tissue called lymph nodes that contain large accumulations of one type of lymphocytes.

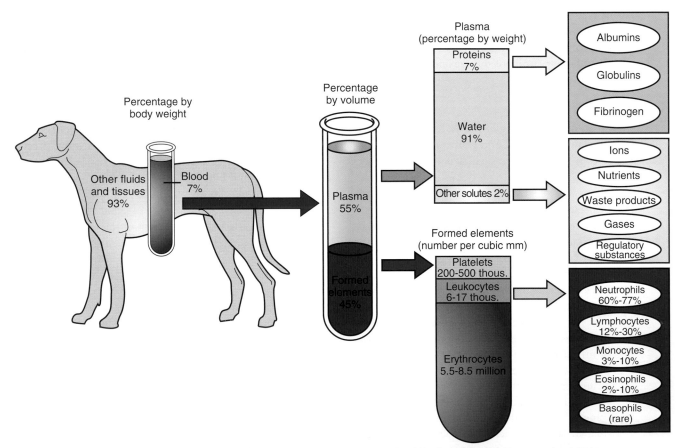

FIGURE 1.2 Composition of blood. Values are approximate for blood components in normal adult dogs. (From Colville TP: *Clinical anatomy and physiology for veterinary technicians*, ed 2, St Louis, 2008, Mosby.)

- The spleen, a large, tongue-shaped organ located near the stomach, is a blood-storage organ, but it also contains large accumulations of lymph nodules.
- The thymus is a lymphoid organ located in the caudal cervicocranial thoracic region.
- Accumulations of lymph nodules are also found in the tonsils and scattered in the lining of the intestines.

Respiratory System

- Primary function of the respiratory system is to exchange O_2 in oxygenated blood for CO_2.
- Secondary functions include vocalization (e.g., barking, mooing), body temperature regulation, and acid–base regulation.
- Internal respiration involves gas exchange between the blood and the body's many cells and tissues, and it occurs at the cellular level within capillaries throughout the body.
  - O_2 carried in the RBCs is exchanged for CO_2 produced by tissue cells.
- External respiration involves the exchange of gases between blood and the outside air, and it occurs in the lungs.
  - Carbon dioxide in the blood is exchanged for O_2 from the air.
- The respiratory system is composed of the upper respiratory tract, which consists of a series of tubes that connect the lungs with the external environment, and the lower respiratory tract, which consists of structures within the lungs (Fig. 1.3).
  - The upper respiratory tract starts at the tip of the nose.
    - The lining of the nasal passages contains extensive networks of blood vessels and a ciliated epithelium coated with watery mucus.
    - Blood circulating throughout the nasal lining warms the incoming air, the watery mucus humidifies it, and the cilia sweep foreign material that has become trapped in the mucus out of the nasal passages.
  - From the nasal passages, inhaled air passes through the pharynx, or throat.
    - This is a common passageway for the digestive and respiratory systems.
  - The larynx, commonly called the voice box, is a short, irregular tube of cartilage and muscle that connects the pharynx with the trachea.
    - At the junction of the pharynx and larynx is the epiglottis, a flap of cartilage that acts as a trap door to cover the opening of the larynx during swallowing.
  - The trachea carries air from the larynx to the lungs.
    - The trachea is composed of several C-shaped incomplete rings of hyaline cartilage, which prevent it from collapsing during inhalation.
    - At its caudal end, the trachea divides into the left and right bronchi, which enter the lungs.

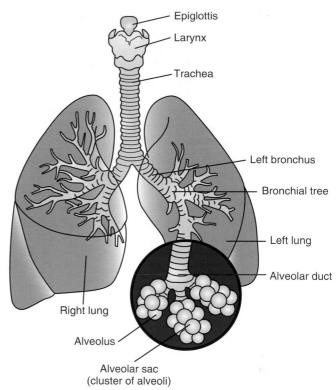

FIGURE 1.3 Lower respiratory tract. (From Colville TP: *Clinical anatomy and physiology for veterinary technicians*, ed 2, St Louis, 2008, Mosby.)

- The bronchi enter the lungs and branch into smaller and smaller air passageways that eventually lead to tiny, grapelike clusters of thin cells called alveoli.
  - The alveolus is the actual site of gas exchange in the lungs.
  - Each alveolus consists of a tiny, extremely thin-walled sac surrounded by elastic fibers and a network of capillaries.
- Inspiration is the process of drawing air into the lungs; it is accomplished by contractions of the diaphragm and other muscles.
- Expiration occurs as muscular contractions compress the thoracic cavity and elastic lung tissue returns to its original shape, expelling air from the lungs.
- Thorax: the area between the neck and diaphragm
- Diaphragm: dome-shaped, sheetlike muscle that completely separates the thoracic cavity from the abdominal cavity
  - Contraction of the diaphragm pushes the abdominal organs down and increases the volume of the thoracic cavity.
  - The lungs expand passively as the thoracic cavity enlarges, and air is drawn into them through the upper respiratory passages.
- Exchange of gases: oxygen diffuses from the alveoli to the blood in the alveolar capillaries; carbon dioxide diffuses in the other direction, from the blood of the alveolar capillaries to the alveoli.

- Control of breathing: two systems control the process of respiration, a mechanical control system and a chemical control system.
  - The inspiratory center in the brain initiates impulses that travel to the diaphragm, allowing it to contract and the lungs to inflate.
  - Stretch receptors in the lungs sense when the preset limit of inflation has been reached.
    - They initiate impulses that travel to the respiratory centers in the brain, stopping inspiration and starting passive expiration.
  - The chemical control system monitors the chemical composition of the blood and initiates adjustments in respiration if it senses fluctuations in O_2 and CO_2 levels or pH.

Digestive System

- The digestive or alimentary system converts food eaten by an animal into nutrient compounds that body cells can use for metabolic fuel.
- Consists of a tube running from the mouth to the anus, with accessory digestive organs attached to it (Fig. 1.4)
- Food moving through the tube is broken down into smaller, simpler compounds through the process of digestion.
  - These simple compounds then pass through the wall of the digestive tract into the bloodstream through the process of absorption for distribution of nutrients to body cells.
- The structure of a species' digestive system is largely dependent on its diet.
  - Herbivores depend on the help of microorganisms, such as protozoa and bacteria, to help break down cellulose through a process called microbial fermentation.
  - Carnivores (meat eaters), such as dogs and cats, depend on enzymes to break down easy-to-digest animal-source nutrients through the process of enzymatic digestion.
- Mouth: food is chewed and mixed with saliva in preparation for swallowing.

- Muscular movements of the tongue and pharynx move the bolus of food back through the pharynx to the opening of the esophagus.
  - Four types of teeth, arranged into upper and lower dental arcades, begin the process of digestion by cutting and crushing the food.
    - The most rostral teeth are the incisors (I); ruminants, such as cattle and sheep, have a firm, fibrous dental pad instead of upper incisors.
    - The four canines (C), if present, are located at the rostral lateral corners of the mouth, adjacent to the incisors.
    - The premolars (PM) are the rostral cheek teeth.
    - The molars (M) are the caudal cheek teeth.
  - Each tooth is composed of three different kinds of firm connective tissue.
    - Crown: the exposed portion of the tooth; covered by enamel
    - The bulk of the tooth is composed of a dense material called *dentin*.
    - The root, which helps anchor the tooth in its bony socket, is covered by cementum.
    - The fibers that connect the cementum to the bony socket are called *periodontal ligaments*.
- Esophagus: muscular tube that connects the pharynx with the stomach
  - The opening of the esophagus into the stomach is regulated by the cardiac sphincter, a muscular ring that functions as a valve to seal the esophagus off from the stomach.
  - The cardiac sphincter opens only to allow swallowed food to pass into the stomach; also relaxes to allow food to pass back up the esophagus in species that can vomit or ruminate.
- Stomach: enlarged chamber in which swallowed food is mixed with hydrochloric acid and digestive enzymes
  - Simple stomach of monogastric animals is a single chamber lined with large folds, the rugae, and dense accumulations of gastric glands.
    - Gastric glands secrete hydrochloric acid and various digestive enzymes, which begin the digestion

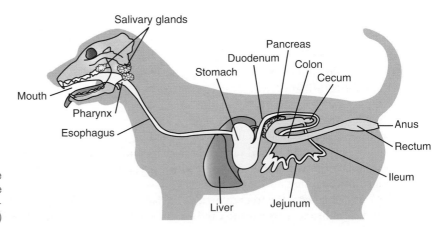

FIGURE 1.4 Schematic representation of the digestive apparatus of the dog. (From Colville TP: *Clinical anatomy and physiology for veterinary technicians*, ed 2, St Louis, 2008, Mosby.)

process, and mucus, which coats the stomach lining and keeps it from being digested along with the food.

- When the food leaves the stomach through the pyloric sphincter to enter the small intestines, it has been converted into a semiliquid homogeneous material called chyme.
- The chyme is moved through the intestine by muscular contractions and further digested by mixing with secretions from the pancreas, liver, and glands in the intestinal wall.
  - Most absorption of nutrients takes place in the intestines.
  - Small intestine has three segments: the duodenum, jejunum, and ileum.
- The large intestine receives undigested and unabsorbed food material from the ileum.
  - Water is absorbed from the chyme and any nutrients not previously absorbed by the small intestine.
- The large intestine segments are the cecum, the colon, and the rectum.
- The anus is the caudal opening of the digestive system to the outside world; surrounded by ringlike sphincter muscles that allow the animal to control defecation consciously.
- Accessory digestive organs: salivary glands, pancreas, liver
  - Several sets of salivary glands produce saliva, a watery fluid that is carried from the salivary glands to the mouth by ducts; primary function is to moisten and lubricate food as it is chewed.
  - Pancreas is located near the duodenum and has endocrine and exocrine functions.
    - The exocrine secretion of the pancreas, called pancreatic juice, is involved with digestion and is carried to the duodenum through the pancreatic duct(s).
  - Liver: assembles simple nutrient molecules into larger compounds, which can be used by the body's cells
    - Also secretes bile, a greenish fluid that carries waste products of hemoglobin metabolism out of the body and aids in the breakdown and absorption of fats and fat-soluble vitamins from the intestine

Nervous System

- Nervous system: detects and processes internal and external information and formulates appropriate responses to changes, threats, and opportunities that the animal continually faces
- The basic structural and functional unit of the nervous system is the nerve cell, the neuron, specialized cells that respond to stimuli and conduct impulses from one part of a cell to another.
- Two types of fiberlike processes extend from the cell bodies of neurons: dendrites and axons.
  - Dendrites conduct impulses received from other neurons toward the nerve cell body.
  - Axons conduct impulses away from the cell body to other neurons or the effector organs, such as muscle cells.
  - The junction of an axon with another nerve cell is called a synapse.
- When a nerve impulse reaches the branched end of an axon, it causes the release of tiny sacs of chemicals called neurotransmitters into the narrow synaptic space.
- When neurotransmitter molecules diffuse across the synapse to contact the cell membrane of the adjacent nerve cell, they induce a change in the other nerve cell.
- Neurons have three unique physical characteristics: they do not reproduce, their processes are capable of limited regeneration if damaged, and they have an extremely high oxygen requirement.
- The main divisions of the nervous system are the central nervous system, the peripheral nervous system, and the autonomic nervous system.
  - **Central nervous system:** nerve cell bodies, nerve fibers (axons), and supporting cells in the brain and spinal cord
    - Brain: cerebrum, cerebellum, and brainstem; housed in the skull
    - The spinal cord is housed in the vertebral canal formed by the vertebrae.
  - Peripheral nervous system: cordlike nerves (bundles of axons) that carry impulses between the central nervous system and the rest of the body; includes the cranial nerves and spinal nerves.
    - Sensory nerves carry information toward the central nervous system.
    - Motor nerves carry instructions from the central nervous system out to the body.
    - Most nerves are mixed nerves, a combination of sensory and motor nerves.
    - Spinal nerves mainly innervate the striated muscles.
    - Cranial nerves: 12 pairs of cranial nerves, mainly arising from the ventral surface of the brain (Table 1.1).
  - **Autonomic nervous system** operates independently of conscious thought to maintain homeostasis, a constant internal environment in the body.
    - Consists of two parts, the sympathetic system and parasympathetic system, which have opposite effects and are in constant balance with each other
      - Sympathetic system produces the fight-or-flight reaction in response to real or perceived threats.
        - In a time of crisis or physical threat, the heart rate and blood pressure increase, the air passageways in the lungs and the pupils of the eyes dilate, digestive tract activity decreases, and the hairs stand on end, producing what is known as raised hackles.

TABLE 1.1 Functions of the 12 Cranial Nerves

Number	Name	Type	Key Functions
I	Olfactory	Sensory	Smell
II	Optic	Sensory	Vision
III	Oculomotor	Motor	Eye movement, pupil size, focusing lens
IV	Trochlear	Motor	Eye movement
V	Trigeminal	Both sensory and motor	Sensations from the head and teeth, chewing
VI	Abducent	Motor	Eye movement
VII	Facial	Both sensory and motor	Face and scalp movement, salivation, tears, taste
VIII	Vestibulocochlear	Sensory	Balance, hearing
IX	Glossopharyngeal	Both sensory and motor	Tongue movement, swallowing, salivation, taste
X	Vagus (wanderer)	Both sensory and motor	Sensory form gastrointestinal tract and respiratory tree; motor to the larynx, pharynx, parasympathetic; motor to the abdominal and thoracic organs
XI	Accessory	Motor	Head movement, accessory motor with vagus
XII	Hypoglossal	Motor	Tongue movement

From Colville TP: Clinical anatomy and physiology for veterinary technicians, ed 2, St Louis, 2008, Mosby.

- The parasympathetic system has the opposite effect and is the rest and restore system.
  - The heart rate and blood pressure decrease, the air passageways in the lung and the pupils of the eyes constrict, and digestive tract activity increases.

Senses

- General senses: distributed generally throughout the body or over the entire skin surface; receptors are fairly simple modified nerve endings.
  - The tactile sense: sense of touch, perceives mechanical contact with the surface of the body
  - The temperature sense is a thermal sense that perceives hot and cold.
  - Kinesthetic sense monitors the position of the limbs.
  - The sense of pain can be set off by overloads of mechanical, thermal, or chemical stimuli.
- Special senses: sensory receptors are concentrated in certain areas; all receptors for the special senses are located in the head.
  - Gustatory sense: the sense of taste; detects chemical substances in the mouth that are dissolved in saliva; receptor cells are located in taste buds found mainly on the tongue.
  - Olfactory sense: the sense of smell; detects chemical substances in inhaled air: receptor cells are located in the epithelium of the nasal passages.
  - Auditory sense: the sense of hearing detects mechanical vibrations of air molecules and converts them into impulses that the brain decodes as sounds (Fig. 1.5).

- External ear: the pinna (ear flap), external auditory canal, and tympanic membrane (eardrum)
- Middle ear cavity: medial to the tympanic; transmits vibrations of the tympanic membrane to the inner ear via three tiny bones called *ossicles* (malleus, the incus, the stapes)
- Inner ear: the cochlea, vestibule, and semicircular canals
  - The cochlea is responsible for the sense of hearing.
  - The vestibule and semicircular canals help in monitoring balance and head position.
- Visual sense: the sense of sight
  - The eye contains sensory cells that generate impulses to the brain through the optic nerve.
  - Components: cornea, sclera, anterior chamber, iris, pupil, lens, ciliary body, retina (containing photoreceptor cells, the rods and cones)
  - Accessory structures: the conjunctiva, eyelids, and lacrimal apparatus, nictitating membrane (in some species)

Endocrine System

- Glands of the endocrine system secrete hormones directly into the bloodstream.
- Partners with the nervous system in regulating and controlling functions in an animal's body
- Major endocrine glands are the anterior pituitary, posterior pituitary, thyroid, parathyroid, adrenal cortex, adrenal medulla, pancreas, testes, and ovaries.
- Table 1.2 summarizes some of the hormones produced by the major endocrine glands.

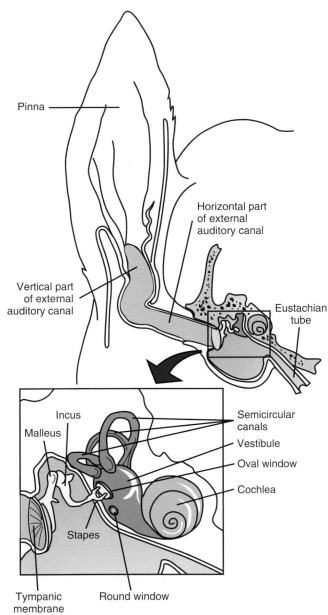

FIGURE 1.5 Cross-section of the dog's ear structures, with middle and inner ear regions enlarged. (From Colville TP: *Clinical anatomy and physiology for veterinary technicians,* ed 2, St Louis, 2008, Mosby.)

Urogenital Systems

Urinary System

- Eliminates harmful waste products from the body
- Consists of two kidneys, two ureters, the urinary bladder, and the urethra
  - Kidneys: paired organs located in the dorsal part of the abdominal cavity, just ventral to the most cranial lumbar vertebrae
    - Nephron: functional unit of the kidneys; consist of the renal corpuscle (glomerulus and Bowman capsule); proximal convoluted tubule; loop of Henle; distal convoluted tubule; and collecting tubule
  - Ureters: muscular tubes that transport the urine by smooth muscle contractions from the renal pelvis to the urinary bladder
  - Urinary bladder: muscular sac that stores urine and releases it periodically to the outside in a process called urination
    - As urine accumulates in the urinary bladder, the bladder enlarges, and stretch receptors in the bladder wall are activated when the volume reaches a certain point.
    - A voluntarily controlled sphincter muscle around the neck of the urinary bladder enables conscious control of urination.
  - Urethra: carries urine from the urinary bladder to the outside of the body
    - In females, it is relatively short, straight, and wide and has a strictly urinary function.
    - In males, it is relatively long, curved, and narrow and serves both urinary and reproductive functions.

Reproductive System

- Main function of the reproductive system is to help maintain the species.
- Male reproductive system: components are the testes, epididymis, vas deferens, accessory sex glands, and penis.
  - Testes produce male reproductive cells (spermatozoa) and male sex hormones.
  - Accessory sex glands: prostate gland is found in all mammals; other glands, such as the seminal vesicles and bulbourethral glands, are present only in certain species.
- Female reproductive system consists of the ovaries, oviducts, uterus, cervix, vagina, and vulva.
  - Ovaries: produce the female reproductive cells (ova) and hormones
    - Under the influence of follicle-stimulating hormone (FSH) and luteinizing hormone (LH) from the pituitary gland, a few ova at a time develop in the follicles of the ovary.
    - As the follicle develops, it secretes increasing amounts of estrogen, which causes the physical and behavioral signs of heat, or estrus.
  - Oviducts: convoluted, tubular extensions of the uterus
    - At its ovarian end, each oviduct is flared to form the funnel-like infundibulum, which catches ova as they are released from the follicles.
  - Uterus: hollow, muscular organ that is continuous with the oviducts cranially and opens, via the cervix, into the vagina caudally
    - In most common domestic mammals, the uterus consists of two cranial uterine horns that unite in a caudal uterine body.

TABLE 1.2 Major Endocrine Glands

Gland	Hormone	Target	Action
Anterior pituitary	Growth hormone	All body cells	Growth, metabolic regulation
	Prolactin	Female—mammary gland	Lactation
		Male—no known effect	None
	Thyroid-stimulating hormone	Thyroid gland	Thyroid hormone production
	Adrenocorticotropic hormone	Adrenal cortex	Adrenocortical hormone production
	Follicle-stimulating hormone (FSH)	Female—ovary (follicles) Male—testis (seminiferous tubules)	Oogenesis Spermatogenesis
	Luteinizing hormone (LH)	Female—ovary (follicle/ corpus luteum)	Ovulation and corpus luteum production
		Male—testis (interstitial cells)	Testosterone production
Posterior pituitary	Antidiuretic hormone	Kidney	Water conservation
	Oxytocin	Female—uterus	Contraction at parturition
		Mammary gland	Milk let-down
Thyroid	Thyroid hormone	All body cells	Growth, metabolic regulation
	Calcitonin	Bones	Prevents hypercalcemia
Parathyroid	Parathyroid hormone	Kidneys, intestines, bones	Prevents hypocalcemia
Adrenal cortex	Glucocorticoid hormones	Whole body	Increased blood glucose, blood pressure maintenance
	Mineralocorticoid hormones	Kidneys	Sodium and water retention, potassium elimination
Adrenal medulla	Epinephrine and norepinephrine	Whole body	Part of fight-or-flight response
Pancreas (islets)	Insulin	All body cells	Movement of glucose into cells and its use for energy
	Glucagon	Whole body	Increased blood glucose
Testis	Androgens	Whole body	Anabolic effect, development of male secondary sex characteristics
Ovary	Estrogens	Whole body	Preparation for breeding and pregnancy
	Progestins	Uterus	Preparation for and maintenance of pregnancy

- Cervix: powerful smooth muscle sphincter that functions to close off the lumen of the uterus from the lumen of the vagina most of the time
- Vagina: the canal from the cervix to the vulva
- Female reproduction physiology: Nonpregnant animals
  - Mammals commonly encountered in veterinary medicine have an estrous cycle, in which the period of sexual receptivity, estrus (heat), is concentrated during a short period, lasting from one to several days.
- The estrous cycle is composed of four or five stages, depending on the species and whether the animal is polyestrous (cycles repeatedly) or monestrous (cycles only once during the breeding season).

- The stages of estrus are anestrus, proestrus, estrus, metestrus, and diestrus.
  - Anestrus is the period of ovarian inactivity, with no behavioral signs of heat or estrus.
  - Estrus is the period of true heat, during which the female allows mating.
  - Metestrus is the short stage during which the female may still attract males but no longer allows mating.
  - Diestrus is a stage of ovarian activity without signs of heat.
- Reproductive physiologic patterns
  - The bitch (female dog) is a seasonally monestrous animal with a definite anestrous period between cycles.
  - Most bitches come into season approximately once every 6 to 7 months.
  - The queen (female cat) is an induced ovulator, meaning coitus (mating) is necessary to stimulate ovulation.
- Fertilization and pregnancy
  - Spermatozoa rapidly move through the cervix, into the uterus, and up the oviducts through a combination of their own swimming actions and contractions of the female reproductive tract.
  - When the ovum arrives in the oviduct, spermatozoa swarm around it, but only one sperm cell is allowed to penetrate the ovum and fertilize it.
  - Soon after fertilization, the nucleus of the ovum and nucleus of the spermatozoon fuse, or combine.
    - The fertilized ovum now has the full complement of chromosomes and is called a *zygote*.
    - After implantation, the placenta, the life support system of the developing fetus, develops.
      - The placenta is a multilayered, fluid-filled sac in which the embryo develops.
      - It attaches to the uterine wall so that its blood vessels and the uterine blood vessels are intertwined.
      - Nutrients and gases are exchanged between these maternal and fetal blood vessels.
      - The developing fetus is linked with the placenta via the umbilical cord, through which blood in the umbilical arteries and vein flows to and from the fetus.
  - Gestation period: the time from fertilization of the ovum to delivery of the newborn; varies among species (Table 1.3)
- Parturition: giving birth
  - Parturition in the bitch is called whelping. In the cat, it is called kittening or queening.
  - Stage 1 is preliminary to expulsion of the fetus; uterine muscles undergo rhythmic contractions,

TABLE 1.3 Gestation Periods of Some Common Species

Species	Range	Approximate Gestation Period
Cats	55–69 days	2 mo
Cattle	271–291 days	9 mo
Dogs	59–68 days	2 mo
Hamsters	19–20 days	3 wk
Horses	321–346 days	11 mo
Pigs	110–116 days	3 mo, 3 wk, and 3 days
Rabbits	30–32 days	1 mo
Sheep	143–151 days	5 mo

which reposition and advance the fetus toward the cervix.
- Stage 1 ends with delivery of the fetus into the pelvic canal and rupture of the fetal membranes.
- Stage 2 is the stage of expulsion of the fetus from the birth canal.
- Stage 3 of parturition is characterized by expulsion of the placenta.
- In polytocous (litter-bearing) species, the cycle of stages 1 to 3 repeats itself with each fetus.
  - Stages 1 and 2 may occur several times and result in the passage of several fetuses before a placenta is passed in stage 3 in these species.

Milk production
- The mammary glands are specialized skin glands that produce secretions essential for nourishment of the newborn.
- Mammary glands are found in males and females, but the hormone environment necessary for their full development and milk secretion only occurs near the end of pregnancy in females.
- Lactation: the process of milk production; begins toward the end of pregnancy
  - Several hormones are involved, chiefly prolactin.
- The initial mammary secretion after parturition is called colostrum and differs from normal milk in composition and appearance.
  - Colostrum has a laxative effect on the newborn and is important in transferring antibodies from the mother to the offspring.
- Suckling or milking stimulates continued production of milk.
  - Stimulation of the teat or nipple causes immediate release of oxytocin from the posterior pituitary gland.
    - Oxytocin has the effect of squeezing milk out of the alveoli and small ducts of the mammary gland into the large ducts and sinuses, where the newborn can extract it by suckling.

MEDICAL TERMINOLOGY

Word Parts and Combining Forms

- Prefix: syllable, group of syllables, or word joined to the beginning of another word to alter its meaning or create a new word
  - May indicate position, time, amount, color, or direction to a root word
- Root word: subject part of the word consisting of a syllable, group of syllables, or word that is the basis (or word base) for the meaning of the medical word
- Combining form: word or root word that may or may not use the connecting vowel *o* when it is used as an element in a medical word formation
  - Combination of the root word and the combining vowel
- Combining vowel: usually an *o*, used to connect a word or root word to the appropriate suffix or to another root word
- Suffix: syllable, a group of syllables, or a word added at the end of a root word to change its meaning, give it grammatical function, or form a new word
- A compound word is two or more words or root words combined to make a new word.

Using Word Parts to Form Words

- A prefix is attached to the beginning of a root word to form a new word.

Prefix	Root Word	Combined	Definition
de-	horn	DEhorn	To remove the horns
semi-	PERmeable	semiPERmeable	Allowing only certain elements or liquids to pass through a membrane

- A suffix is attached to the end of a root word to form a new word.

Root Word	Suffix	Combined	Definition
TONsil	-itis	TONsillitis	Inflammation of the tonsils
THYroid	-ectomy	THYroid**EC**tomy	Removal of the thyroid gland

- Compound word: Two words are joined together to form a new word.

Word 1	Word 2	Combined	Definition
lock	jaw	LOCKjaw	Common name for the disease tetanus
blood	worms	BLOODworms	Worms (nematodes) that inhabit a main artery of the intestines in horses

- Rules related to the use of combining forms and the combining vowel *o*:
  - If a suffix begins with a consonant, use the combining vowel *o* with the root word (the combining form) to which the suffix will be added.
  - Do not use the combining vowel *o* when a suffix begins with a vowel.
  - If the suffix begins with the same vowel with which the combining form ends (minus the combining vowel *o*), do not repeat the vowel when forming the new word.

Combining Forms	Suffix	Combined	Definitions
cardi/o	-logy	CARdiOLogy	Study of heart diseases
mast/o	-itis	masTItis	Inflammation of the mammary glands

Prefix	Suffix	Combined	Definition
dys-	-uria	dysUria	Trouble urinating
POLy-	-phagia	POLyPHAgia	Eating to excess

Combining Forms for Body Parts and Anatomy

- Words for some body parts have more than one combining form.
  - mouth = or/o, stomat/o
  - teeth = dent/o, odont/o

Combining Form	Body Part
abdomin/o	abdomen
aden/o	gland
adren/o	adrenal gland
angi/o	vessel
arteri/o	artery
arthr/o	joint
bronch/o	bronchus
cardi/o	heart
cephel/o	head
chol/o, chole-	bile
cholecyst/o	gallbladder
chondr/o	cartilage
col/o	colon
cost/o	rib
crani/o	cranium, skull
cyst/o	bladder
cyt/o	cell
dactyl/o	digit, toe

Combining Form	Body Part
dent/o	tooth, teeth
derm/o, dermat/o	skin
duoden/o	duodenum
encephal/o	brain
enter/o	intestines
esophag/o	esophagus
gastr/o	stomach
gingiv/o	gums
gnath/o	jaw
hem/o, hemat/o	blood
hepa-, hepat/o	liver
hist/o	tissue
hyster/o	uterus
jejun/o	jejunum
kerat/o	cornea or horny tissue
lapar/o	flank, abdomen
laryng/o	larynx
lip/o	fat
lymph/o	lymph
mast/o, mamm/o	mammary glands
mening/o	meninges
muscul/o, my/o, myos-	muscle
myel/o	bone marrow or spinal cord
nephr/o	kidney, nephron
neur/o	nerve
ocul/o	eye
odont/o	tooth, teeth
onych/o	claw, hoof
ophthalm/o	eye
orchi/o, orchid/o	testes
or/o	mouth
oste/o, oss/eo, oss/i	bone
ot/o	ear
ovari/o	ovary
peritone/o	peritoneum
pharyng/o	pharynx
phleb/o	vein
pil/o	hair
pneum/o	lung, air, breath
pulmo-, pulmon/o	lung
rect/o	rectum
ren/o	renal (kidney)
rhin/o	nose
splen/o	spleen
stomat/o	mouth
thorac/o	thorax
thyr/o, thyroid-	thyroid gland
trache/o	trachea
tympan/o	tympanum (middle ear), tympanic membrane, eardrum
ureter/o	ureter
urethr/o	urethra
uter/o	uterus
vas/o	vessel or duct
ven/o	vein
ventricul/o	ventricle
vertebr/o	vertebra

Suffixes and Prefixes

- Suffixes for surgical procedures

Suffix	Meaning	Example and Definition
-centesis	to puncture, perforate, or tap—permitting withdrawal of substances (e.g., fluid, air)	AbDOMinocenTEsis = surgical puncture of the abdomen to remove fluid from the peritoneal cavity
-ectomy	to excise or surgically remove	CHOLecysTECtomy = surgical removal of the gallbladder
-ize	use, subject to	AnEStheTIZE = subject to anesthesia
-pexy	fixation or suturing (a stabilizing type of repair)	GAStroPEXy = fixation of the stomach to the body wall
-plasty	to shape, the surgical formation of, or plastic surgery (meaning "to improve function, to relieve pain, or for cosmetic reasons")	CHElloPLASty = plastic repair of the lips (to improve looks and function)
-rrhaphy	to surgically repair by joining in a seam or by suturing together	HERniORRhaphy = surgical repair of a hernia
-stomy	to make a new, artificial opening in a hollow organ (to the outside of the body), or to make a new opening between two hollow organs	CoLOStomy = surgical creation of a new opening between the colon and the outside of the body. GAStroDUodeNOStomy = to create a new opening between the stomach and the duodenum
-tomy	to incise or cut into (making an incision)	LAPaROTomy = surgical incision into the abdomen

- Suffixes for diseases or conditions

Suffix	Meaning	Example and Definition
-algia	pain	MyALgia = muscular pain
-emesis	vomit	HemateMEsis = vomiting blood

Suffix	Meaning	Example and Definition	Prefix	Meaning	Example and Definition
-emia	blood condition	AnEmia = lack of blood	brachy-	short	BRAchycePHALic = short head
-esis, -iasis, -asis	infestation or infection with, a condition characterized by	ParEsis = partial paralysis LithIasis = condition characterized by formation of calculi	brady-	slow	BRAdyCARdia = excessively slow heart rate
-genesis	development, origin	CarCINoGENesis = development of cancer	cata-	down, under, lower, against	CaTAbolism = breaking down
-ism	a state or condition, a fact of being, result of a process	HyperCORtiSONism = condition resulting from excessive cortisone	contra-	against, opposed	CONtraINdiCAted = something that is not indicated
-itis	inflammation of	TONsilItis = inflammation of the tonsils	crypt/o	hidden	CryptORCHidism = hidden or undescended testis
-megaly	enlarged	HePAtoMEGaly = enlarged liver	de-	remove, take away, loss of	deHYdrated = excessive loss of body water
-oma	tumor	LEIomyOMa = tumor of smooth muscles	dis-	apart from, free from	DISinFECtion = to free from infection
-osis	abnormal condition or process of degeneration	NePHROsis = degenerative disease of the kidneys	dys-	difficult, painful, abnormal	DysPHAgia = difficulty eating or swallowing
-path, -pathy	disease	pathogenic = disease causing	e-, ec-, ex-	out of, from, away from	ecTOPic = out of place
-penia	deficiency or lack of	LEUkoPENia = deficiency of white blood cells	glyc/o-, gluc/o-	sugar, sweet	HyperglycEMia = a condition of excessive sugar in the blood
-phage, -phagy	eating	COproPHAgy = eating feces	hem/a-, hemat/o-, hem/o-	blood	HEmatURia = blood in the urine
-plasia, -plastic, -plasty	forming, growing, changing	ANaPLAsia = changing structure of cells-RHInoPLASty = surgical change to the nose	hemi-	half	hemiPLEgia = paralysis of one side of the body
			hydr/o-	water, fluid	HYdroCEPHalus = fluid in the brain
-pnea	breathing	DYSpnea = difficulty breathing	hyper-	high, excessive	HYperTHERmia = body temperature higher than normal
-rrhea	flow or discharge	DIarRHEa = discharge of feces	hypo-	low, insufficient	HYpoTHYroidism = deficiency of thyroid activity
			macro-	large	MAcrocyte = large cell

Prefixes for Diseases or Conditions

Prefix	Meaning	Example and Definition			
			mal-	bad, poor	MALocCLUsion = poor fit of upper and lower teeth when jaws close
a-, an-	without or not having	aNEmia = not having enough red blood cells	meg/a-, meg/alo-	large, oversized	MEgaCOLon = abnormally enlarged colon
anti-	against	AntibiOTic = drug that acts against bacteria	micro-	small	MIcrophTHALmos = abnormally small eye

Prefix	Meaning	Example and Definition
necr/o-	death	NEcropsy = examination of dead animal
neo-	new	NeoPLAStic = new tissue growth
olig/o-	few, little	OLigURia = scant urine production
pan-	all, entire	PanzoOtic = throughout an animal population
poly-	many, much	POLyPHAgia = excessive eating
pseudo-	false	PSEUdocyEsis = false pregnancy
py/o-	pus	PYoMEtra = pus in the uterus
tachy-	fast, rapid	TACHyCARdia = excessively fast heart rate
ur/e-, ur/ea-, ur/eo-, ur/in-, ur/ino, ur/o	urine or urea	GlucosURia = sugar in the urine UrEMia = urea in the blood

Suffixes for Instruments, Procedures, and Machines

Suffix	Meaning	Example and Definition
-graph	Instrument or machine that writes or records	ELECtroCARdio-graph = machine that records electrical impulses produced by the beating heart
-graphy	procedure of using an instrument or machine to record	ELECtroCARdiOG-raphy = procedure of using an electrocardiograph to produce an electrocardiogram
-gram	product, written record, "picture," or graph produced	ELECtroCARdio-gram (ECG, EKG) = graphic tracing of the electrical currents flowing through the beating heart
-meter	instrument or machine that measures or counts	TherMOmeter = instrument used to measure body temperature
-metry -imetry	procedure of measuring	doSIMetry = act of determining the amount, rate, and distribution of ionizing radiation

Suffix	Meaning	Example and Definition
-scope	instrument for examining, viewing, or listening	OtoSCOPE = instrument for looking into the ears
-scopy	act of examining or using the scope	LAPaROScopy = procedure of using a laparo-scope to view the abdominal cavity
-tome	instrument for cutting, such as into smaller or thinner sections	MicroTOME = instrument for cutting tissues into microthin slices or sections

TERMS FOR DIRECTION, POSITION, AND MOVEMENT

- Many directional terms come in pairs that mean they are opposite of each other.
- Most terms are relative terms that mean they are used in relation to other parts.
- Left and right always refer to the animal's left and right.

Veterinary Position or Direction	Definition
right and left	the animal's right side and left side
median plane	an imaginary plane that runs down the center of the body length-wise and divides it into equal left and right halves
medial	toward the median plane
lateral	away from the median plane
rostral	toward the tip of the nose when referring to the head
cranial	toward the head end of the body or in a direction toward the head AND on the front of the forelegs above the carpus (the joint corresponding to the human wrist) and on the front of the back legs above the tarsus (the joint corresponding to the human ankle)
caudal	toward the tail end of the body or in a direction toward the tail AND on the back of the forelegs above the carpus (the joint corresponding to the human wrist) and on the back of the rear legs above the tarsus (the joint corresponding to the human ankle)
proximal	a position on a limb that is closer to the point of attachment to the body

Veterinary Position or Direction	Definition
distal	a position on a limb that is farther away from the point of attachment to the body
dorsal	toward the animal's back AND the top/front surface of the forelimb distal to the carpus (the joint corresponding to the human wrist) and the top/front surface of the rear legs distal to the tarsus (the joint corresponding to the human ankle)
ventral	toward the animal's belly
palmar	the back of the forefeet distal to the carpus (the joint corresponding to the human wrist)
plantar	the back of the rear feet distal to the tarsus (the joint corresponding to the human ankle)
superficial or external	toward the surface of the body or body part
deep or internal	toward the center of the body or body part
recumbency	lying down
supine	lying face up, in dorsal recumbency
extension	the act of straightening, such as a joint; also, the act of pulling two component parts apart to lengthen the whole part
flexion	the act of bending, such as a joint

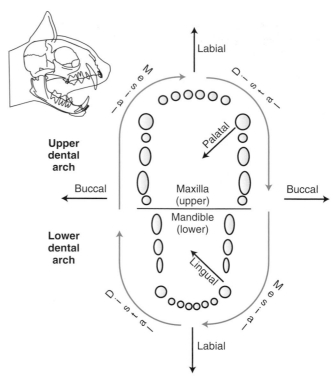

FIGURE 1.6 Positional terminology—the oral road map. (From Colville TP, Bassert JM: *Clinical anatomy and physiology laboratory manual for veterinary technicians*, St Louis, 2009, Mosby.)

DENTAL TERMINOLOGY

- The teeth have their own set of positional terms (Fig. 1.6):
- ocCLUsal: The chewing or biting surface of teeth; toward the plane between the mandibular and maxillary teeth
- BUccal: Toward the cheek; tooth surface toward the cheek
- LINGual: Pertaining to the tongue; tooth surface toward the tongue
- CONtact: Tooth surface facing an adjacent or opposing tooth

- MEsial: Tooth surface closest to the midline of the dental arcade
- A **dental formula** places the teeth in the upper arcade in the numerator position and the teeth in the lower arcade in the denominator position. To get the entire mouth, multiply by 2:

$$\text{Dog}: 2\left(\text{I}\frac{3}{3},\ \text{C}\frac{1}{1},\ \text{PM}\frac{4}{4},\ \text{M}\frac{2}{3}\right) = 42$$

$$\text{Cat}: 2\left(\text{I}\frac{3}{3},\ \text{C}\frac{1}{1},\ \text{PM}\frac{3}{2},\ \text{M}\frac{1}{1}\right) = 30$$

COMMON ABBREVIATIONS

Many common terms are written as abbreviations in medical records. This includes terms for body direction, physical status, specific diseases, and diagnostic procedures. Table 1.4 contains some commonly used abbreviations.

TABLE 1.4 Common Abbreviations

Abbreviation	Definition	Abbreviation	Definition
ad lib	As much as needed	bpm	Beats per minute
BAR	Bright, alert, responsive	BUN	Blood urea nitrogen
Bid	Twice a day	BW	Body weight
BM	Bowel movement	bx	Biopsy

TABLE 1.4 Common Abbreviations—cont'd

Abbreviation	Definition	Abbreviation	Definition
CBC	Complete blood count	NPO	Nothing by mouth
CC	Chief complaint	O	Owner
cc	Cubic centimeter	PCV	Packed cell volume
CHF	Congestive heart failure	PD	Polydipsia
CNS	Central nervous system	PE	Physical exam
COHAT	Comprehensive oral health assessment and treatment	PO	By mouth
CPCR	Cardiopulmonary-cerebral resuscitation	PRN	As often as needed
		pt	Patient
CPR	Cardiopulmonary resuscitation	PU/PD	Polyuria/polydipsia
CSF	Cerebrospinal fluid	q24h	Once a day
CVP	Central venous pressure	qh	Every hour
Cysto	Cystocentesis	qid	Four times a day
ddx	Differential diagnosis	QNS	Quantity not sufficient
Diff	Differential white blood cell count	R/I	Rule in
DLH	Domestic longhair (cat)	R/O	Rule out
DSH	Domestic shorthair (cat)	RBC	Red blood cell
dx	Diagnosis	Rx	Prescription
FLUTD	Feline lower urinary tract disease	SF	Spayed female
FUO	Fever of unknown origin	SC	Subcutaneous
fx	Fracture	SG	Specific gravity
GI	Gastrointestinal	sid	Once a day
Hb	Hemoglobin	SQ	Subcutaneous
HBC	Hit by car	sx	Surgery
Hct	Hematocrit	tid	Three times a day
HR	Heart rate	TNTC	Too numerous to count
hx	History	TPN	Total parenteral nutrition
ID	Intradermal	TPR	Temperature, pulse, respiration
IM	Intramuscular	tx	Treatment
IP	Intraperitoneal	UA	Urinalysis
IV	Intravenous	URI	Upper respiratory infection
K9	Canine	UTI	Urinary tract infection
MM	Mucous membrane	WBC	White blood cell
NM	Neutered male		

RECOMMENDED READING

Colville, J, Oien, S: *Clinical veterinary language*, St. Louis, 2014, Elsevier.

Colville TP, Bassert JM: *Clinical anatomy and physiology for veterinary technicians*, ed 3, St Louis, 2015, Mosby.

Dyce KM: *Textbook of veterinary anatomy*, ed 4, St Louis, 2010, Saunders.

Saunders veterinary anatomy coloring book, St Louis, 2011, Saunders.

Office and Hospital Procedures

CHAPTER OUTLINE

KEY TERMS

Anesthetic consent form
Client and patient
  information sheet
Copay
Deductible
Dispensing fee
Etiquette

Euthanasia release form
Fair Debt Collections
    Practices Act
Indemnity insurance
Informed consent
Interstate health certificate
Markup

Master problem list
Medical records
Minimum prescription fee
Premium
Problem-oriented medical
  record (POMR)
Rabies certificates

Reorder point
Shrinkage
Standard operating
  procedure (SOP)
Subjective, objective,
  assessment, and plan
  (SOAP)

LEARNING OBJECTIVES

After reviewing this chapter, the reader will be able to:

1. Describe the importance of informed consent.
2. Clarify admitting and discharge instructions.
3. Identify effective and professional discharge sheets.
4. Define and educate clients regarding pet health insurance.
5. Identify a completed medical record.
6. Identify and use problem-oriented medical record (POMR) and subjective, objective, assessment, and plan (SOAP) record formats.
7. Identify methods used to maintain inventory accurately and efficiently.
8. Identify techniques for handling multiple phone lines.
9. Differentiate forms used in the veterinary practice.
10. Discuss features of appropriate housing for animals.
11. Describe basic sanitation needs for veterinary facilities.

FRONT OFFICE PROCEDURES

- A client's experience starts with the first impression and ends when the practice has followed up with the visit.
- For clients who have made an appointment, the second impression begins when they enter the practice.
- Clients should be greeted by a warm, sincere individual who has a genuine concern for them and their pet.
  - If a receptionist is on the phone, a wave and a smile let clients know that they have been recognized and that a team member will help them shortly.

- A negative impression may be developed if clients are ignored or have to wait an excessive amount of time, or if the practice exhibits a dirty appearance.
- Clients perceive a positive atmosphere in a practice when a team works together.

Telephone Etiquette

- The receptionist should answer the phone within three rings; if the receptionist team is busy, another member of the team should receive the phone call.
- The receptionist should speak slowly and clearly, with correct enunciation.
- The human voice has four components—volume, tone, rate, and quality.
  - Correct volume is essential to a successful phone experience; if a person's voice is too loud, listeners (in this case, clients) may pull the phone away from their ear, preventing them from hearing all of a conversation. If a receptionist's volume is too low, clients may be too embarrassed to ask for clarification of something that they did not hear well.
  - The tone of a voice is also referred to as *pitch*.
    - A low, comforting tone increases the quality of the conversation.
    - Team members should smile as they answer the phone; the tone of that smile will come across the phone line
  - Speaking rate: The receptionist must be efficient and knowledgeable and speak slowly and clearly.
- Team members should answer the phone by introducing themselves.
- If a client asks a question that the receptionist cannot answer, the receptionist should ask the client if the call can be placed on hold, allowing the correct answer to be determined.
- It is important not to leave callers on hold for longer than 1 minute.
  - If the client will be on hold more than 1 or 2 minutes, the client should be asked if a team member can return the call as soon as the requested information is available.
- A pet's condition cannot be diagnosed over the phone, and team members cannot recommend treatments to clients without illegally diagnosing a disease or condition.

Scheduling Appointments

- Veterinary practice management software systems usually have a template that has already been created to accommodate the schedule that the practice has deemed appropriate.
- Appointment schedules should be developed to maximize production while minimizing client wait time.
- If the appointment schedule is running behind, clients should be notified immediately.
- The length of time for an appointment should depend on the reason for the appointment.
  - An orthopedic appointment (e.g., limping dog) will likely take longer for the examination and radiographs than a yearly examination with vaccinations.

- A senior patient's wellness examination may take longer than a standard regular examination because recommendations for laboratory diagnostics may be made.
- Appointments for client education, nail trims, and anal gland expressions can be made with veterinary technicians, allowing the veterinarian(s) to see cases that need to be diagnosed.
- Appointments should contain the client's first and last names, phone number, pet's name, and reason for the appointment.
- All those scheduled for appointments and surgeries should be called and reminded of their appointment 1 day prior.
- If a recheck, follow-up appointment, or booster vaccination is required, the appointment should be made for the client before she or he leaves the practice.

Reminders and Recall Systems

- Many software programs can automatically generate reminders and recalls for the veterinary team.
- Practices may elect to send out reminders for a variety of services, including yearly examinations and vaccines, heartworm testing, or a fecal analysis.
- Practices may also send out reminders for annual laboratory work, including testing of patients that are on long-term medications that may have potential side effects if not monitored closely.
- Communications can also be sent to remind clients to refill their pets' medication, including heartworm prevention and medications that treat hypothyroidism or hyperthyroidism, seizures, and allergies.
- Reminders must be clear, concise, and to the point.
- Reminders can also come in the form of phone calls.
- Reminder systems must be programmed to remove patients once they have died.
- Veterinary practices can send reminders by email or via text message.
- Recalls are lists that are generated by veterinary software systems to remind staff to call certain clients to check on patients.
- Recalls can be created for surgical patients, pets that have received vaccines, or any patient that has been in the hospital for a period of time.

Cleanliness

- The receptionist team is responsible for maintaining the reception area.
- Hair and dirt should also be swept up immediately.
- Sweeping and mopping of the reception floor should occur more than once a day because odors will penetrate the walls and disseminate rapidly throughout the practice.
- Products, shelves, and pictures must be dusted regularly, along with ceiling fan blades, blinds, and windowsills.
- Walls should be washed on a regular basis and chairs cleaned each night.

Commonly Used Forms

- Client form: signed by the client; contains the name, contact information, and driver's license number and a statement indicating that the client is financially responsible for the patient and understands that all services must be paid for once they are rendered
- Patient history forms should include the name of the client and patient's name, age, breed, gender, whether the pet has been spayed or neutered, and a medical history, including current medications that the pet is receiving.
- Release forms for any treatment or procedure that is authorized
  - Include anesthesia consent forms, treatment forms, and euthanasia forms
  - All consent forms must state the client's name, patient's name, name of the procedure, and date.
  - Euthanasia release forms must be signed by the owner of the patient and state that the pet's death will result.
    - If a necropsy is requested by the pet's owner, the consent form may include the appropriate information, as well as the request for disposal of the body.
- An informed consent form is signed by the client after all information regarding the procedure has been provided and the client has had the opportunity to ask questions (Fig. 2.1).
  - Information that must be documented for clients includes any risks of the procedure (including death, if that is a risk), the potential outcomes of the procedure, and any alternative procedures that are available, along with an estimate of the costs associated with those procedures.
- Blanket consent forms authorize any procedure but do not include the risks, benefits, outcomes, or estimates.
  - Blanket consent forms are not recommended in practice but are often the sole source of consent forms used.
- Rabies certificates include the client's name, contact information, patient's name, species, breed, gender, and age (Fig. 2.2).
  - Vaccination information, including the manufacturer of the vaccine, vaccine expiration date, lot number, and tag number, is also included.
  - The veterinarian administering the vaccination must sign the certificate.
- Health certificates are issued by the state and the U.S. Department of Agriculture (USDA).
  - Small animals flying within the United States may require an interstate health certificate, whereas

FIGURE 2.1 Informed consent form. (From Sirois M: *Principles and practice of veterinary technology*, ed 3, St Louis, 2011, Mosby.)

OWNER'S COPY **RABIES VACCINATION CERTIFICATE**

NASPHV Form #51

Rabies Tag Number

Owner's Name and Address **Print - use ball point pen or type**

PRINT - Last First M.I. Telephone

No. Street City State Zip

Species:	Sex:	Age:	Size:	Predominant Breed:	Colors:
Dog ☐	Male ☐	3 mo to 12 mo ☐	Under 20 lbs. ☐		
Cat ☐	Female ☐	12 mo or older ☐	20 - 50 lbs. ☐		
Other: ☐ (Specify)	Neutered ☐	Actual Age_____	Over 50 lbs. ☐	Name:	
			Actual_____lbs.		

DATE VACCINATED:	Producer: ☐☐☐ (First 3 letters)	Veterinarian's: # _____ (License No.)
Month Day Year	☐ 1 yr. Lic./Vacc.	(Signature)
VACCINATION EXPIRED:	☐ 3 yr. Lic./Vacc.	Address:
	_____ Other	
Month Day Year	Vacc. Serial (lot) no.	

FIGURE 2.2 Handwritten rabies certificate. (From Sirois M: *Principles and practice of veterinary technology*, ed 3, St Louis, 2011, Mosby.)

those traveling outside the United States will be required to have an international health certificate.

Invoicing Clients

- Estimates should always be given to clients, whether on the phone or in the hospital, for every procedure.
- When invoices are needed, they should be detailed for clients.
  - For example, many clients perceive that a DHLPP injection has only one component because it is only one injection. The invoice should list all five vaccine components of the injection—distemper, hepatitis, leptospirosis, parainfluenza, parvovirus—allowing the client to understand the value of this injection.
- Because of the number of outstanding accounts in veterinary medicine, extending credit to clients should not be allowed.
- Accounts receivable totals should never exceed 2% to 3% of the total gross revenue amount for the practice.
- Most practices accept cash, checks, debit cards, and credit cards.
  - Businesses must pay a percentage of the total month's charges of each credit card accepted to the credit card agency.
  - This is a hidden overhead expense that the practice must recover.
- CareCredit is a type of third-party payment system used exclusively for medical expenses.
  - Clients must fill out an application in the practice, and team members must verify identification before application acceptance.

Monthly Statements

- Monthly statements must be sent for clients who are allowed to charge.
- These statements should include a statement charge, which covers the time required for the team to print and send statements.
  - A minimum of $5.00 should be charged for this.
- Many practices may also institute a finance charge, which charges the client a percentage of the total amount due.
  - Regulations vary regarding finance fees; therefore regulations must be confirmed before the institution of such fees.
  - Notice of such fees must also be clearly posted for clients to see, and they should be documented in the statement.

Outstanding Debt Collection

- Accounts that are allowed to age to 30, 60, or 90 days postservice can become difficult to collect.
- Those responsible for collecting accounts should become familiar with the Fair Debt Collections Practices Act, which prevents someone from using unruly tactics when trying to collect on an overdue account.
  - Phone calls cannot be made before 8 AM or after 9 PM, and the account balance cannot be discussed with anyone other than the person who owes on the account (Box 2.1).
- Accounts that cannot be collected by team members must be turned over to a collection agency.
- The sooner the overdue amount is turned in to collection agents, the easier they can collect the account.

THE OFFICE VISIT

- After clients have been greeted by the receptionist team, they are generally placed in an examination room.
  - Usually, an assistant or technician will take a medical history of the patient.
  - A medical history includes each patient's weight and vital signs, which should include the temperature, pulse, and heart and respiratory rates.
  - Additional information would include the patient's nutritional and environmental history.
  - If any laboratory samples will be needed, the veterinary health care team may confirm the proper sampling technique, equipment, or products needed and ask the veterinarian for authorization to obtain the samples.
- Puppy and kitten owners should be informed about vaccination schedules, heartworm and intestinal worm prevention, flea and tick disease and prevention, dental disease, and nutrition.
  - Information can be spread over several visits so that the client is not overwhelmed with too much information.
- Clients with adult patients arriving for yearly examinations must be reminded of heartworm, flea and tick disease and prevention, provided with nutrition guidance, and given information on dental disease prevention.

Admitting and Discharging Patients

- A treatment consent form must be given to the owner to sign.
- The client must be informed of risks, prognosis, and alternative treatments that are available.
- An estimate should also be provided for the client, highlighting all possible treatments, procedures, medications, or services that are recommended for the owner.
- Once the client has been informed, she or he can sign the consent form and estimate, indicating the services that the client authorizes.

- If a patient is being admitted for boarding, a separate form should be available for clients to complete.
  - These forms should include emergency and alternative contact information, as well as any pertinent information regarding the pet.
  - This information should include current diet, amount fed per feeding, when the pet is fed, what medications the pet receives, and at what time those mediations are administered.
  - If a blanket, toy, collars, or leash is left, a clear description should be indicated on the admitting sheet.
- Clients may also be asked if they would prefer any additional services or treatments to be performed on their pet while in the boarding facility, such as bathing, dipping, or grooming services.
- Patients discharged from the hospital must be released with written instructions (Fig. 2.3).
- Invoices and discharge instructions should be detailed with clients before the pet is brought to the owner.
  - Once a pet has been brought to the owner, the owner is more interested in the pet than the release instructions.
- Discharge instructions must include any recommended restrictions for food, activity, or therapy and should indicate when to start medications.
  - Doses and instructions for medications should also be included.

ABC Veterinary Clinic
123-456-7890
Dr. Roe, Dr. Morton, Dr. Larsen
Post Anesthesia Release Sheet

Please provide clean, dry bedding and a quiet place for your pet to recuperate. Please notify the hospital with any concerns.
DIET:
( ) Wait a few hours after arriving home to offer your pet water. Please give only a small amount. If no vomiting occurs, you may offer more water about an hour later. You may feed a small amount (1/4 normal amount) if water stays down.
( ) You may continue to feed your pet normally.
( ) Special diet instructions _____
ACTIVITY:
( ) Restrict exercise for 1 day. NO RUNNING, JUMPING, CLIMBING, OR BATHING.
( ) Restrict exercise for 7 days. NO RUNNING, JUMPING, CLIMBING, OR BATHING.
( ) Other _____
OTHER:
( ) Please use paper strips or pinto beans in place of litter for 7 days.
( ) Please return for booster vaccines in 3-4 weeks.
( ) Your pet's metabolism may permanently decrease after surgery. You may need to decrease the amount of food you feed in order to prevent obesity.
INCISION:
( ) Watch for swelling, redness, or drainage. Prevent scratching, rubbing, and licking of the incision. Please ask for an E-collar if you think your pet will lick the site.
( ) Ice incision for 5 minutes, 3 to 4 times daily for the first 72 hours.
MEDICATION:
( ) Give pain medication _____
( ) Give antibiotics _____
( ) Give other medication _____
( ) Start medication _____
FOLLOW UP VISITS:
( ) Recheck in _____ days.
( ) There is no need to return for suture removal; the skin was closed with absorbable suture or tissue adhesive.
( ) Not necessary unless you feel there is a problem.
Comments:

Doctor _____ Tech _____ Client _____ Date _____

FIGURE 2.3 Discharge instructions. (From Sirois M: *Principles and practice of veterinary technology*, ed 3, St Louis, 2011, Mosby.)

- If a pet has been diagnosed with a particular disease or condition, the client should also be given written materials regarding the diagnosis.

PET HEALTH INSURANCE

- Pet health insurance is a method whereby pet owners can manage the risks of expensive health care.
- Studies have indicated that the increased use of veterinary pet health insurance could increase the demand for service, therefore decreasing the euthanasia rate in the United States.
- The entire staff should understand the concept of pet insurance and offer it to all clients.
- Clients should be made aware of the various companies that offer pet health insurance.
- Plans and companies vary in different regions; therefore each policy should be reviewed carefully.
- Terms that should be considered include whether hereditary conditions are covered and whether benefit schedules or exclusions are listed in the policy.
- Indemnity insurance offers compensation for the treatment of injured and sick pets.
- Policies are available for comprehensive illness, standard care, and accident coverage and may cover pet species ranging from dogs and cats to small mammals and birds.
- A premium is defined as the amount an owner pays monthly or annually to maintain an insurance policy for a pet.
  - Premium amounts are affected by a number of factors, including the deductible; copay; and per-incident, annual, or lifetime limit payout.
  - The age, species, and breed of the animal also affect the cost of the premium, as well as if the pet is spayed or neutered and geographic location of the owner in the United States.
- A deductible is the amount an owner must pay before the insurance company will offer compensation.
  - Insurance companies vary and offer either a per-incident deductible or annual deductible.
  - Per-incident deductibles refer to the owner paying the chosen deductible amount each time an incident occurs with the pet.
  - An annual deductible refers to an owner paying the chosen deductible once annually.
- A copay is the percentage that the owner is responsible for after the deductible has been met.
- Annual limits refer to the maximum amount that the insurance company will pay for a condition or illness during the policy term.
- Per-incident limits refer to the maximum amount an insurance company will pay each time a new problem or disease occurs.
- Lifetime limits refer to the maximum amount an insurance company will pay during the pet's lifetime.
- A preexisting health condition is defined as any accident or illness contracted, manifested, or incurred before the policy effective date and may be excluded from coverage.

- Purebred pets known to have congenital and hereditary conditions may also have coverage excluded for those conditions, depending on insurance company policy.
- A congenital condition is generally referred to as an abnormality present at birth, whether apparent or not, that can cause illness or disease.
- A hereditary condition is an abnormality that is transmitted by genes from the parent to the offspring, whether apparent or not, that can cause disease or illness.
- Many companies have a list of exclusions: diseases, conditions, or treatments that are excluded from policies.
- Behavior counseling and medications are usually not covered, along with compounded medications, nutraceuticals, or diets.

MEDICAL RECORDS

- Medical records are legal documents that must be complete, legible, and made available to clients at their request.
- Medical records are the legal property of the practice; however, clients may request to have copies for themselves, for a referral, or for a new veterinarian.
  - The practice is permitted to charge a fee to cover the cost of creating duplicate records.
- Inactive client records must be maintained for 3 years.
- Completed records must include client contact information, patient name and information, and the date that the service(s) were rendered.
- The person who made entries in the medical record must initial each entry.
- Illegible records may lead to incorrect treatments, incorrect client diagnosis, or incorrect client education.
  - If a record must be presented in a court of law and a judge cannot read the record, the practice may be at fault and held liable for the presenting claim.
- Medical records and client-patient information is also confidential; cases should never be discussed by name, and client information should never be released to anyone other than the pet owner.
- Medical records may be written, or a practice may be paperless.
  - Paperless medical records must also be complete and initialed by the author.
  - Many programs will automatically time-stamp entries when they are made, along with the team members' initials.
  - Some programs can be programmed with a lockout period, preventing record alteration after a 12- or 24-hour period. If any changes need to be made, a second entry can be made, indicating the change.
- All entries in written medical records must be in permanent ink and cannot be altered; instead, the mistake should be crossed out with a one-line strike.
  - Mistakes should be initialed and dated, with the change to follow (Fig. 2.4).
- Master lists are often used to summarize patient histories.

- An individual patient record should include a master sheet listing species, gender, breed, age, diet, allergies, unique behaviors, and annual vaccination and parasite control documentation.
- The master sheet chronologically lists visits, treatments, and client communications (Fig. 2.5).

> stopped ^TM^
> Owner ~~started~~ antibiotics 5 days ago.

FIGURE 2.4 Example of strike. (From Sirois M: *Principles and practice of veterinary technology*, ed 3, St Louis, 2011, Mosby.)

Record Format

- Written medical records are generally held in a clasp-type 8½- × 11-inch file folder.
- Each client has one folder, and all patients owned by that client are clipped within the folder.
- Patients are separated with color-coded tabs.
- Some hospitals maintain entirely computerized medical and financial records for each client.
- Regardless of the format, the record must be accurate, complete, and secure.
- Storage and retrieval of records must be convenient and well organized.

Master Problem List

Client Name _____ Telephone Number _____

Address _____ Client Number _____

Pet Name _____ Breed _____ Color _____

Sex _____ Altered _____ DOB _____ Age _____

	Date Received	Date Received	Date Received	Date Received
DHLPP				
FVRCP				
FeLV				
Rabies				
HWT				
FeLV/FIV				

Chronic Diseases/Date of Onset: _____

_____

_____

_____

Current Medications and Directions: _____

_____

_____

_____

FIGURE 2.5 Master sheet. (From Sirois M: *Principles and practice of veterinary technology*, ed 3, St Louis, 2011, Mosby.)

POMR and SOAP

- A **problem-oriented medical record** (POMR) is the most commonly used format in veterinary practice.
- Each entry follows a distinct format: defined database, **master problem list** (also referred to as master list), plan, and progress sections.
- Within the progress section, a standard SOAP format is followed.
- SOAP is an acronym that stands for subjective, objective, assessment, and plan.
- Subjective is the most important element and is obtained from the client by the reception staff, veterinary technicians, and assistants.
- Most subjective information is the opinion(s) and perception(s) of the client.
- Objective information is gathered directly from the patient; the physical examination, diagnostic workup, and interpretation are included in this section of the medical record.
- The assessment section includes any conclusions reached by the veterinarian from the subjective and objective sections; it also includes a definitive diagnosis.
  - If there are multiple diagnoses or a tentative diagnosis, this can all be documented here, along with a list of rule-ins or rule-outs (R/I or R/O, respectively).
  - Rule-ins can be classified as any disease that the patient could possibly have.
- A plan is developed by the veterinarian based on the assessment and includes any treatment, surgery, medication, intended diagnostics, or intended communications with the owner.
- Veterinarians must interpret the results of diagnostic testing, not just document the results. Interpretation is defined as analyzing the results and explaining why those abnormalities may be present.
- Animals should have a daily physical examination while they are hospitalized.
- Results of the physical examination; any medications administered; and any urination, bowel movements, or vomiting must be documented in the progress notes.
- Hospitalization sheets should be used to help keep track of patients' status while hospitalized.
- Surgical patients must be examined within 12 hours before administration of anesthesia, and the examination must be documented in the medical record.
- Anesthetic drugs, details of the procedure, and the patient's response to and/or complications from the procedure must also be documented.
- The medical record must clearly state whether the patient prognosis is poor, guarded, fair, or excellent.
- Medication names, strength, and route given must be accurately written in the medical records.
  - Many drugs are available in different strengths, and it is important to identify and document the correct strength of medication.
  - The same drug can also be administered by different routes.
- Some drugs will have a different dose, depending on the route administered.
- Labels can be used for documentation of examinations, dental prophylaxis, or surgeries and be developed by the practice manager or ordered from standard office supply and label catalogues (Fig. 2.6).

STANDARD OPERATING PROCEDURES

- **Standard operating procedure** (SOP) descriptions may be written for all standardized procedures used in the practice, and a loose-leaf binder may be used to store SOP sheets in a central location.
- SOP descriptions may also be used for front office staff, including which type of questions may be answered by staff, check-in and release procedures, and front office record-keeping procedures.
- Annual reviews and updates of SOP descriptions are important.
- Once the SOP binder is in place, one may reference all standardized procedures by "procedure name, SOP" as the patient medical records are completed.

INVENTORY MANAGEMENT

- The goal of inventory management is to maintain inventory costs between 12% and 15% of the overall income of the practice.
- A large amount of money can be lost in inventoried products through shrinkage, product expiration, or missed charges.
  - **Shrinkage** is defined as the loss of a product without explanation.
- The inventory manager should determine a day that is appropriate to place an order. An order should be developed that encompasses the practice's needs for the following 1- or 2-week period.
- Ordering products should be based on the economic order quantity, reorder point, and number of inventory turns that the product takes within a year.
  - Economic order quantity represents the costs related to ordering the item, sales of the item, and purchase price.
  - Inventory turns per year refers to the number of times inventory turns over in a practice, in a specified time. Each practice should set a goal of 8 to 12 turns per year.
  - A **reorder point** is the point that a stock level reaches before reordering.
- The average shelf life of an item should not exceed 3 months.
- If a product is used infrequently and expires before the entire amount can be dispensed, the practice may want to consider writing a prescription for the medication.
- Physical inventory must be taken at the beginning or end of each year, and spot checks should be performed throughout the year.

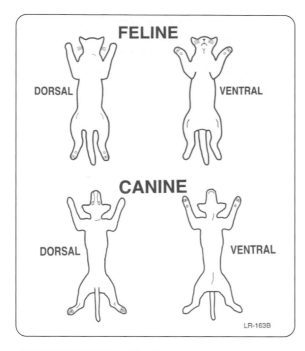

FELINE

DORSAL   VENTRAL

CANINE

DORSAL   VENTRAL

LR-163B

Feline Castration:

Using autoligation technique. No skin closure.
Surgery and recovery uneventful.

Canine and Feline OVH:
Ventral midline incision; _____Polysorb Double ligatures ovarian pedicles; _____Polysorb Double ligature encircling uterine body; _____ Polysorb Simple continuous body wall; _____Polysorb Simple cont. double layer; SubQ / subcut. closure. Surgery and recovery uneventful.

Canine Neuter:
Open/closed technique. Pre-scrotal incision, double ligate testicular artery, vein, and vas deferens with_____Polysorb. Subcutaneous and subcuticular layers closed simple continuous with _____Polysorb. Surgery/recovery uneventful.

Feline Declaw:

Using Roscoe blades, P3 was amputated and sealed with tissue adhesive.

Urinalysis

Source_____		Crystals_____
S.G._____	Glu_____	Casts_____
pH_____	Ket_____	WBC_____
Leuk_____	Uro_____	RBC_____
Nit_____	Bili_____	Epith_____
Protein_____	Blood_____	Bact_____

DENTAL Name _____ Date _____

Canine Upper

Feline Upper

MAXILLA

MANDIBLE

Feline Lower

Canine Lower

KEY: O = Displaced Tooth
X = Missing Tooth
= Caries, Injury, FX

a _____
b _____
c _____
d _____
Gingiva: _____
Occlusion: _____

Salivation: _____

Halitosis: Y N
Periodontal Disease: _____

Other: _____

FIGURE 2.6 Examples of labels. (From Prendergast H: *Front office management for the veterinary team*, ed 2, St Louis, 2015, Saunders.)

- Items should be checked when they are received. Expiration dates, correct product, strength, and count should all be verified against the order book and invoice.

Product Pricing

- The **markup** of a product is the cost of the product multiplied by a percentage to recover hidden costs associated with inventory management.
- Many practices will mark products up by 100% to 200%.
  - Product markup must be at least 40% to break even.
- **Dispensing fee:** the average dispensing fee ranges from $6.00 to $14.00 to cover the cost of the label, pill vial, and time used to count the medication.
- If a full bottle of shampoo or medication is dispensed, the average dispensing fee ranges from $3.00 to $5.00.
- Many practices initiate a **minimum prescription fee** of $11.00 to $13.00 to help recover hidden pharmacy costs.
  - Hidden pharmacy costs include costs associated with expired medications, ordering and shipping costs, and insurance and taxes on products and supplies.

- Pricing for items (e.g., injections, single-dose items) used in the hospital or administered to patients while in the examination room must also be considered.
- Common methods include charging a flat fee for injections (e.g., $12.00 per injection) or adding a surcharge for very expensive drugs, such as some postoperative analgesics.
- In-hospital tablet administration frequently is priced to include drug, labor, and record-keeping costs, such as $3.00 per administration.
- Over-the-counter (OTC) products do not require a prescription and can be sold to clients without a veterinarian-client-patient relationship.
- A prescription product can only be sold on the order of a veterinarian when a current veterinarian–client-patient relationship exists.
  - The veterinarian must be familiar with the case, patient, and client.
- Manufacturers may dictate that some products are not prescription products but can only be sold through

a veterinarian, wherein a veterinarian-client-patient relationship exists.

- Examples of such products include some heartworm preventive medications and therapeutic diets such as Purina NF, Royal Canin SO, and Hills K/D.

Labeling Prescription Items

- Every item that is a prescription product must have a label before it leaves the practice.
- Labels must include the practice name, address, and phone number; veterinarian's name; date of the prescription; client's last name and patient's name; name and strength of the drug (in milligrams [mg] or grams [g]); number of items dispensed (tablets, capsules, or volume in milliliters [mL]); and expiration date of the product.
- The directions for use of the product must be detailed and specific.

COMPUTER AND SOFTWARE MANAGEMENT

- Computers can greatly increase the efficiency of every team member, lower the amount of missed charges, provide professional-appearing client educational materials, maintain inventory and accounts receivable, and provide paperless medical records.
- Many practices use computers in examination rooms, laboratory areas, pharmacy counters, veterinarian's office, and reception area.
  - This allows data to be entered in multiple locations of the practice.
- Pharmacy labels can be generated at any terminal and printed in the pharmacy area. Invoices can also be generated at any location and printed at the reception desk.
- Veterinary software can aid in invoice development, client education, practice management, and digital radiology.
- New computers with large amounts of random access memory (RAM), memory, and storage must be used.
  - Many software companies will not guarantee their products without installation on new computers.
- Fire, theft, or natural disasters can destroy a practice in a matter of minutes, as can computer viruses or a hacked computer system.
- Regular scanning of the system to detect evidence of computer viruses or malware is vital to ensuring the safety and security of records.
- Computer systems should be backed up nightly, on and off premises.
  - On-premise system backup may include a rewritable disk or zip drive.
  - Off-premise system backup can be done through the veterinary software website or another location, such as with cloud computing.
  - Backing up documents offsite prevents thieves from stealing the most current copy of data from the practice if they are removing all the computer equipment.

- If a fire or natural disaster occurs, the data are also protected.
- Many computers function optimally for only 5 or 6 years and then need to be replaced.
  - If the main computer needs to be replaced, the backup data from the previous evening can be uploaded, bringing the system back up and allowing the team to move forward.

ANIMAL HUSBANDRY

Temperature, Light, and Ventilation

- For small animals, such as dogs, cats, birds, and small mammals, the ambient (room) temperature should ideally be 65° to 84°F (18° to 29°C).
- Birds, very young pets, old pets, and those with a sparse hair coat should be maintained at the higher end of this temperature range.
- Those that are well-furred or overweight should be kept at the lower end of this range.
- Smaller animals of any species generally require warmer temperatures, whereas larger animals, with their greater body mass, generally require cooler temperatures.
- Light sufficient for a human is adequate for most animals.
- All species do better when there is a definite difference between day and night.
- Animals should never be kept in direct sunlight without access to shade because they may become sunburned and overheated.
- Ventilation is extremely important in maintaining good health.
- Inadequate air exchange in an enclosure increases urine odors, ammonia levels, and the numbers of airborne bacteria and viruses.
- Drafty conditions or excessive ventilation can also be dangerous.
- Excessive cool airflow can cause chilling. In a low-humidity environment, as with air conditioning, high airflow can dehydrate an animal.
- Small pets caged indoors must be kept away from air-conditioning drafts or heater vents.

Housing

- An important aspect of husbandry is housing, such as cages, pens, or stalls.
- Housing should do the following:
  - Prevent contamination of the animal with feces or urine.
  - Provide for the psychosocial comfort of companion animals.
  - Be appropriate for the species.
  - Be structurally sound.
  - Be free of dangerous surfaces.
  - Be constructed so that the animal cannot escape and vermin are not allowed access.
  - Be easy for the owner to clean.

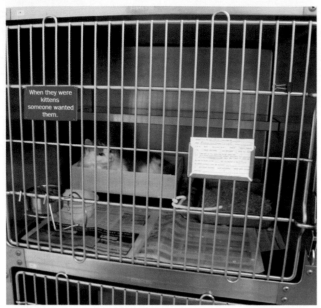

FIGURE 2.7 Cats in cages should be provided with resting boards or boxes elevated above the cage floor. (From August JR: *Consultations in feline internal medicine*, vol 6, ed 6, St Louis, 2009, Saunders.)

- Housed animals should be dry, clean, and protected from environmental extremes.
- Walls and roofing should be sufficient to protect animals from the sun, wind, rain, and snow.
- Accommodation must also be made for species-specific behavior.
  - For example, cats need scratching posts and resting boards (Fig. 2.7).
- A general rule for holding enclosures is that they be a minimum of 10 times the body size of the animal.
  - This recommendation assumes that the animal will be given opportunity to exercise routinely outside the primary enclosure.

- Cages, pens, and stalls that are too small increase the risk of disease and may predispose to abnormal behavior, such as pacing or excessive barking.
- Housing too many animals in a single primary enclosure of insufficient size can increase the risk of stress, aggression, and disease transmission.
- Animals of different species should be housed separately or, in some cases, at least in separate rooms.
  - Do not house natural predators and prey animals in the same room, such as cats with mice or birds, because this leads to stress and possible attack.
  - Medical concerns related to housing of different species.
    - A disease considered inconsequential in one species can be deadly in another species.
    - Disease-causing organisms, such as some species of bacteria, may be part of the normal flora of one species while causing serious disease in a different species.

Animal Identification

- The method of identification depends on the species.
- For pets allowed outdoors, an implanted microchip or tattoo is preferred to a collar with a name tag.
- Permanent identification ensures that a lost pet can be identified for return to its owner.
- When hospitalized, each animal should be adequately identified with cage cards and paper ID neck bands (Fig. 2.8).

Housekeeping

- The floors, flat surfaces, walls, cages, runs, and stalls in the veterinary practice must be kept sparkling clean and odor-free.
- The counters, magazine racks, and pictures need to be organized and dusted frequently.
- The reception room, examination rooms, and public bathrooms must be inspected and cleaned regularly throughout each day.

Owner							Name							
Date in:		Ph #1												
Est. date out:		Ph #2												
	Sunday		Monday		Tuesday		Wednesday		Thursday		Friday		Saturday	
	am	pm	am	pm	am	pm	am	pm	am	pm	am	pm	am	pm
Fed														
Ate														
Water														
Urine														
Stool														
Meds														
Walked														

FIGURE 2.8 Stable hospitalized patients require minimally a daily weight and record of eating, drinking, and elimination. This example of a cage card is conveniently graphed for recording this information. This type is also a sticker that can be applied to the permanent medical record after use. (From Sirois M: *Principles and practice of veterinary technology*, ed 3, St Louis, 2011, Mosby.)

- One of the reasons cleanup in a veterinary practice is so challenging is the large quantity of hair shed by animals.
  - A vacuum system needs to be available and used before general mopping; otherwise, a buildup of hair is simply moved around the facility.
- The lack of cleanliness can result in complaints from clients or in nosocomial (hospital-acquired) infections.
- Appropriate disinfectants need to be used to prevent odor buildup.
- The ventilation system should be capable of exhausting all air within the building within 15 to 20 minutes to facilitate odor control.
- Cages, runs, and other enclosures should be cleaned and sanitized frequently.
- Sanitation is commonly performed with a dilute solution of bleach, using 1 part bleach to 20 parts of water.
- All surfaces should be rinsed thoroughly after cleaning and disinfecting.
- Wet items should be left to dry completely before returning the animal to the cage.

Disinfection and Sanitation

- Disinfection is the destruction of pathogenic microorganisms or their toxins.
- Disinfectants are chemical agents that kill or prevent the growth of microorganisms on inanimate objects, such as surgical equipment, floors, and tabletops.
- Sanitizers are chemical agents that reduce the number of microorganisms to a safe level, without completely eliminating all microorganisms.
- Sterilizers are chemicals or other agents that completely destroy all microorganisms.

- As with antimicrobials, it is important to know against which organisms the antiseptic or disinfectant is effective.
- Chemicals used to clean floors should never be mixed; caustic vapors may result, causing harm to patients and team members.
- Labels must be read clearly to dilute the product to the correct strength to have a solution that kills viruses, fungi, or bacteria.
- Trash cans absorb odors that can also travel through the practice and should be emptied several times a day.
- Rooms must be cleaned after every patient to prevent the transmission of odors and diseases.
- Walls should be cleaned weekly, if not more often.
- Potted plants that sit on the floor must be cleaned frequently because animals often urinate on them.
- Blinds, fans, vents, baseboards, and door frames must be dusted weekly.
- The outside of the practice must remain clean as well.
  - Feces must be removed daily, and common urination areas must be scrubbed with a dilute Clorox solution.
  - Urine stains walls and sidewalks and produces a terrible smell.
- Windows should be washed weekly and dirt swept away from the entrance and exit areas.
- The outside of the building must be as presentable as the inside of the practice.

RECOMMENDED READINGS

Prendergast H, editor: *Front office management for the veterinary team*, ed 2, St Louis, 2014, Saunders.

Sirois M, editor: *Principles and practice of veterinary technology*, ed 3, St Louis, 2011, Elsevier.

3 Communication and Client Relations

CHAPTER OUTLINE

KEY TERMS

Assertive communication
Body language

Conflict management
Nonverbal communication

Nosocomial infections

LEARNING OBJECTIVES

After reviewing this chapter, the reader will be able to:

1. Discuss methods to implement effective communication skills in the veterinary clinic.
2. Identify barriers that prevent successful communication exchanges.
3. Review techniques to reduce conflict and manage difficult situations with team members.
4. Describe the stages of grief.
5. Explain the importance of the human–animal bond to client and coworker interaction.
6. Describe the educational requirements of veterinary team members.
7. Define appropriate nomenclature describing veterinary personnel.
8. Identify the duties of the members of the veterinary health care team.
9. Recognize professional organizations supporting veterinary medicine.
10. Discuss ethical issues and guidelines relevant to the veterinary profession.
11. List and describe general categories of laws relevant to the veterinary profession.

THE COMMUNICATION PROCESS

- Your expertise is most valuable when it can be expressed in a way that is understood; you actively listen to the needs of clients and understand how to serve them, as well as have the ability to build working relationships in cooperation with other team members.
- Effective communication between team members entails a receiver and a sender of a message.
- The receiver is the person listening to the message, whereas the sender is the one who is talking and giving the message.
- Ideal conversations entail having an interaction that allows all team members involved the ability to be both a sender and a receiver.
- The goal of communication is to exchange thoughts and ideas in a flowing two-way manner.
- Communication occurs through four primary methods: listening, speaking, reading, and writing (Fig. 3.1).
- Computerization is increasing the reading and writing component through email, furthering the need to be clearly understood in writing.
- Communication has several dimensions and occurs on many levels simultaneously.

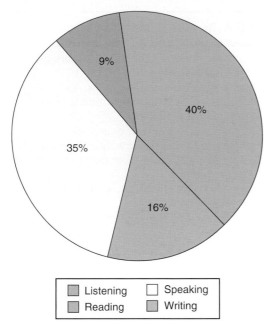

FIGURE 3.1 Legend:
- Listening
- Reading
- Speaking
- Writing

FIGURE 3.1 The communication process. (From Sirois M: *Principles and practice of veterinary technology*, ed 4, St Louis, 2017, Mosby.)

- In the workplace you can use your senses of sight, touch, hearing, and smell to create favorable surroundings, promote positive interaction, and accomplish your tasks. Using more of the different elements in combination will increase the powerful impact when communicating with others.
- People communicate by verbal (spoken and written) and nonverbal means.
- Nonverbal communication is more persuasive than verbal communication and is a substantial part of interactions with others.
- More than 70% of communication is nonverbal.
- Nonverbal communication involves emotions, which alter the interpretation of the message.

Body Language

- Body language is a nonverbal form of communication that plays a key role in client education.
  - It accounts for almost 60% of communication.
- When a person has folded arms, it generally indicates that he or she is defensive and unwilling to accept recommendations or advice.
- A team member can correct this situation easily by handing the client something to hold: a brochure, a model of a joint (e.g., hip, knee, elbow), or anything else that will force the person to unfold the arms.
- Body posture: If a team member enters an examination room slumped over, with head down and shoulders folded in, the client is going to think that the team member lacks confidence and skill and does not enjoy his or her job.
  - Team members who are slumped over are likely to have quiet voices, lack energy, and appear unmotivated.

BOX 3.1 Common Communication Barriers

- Ordering
- Excessive questioning
- Labeling (name calling)
- Falsely praising
- Excessive logical argumentation
- Advising
- Threatening
- Excessive reassuring
- Diagnosing
- Moralizing

- Team members should enter examination rooms with their heads up, a straight body posture, and shoulders back.
- While educating clients, maintain eye contact with them at all times.
- Lack of eye contact is perceived as diminished skill, knowledge, and confidence.

Barriers to Communication

- Communication barriers are best identified as responses that hold a high possibility for affecting a discussion in a negative manner (Box 3.1).
- These barriers have been shown to increase the chance that collaboration will not occur and that a greater distance can exist between individuals.
- Communication barriers can be placed into three primary categories: (1) solution sending, (2) judging, and (3) failure to respond to concerns.
- Awareness of communication barriers is the first important step in reducing their impact.
- It is also important to consider that these elements are assumptions based on what you believe about someone.

Effective Listening Skills

- In the fast-paced environment of the veterinary practice, veterinary team members will be faced with a great need to understand and retain information coming from many directions—the client, the practice owner, the sales representative, the practice manager, and the other health care team members.
- A recent study demonstrated that around 75% of oral communication is ignored.
- Hearing is the physiologic action of capturing auditory waves, whereas listening includes engaging the psychologic process to evaluate and consider the message of another person.
- Active listening requires focus and engagement.
- The message you are sending to the client or your peer is that what they are saying is important and you want to understand their needs. (Box 3.2).
- Clients who know that someone truly has taken the time and made the effort to accurately understand their

---

BOX 3.2 Active Listening Traits

- Strong eye contact
- Positive head nodding
- Thoughtful silence
- Appropriate environment
- Paraphrasing ("What you are saying is ...")
- Meaningful reflection ("If I understand you ...")
- Avoid distracting behavior
- Leaned/faced toward speaker

BOX 3.3 Three Steps to Active Listening

1. **Receive the message**—Listen and look for the total visual and auditory message. Listen for the entire message; if you are thinking about what to say, you are not actively listening.
2. **Process the message**—Evaluate and analyze; ask yourself, "What does the speaker want me to know?" This takes concentration and focus. As emotions escalate, this becomes even more essential.
3. **Respond to the message**—Let the speaker know you have not only heard but you understand the visual message as well. Be sure to avoid responses that are based on communication barriers.

BOX 3.4 Benefits of Assertive Communication

- Expresses your needs and ideas more clearly
- Enhances self-esteem
- Improves confidence level
- Increases respect for others' points of view
- Enhances your character
- Decreases sense of guilt or anxiety
- Enables you to be direct without being blunt
- Increases constructive over destructive communication patterns
- Identifies how to be positive without "sugarcoating" messages
- Emphasizes what you can do, not what you cannot do

---

needs and concerns have a stronger relationship with the practice and are more likely to recommend the practice to other pet owners.

- The entire message is not just in words but in the tone of voice and the body language as well.
- Body language and tone of voice are particularly effective in conveying the total message of the words spoken.
- To adapt better listening skills, it is vital to understand the three stages of listening and to take a proactive position to build this skill over time (Box 3.3).
- Listening skills such as direct eye contact and focused attention convey interest and a desire to understand.
- Along with effective listening skills is the development of empathetic listening—a critical skill of particular importance in the veterinary practice.
- Clients are faced with a broad spectrum of emotions surrounding the serious illness or loss of their pet, and empathetic listening is a less intimidating way to establish a respectful and understanding environment.
- Judgment must be eliminated in communication with clients in these emotional situations.

Assertive Communication Strategies

- **Assertive communication** is a proven method to increase the understanding of thoughts and feelings and

help break the secret code of others, among other benefits (Box 3.4).

- This style of communication also influences how others receive and interpret your messages.
- Focus in this style is placed on speaking in a positive, proactive manner and sharing your concepts and issues in the most effective way possible.
- There is an eight-step process to follow to integrate assertiveness into your communication style; it is called the DISCOVER Method.
  - Decide What You Want
  - Identify Negative Tendencies
  - Substitute Positive Thoughts
  - Choose a Technique
  - Own the Changes
  - Victory Celebration
  - Evaluate the Experience
  - Remember It in the Future

Conflict Management

- To many team members in a clinic, the idea of conflict brings to mind angry words, heated exchanges, name calling, tension, and hurt feelings.
- By facing and managing conflict directly, it is possible to eliminate tension and angry emotions along with strengthening coworker relationships.
- Conflict is based on different perspectives in a situation.
- It is not realistic to believe that avoiding conflict is a successful way to deal with this issue.
- The foundation of conflict resolution is to accept the idea that discord does not always mean negative, but can be positive, perhaps even enlightening, if effectively handled with easily learned skills and techniques.
- Veterinary health care teams face team interactions and conflict situations that exhaust their energy, create stress, and lessen their job satisfaction.
- Usually the biggest obstacle in communication is the use of inflammatory remarks or statements (Box 3.5).

BOX 3.5 Inflammatory Statements and Phrases

Avoid these when resolving conflict:
- "You never/always ..."—This is an extreme statement; things are rarely all or none
- "But ..."—Can be read as negating everything said before "but"; try to substitute "and" instead
- "You make me so ..."—Placing blame
- "You should ..."—Placing blame
- "I can't ..."—May be read as unwilling to cooperate

- Avoidance of these common phrases and barriers will allow discussion and focus on the issues at hand.
- Full use of active listening skills is also an essential part of the resolution strategy.
- In situations involving heightened emotions, our mind engages what we want to say while the other person is speaking.
- This action almost assures you will miss important information that is being shared, and the chance to grasp an understanding of the other person's position is lost.
- Before replying to the other person, wait 3 seconds after they have stopped speaking.
- The five-step plan of conflict resolution will work out the majority of conflict circumstances in the veterinary practice.
  - Step 1: Create a solution setting
  - Step 2: Clarify each person's perspective on the problem
  - Step 3: Develop a resolution plan with action steps
  - Step 4: Implement the plan
  - Step 5: Celebrate success

CLIENT RELATIONS

- Clients draw preliminary conclusions about a practice within the first 2 to 5 minutes of entering the building.
- Team members should always greet clients as they enter the facility, regardless of what other tasks they may be doing.
  - If a receptionist is on the phone, acknowledging clients with a smile and a wave is acceptable.
- Greeting clients by their names and addressing their pets create a positive first impression.
- Communication is one of the most important aspects of working with veterinary clients.
- It is extremely important that clients fully understand procedures that are being performed on their pets.
  - They must also be educated on the proper care of their animals throughout the various life stages.
- Communication includes verbal and written forms in the examination room.
- The veterinary health care team must educate the client with words that can be understood; many clients do not understand medical terminology.

- Written communication includes all client educational materials.
  - After puppy and kitten examinations, clients should be sent home with material informing them about internal parasites and vaccination schedules.
  - Clients bringing pets in for follow-up booster examinations may be sent home with information on nutrition and the benefits of spaying and neutering, as well as information on the prevention of obesity and dental disease.
- Yearly examination patients may need to be educated on weight loss programs and nutritional and behavioral issues.
- Senior patients should be educated about the importance of monitoring blood work and frequent regular examinations.
- Surgical patients must receive postoperative discharge instructions; these instructions vary by procedure, but all clients must be informed about when to start food, medications, and activity.
- Clients of pets diagnosed with a disease or condition should be given information to take home and review regarding the disease and any treatments available.
- Clients can be pleasant or difficult, depending on the type of person they are, type of day they have had, or type of situation presented to them once they arrive at the practice.
- Receptionists must effectively handle hostile clients on the phone.
- Always listen to the client; once the client has finished her or his portion of the conversation, the receptionist should review the facts, ensuring that a miscommunication does not occur.
  - If a manager is available to take the telephone call, the manager and client can discuss the case.
- Angry clients at the practice should be taken into an examination room and allowed to vent in private.
- A team member who simply listens to the client often defuses the situation.

The Human–Animal Bond

- Over the last century, veterinary medicine has evolved from a focus predominantly on food animals to a companion animal orientation.
- Pets are perceived as members of the family.
- Client expectations are changing as medicine changes and more is learned about the human–animal bond.
- Clients who are not well informed about the human–animal bond may not consider the impact on household members when making decisions about veterinary care.
- If there is little bond with the animal, financial considerations may influence the decision more.
- It is critical for the veterinary team to help the decision maker understand the impact of the human–animal bond and how it may affect household members.
  - It is equally important to involve household members in decisions about pet care.

- Clients are best served if they consider the human–animal bond in their decisions, but they must not be made to feel guilty or inadequate if financial realities keep them from doing everything that can be offered.
- The veterinary team's responsibility is to help the animal and prevent suffering, as well as serve the client.
- Educating clients about the human–animal bond long before there is a crisis and encouraging them to have pet health insurance can help ease the difficult passages.
- The opposite extreme from clients who have little appreciation for the human–animal bond is clients who are extremely bonded.
  - These clients may seek or demand services that have never been requested and that the hospital is not prepared to deliver.
  - Clients such as these actually lead those in the profession to offer new levels of service and veterinary care.
- Clients consider companion animals to be members of the family or household, in a role comparable to that of children.
- Part of your role in nurturing the human–animal bond is to help clients have realistic expectations of behavior in relation to the species and breed of pet.
- The greatest number of pets left in animal shelters are there because of behavior problems.
  - These problems are mostly preventable or treatable with client education and animal training.
  - Behavior that goes uncorrected for too long prevents the human–animal bond from forming or breaks the bond and results in the pet being surrendered.
  - Recognizing and correcting problem behaviors early in a relationship can be lifesaving for the pet.
- It is important to recognize and honor the bond between the client and pet by treating the pet as an individual, not as an example of a particular species or breed.
- The careful use of gentle but firm physical restraint, and chemical restraint when needed, will protect you and the animal, and reassure the client that the pet is precious to you as well.
- Assistance animals such as guide dogs and hearing ear dogs require special care on the part of the veterinary team in recognition of the dependency of the client on the animal and the deep bond between them.
  - Avoid separating the person and the animal if at all possible.
  - You must also discuss in great detail any procedure that may temporarily incapacitate the assistance animal and prevent it from working.
- Hospitalization, which is a routine to people who work in animal hospitals, is stressful to clients who are highly bonded to their pets.
  - The veterinary team can relieve this strain on the patient and client by making patient visits possible and convenient. Frequent calls to give progress reports also help ease the client's mind.

Grief Counseling

- As pets approach the end of life, clients may begin to recognize how strongly they are bonded and anticipate the loss that they will experience when the pet dies.
- The mission of the veterinary team is to prevent suffering and support the highest quality of life possible during this time before the pet dies or is euthanized.
- Veterinary hospice endeavors to keep patients in their homes, surrounded by family and friends, pain-free, with their symptoms controlled, so that their last days can be good ones.
  - The patient and family are supported with skilled nursing and bereavement support.
  - A number of veterinary hospice companies exist that are focused on providing these services.
  - The International Association for Animal Hospice and Palliative Care (IAAHPC) is dedicated to promoting knowledge of and developing guidelines for comfort-oriented care to companion animals as they approach the end of life.
- Clients can be assisted in the bereavement process by suggesting ways to memorialize and honor the special relationship they had with their pet.
  - Funeral and burial ceremonies, donations, clay paw prints, pictures, and plantings are all ways of recognizing a special and meaningful relationship (Fig. 3.2).
- Clients who are most bonded with their animals are at risk of suffering the most grief over their loss.
- Loss of a pet elicits a wide range of emotions in clients, which can be associated with certain stages of the grieving process.

Stages of Grief

- By familiarizing yourself with the characteristics of each stage, you will recognize where your client is in this process and be able to shape your responses appropriately.
- The stages of grief include denial, bargaining, anger, guilt, sorrow, and resolution.

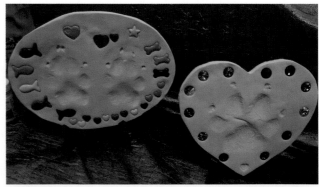

FIGURE 3.2 ClayPaws can be provided to assist clients in memorializing their pet. (From Sirois M: *Principles and practice of veterinary technology*, ed 3, St Louis, 2011, Mosby.)

- These stages frequently occur in this order but can occur in other sequences, and some stages may be repeated.

Denial
- Denial, the first stage of grief, may be played out during the first 24 hours if the animal's death is sudden, or for several days if a terminal illness has been diagnosed.
- Denial is a coping mechanism that cushions the mind against the shock it has received.

Bargaining
- Clients may bargain with God or another higher entity for the life of a pet, or bargain with the pet itself, trying to make it live.
- They may offer the pet vitamins, tempt it with its favorite foods, and promise never to scold or neglect it again.
- When bargaining does not yield the desired results, anger is a natural response.

Anger
- When faced with the loss of a treasured pet, clients may become angry with the veterinarian, practice staff, family, friends, and themselves.
- If clients are angry with themselves for overlooking clinical signs or waiting too long to seek care, this self-directed anger, once dissipated, gives way to guilt.

Guilt
- Guilt is an unproductive, debilitating emotion that often inhibits progress toward resolution of the loss.
- It is the enemy of healing and closure and, if excessive, may require the attention of a mental health professional.
- When guilt subsides, it opens the door for sorrow.

Sorrow
- Sorrow, or deep sadness, is the core of the grieving process.
- Sorrow eventually settles in and permeates all aspects of life and is, in fact, a healing emotion.
- Clients feel relief and release from the pent-up emotions of previous days or weeks.
- Tears flow freely and may come at work, in the supermarket, or while driving.
- Clients may report sleep and appetite disturbances at this time.
- With time, sorrow dissipates, and everyday tasks begin to dominate awareness.

Resolution
- In the resolution phase of grieving, clients realize that the pet is gone, that no amount of wishing will make it different, and that they will survive the loss that previously seemed engulfing.
- Now they can look at photographs of the pet and smile rather than cry, and happy times can be recalled with tenderness rather than despair.

Loneliness
- Regardless of how a loss occurs and how well prepared a client is, all clients feel their lives touched by loneliness.
- This can occur in the presence of family and friends, as well as in the company of remaining pets at home.
- Loneliness arises from this space, and the space fills slowly as the grief process unfolds.

Replacement
- The decision to replace a deceased pet with a new one should be left solely to the individual experiencing the loss.
- The veterinary staff should not influence the decision in any way.
- Some pet owners choose to bond with new pets before their older pets die.
- Others decide that the presence of a new pet in their home would be stressful for the older pet and decide to wait.
- If a client is trying to avoid the experience of loss by finding a replacement for the pet, bonding with the new pet usually does not occur.

THE VETERINARY HEALTH CARE TEAM

- The veterinary health care team involves all members of the staff.
  - Each person plays a significant role in a successful practice.
  - Roles and duties vary by practice and typically are defined in an employee manual.
  - Larger practices may have a structured hierarchy, with each team member having a specific role in the practice.
  - Smaller practices have assistants and technicians assigned to all areas of the practice at the same time.

Members of the Veterinary Health Care Team
Veterinarians
- Veterinarians are the only members of the team allowed to diagnose disease, prescribe treatment, and perform surgery on patients.
- They have completed a professional course of study at an accredited college of veterinary medicine.
- Veterinarians must be licensed in the state where they work and must pass national and state examinations before receiving licensure.

Veterinary Technicians
- A credentialed technician is a graduate of a veterinary technology program approved by the American Veterinary Medical Association (AVMA).
- Most veterinary technology programs are 2 years long and award a college associate's degree.
- A technician must pass the Veterinary Technician National Examination (VTNE) and may be required to pass a state examination before receiving a license.
- Depending on the state, the graduate may be considered registered, certified, or licensed, or may be known as an animal health technologist. Credentialed technicians are allowed to perform certain duties under the direct supervision of a veterinarian.

Veterinary Technologists
- A veterinary technologist can be a graduate of a 4-year bachelor of science program in veterinary technology accredited by the AVMA.

- A veterinary technologist may also hold an associate's degree in veterinary technology along with a bachelor's degree in another program, such as business, management, or health science.
- Technologists tend to work in positions that require a higher level of education and may hold teaching positions within technology programs or veterinary schools.

Veterinary Technician Specialists

- Veterinary technicians may decide to focus on a specific area of care and are designated as veterinary technician specialists once they complete the requirements.
- Technicians who choose to specialize must accumulate a specific number of hours within a particular specialty during a set number of years.
- Candidates are also expected to have a minimum of 40 hours of continuing education related to their specialty before application submission.
- Candidates also submit case reports and case logs to document their advanced skill level. Once all requirements are met, the technician is permitted to take the examination in the specialty area.

Veterinary Assistants

- Veterinary assistants may help a veterinary technician and/or veterinarian.
- They should excel at physical restraint, laboratory skills, patient care, and client relations.
- Assistants can be trained on the job by veterinary technicians or practice managers or attend veterinary assistant classes.
- Veterinary assistants are not licensed, and in most states, their role is not clearly defined.

Receptionists

- Receptionists play a significant role in the success of a practice and must appear professional, polite, and caring.
- Receptionists greet clients, detail and clarify invoices, and receive money.
- They answer the phone and can turn an inquiring phone call into an appointment.

Office Managers

- The office manager is generally responsible for overseeing the front office staff and training receptionists to excel at customer service and public relations.

Practice Managers

- A practice manager helps keep the entire team working together and often reports to a hospital administrator.
- Practice managers generally handle client and personnel issues, supervise training sessions for team members, and hold team members accountable for their actions.
- Duties may also include reviewing records for completeness, observing for missed charges, and ensuring that policies are followed correctly.

- Most practice managers hold a bachelor's degree in science or business administration; others hold an associate's degree in veterinary technology.
- Some practice managers choose to become Certified Veterinary Practice Managers (CVPM) through the Veterinary Hospital Managers Association.

Hospital Administrators

- A hospital administrator may be a veterinarian, veterinary technician, or a business manager.
- This position is responsible for setting budgets, paying bills, creating organizational structure, and planning events.
- A typical administrator is responsible for all the duties of the office manager and practice manager.
- A hospital administrator may report to the owner or shareholders if multiple members own the practice.

Students

- Students may function as observers or hold paid positions within a hospital.
- Many students must complete externships as part of an educational program.
- Veterinary assistant and technician students may fulfill hours required for their coursework.
- Many veterinary schools and some veterinary technician schools have in-clinic prerequisites that must be completed before application and/or admission.
- Veterinary students can also complete an externship in a private practice to obtain more experience before graduating from a professional program.

Groomers

- Groomers perform technical skills that they have acquired to care for patients and satisfy clients.
- Several courses are available to learn how to groom; on-the-job training is also available.
- The National Dog Groomers Association works with groomers throughout the country to promote and encourage professionalism and education to maintain the image of the pet grooming profession.

Kennel Assistants

- Kennel assistants keep the patients clean and alert the team of any changes in patient status. Most kennel assistants receive on-the-job training, learning procedures and protocols while they gain proficiency.
- Kennel assistants should become familiar with cleaning protocols and any harmful and potentially fatal cleaning products.
- Kennel assistants should be trained to detect emergency situations that may occur while a patient is hospitalized, including anaphylactic shock and seizures.
- They must also receive education on the prevention of disease transmission.
  - Many diseases can be transmitted by fomites (e.g., bowls, litter pans) that are not properly cleaned.

- Kennel assistants must be able to interpret nutritional instructions correctly, feed the correct diet and amount, and remove food from preoperative patients.
- This important team member reports any and all behavior and condition changes to the immediate patient supervisor.

Personal Qualifications

- The veterinary practice provides both care of animals and service to clients; veterinary health care team members must also enjoy working with people.
- The veterinary clinic can be a stressful environment, and the team must be ready to handle the emotional stress of working with animals that cannot be cured.
- Compassion fatigue, depression, and suicide are serious problems that occur in veterinary workers.

- All veterinary staff members must focus on their own well-being and take steps to minimize sources of tension and stress in the workplace.
- Veterinary work can also be physically demanding.
  - Walking and standing for long periods, reaching, bending, climbing, and the ability to lift and carry 50 pounds without assistance are common requirements.

Professional Organizations and Resources

- State and national organizations have defined purposes and goals.
- Box 3.6 lists a few of the national groups, organizations, and sites that support veterinary medical professionals and a brief synopsis of the benefits to members.

BOX 3.6 Groups, Organizations, and Websites That Support the Veterinary Health Care Team

AAHA: Created in 1933, the American Animal Hospital Association accredits almost 14% of veterinary hospitals serving approximately 6000 practice teams. The standards of excellence expected in veterinary medicine and practice management are high. Students and veterinary technicians can also become members of AAHA, even if the veterinary hospital where they work is not a member. Continuing education, career center, and bookstore discounts are a few of the benefits of membership (http://www.aahanet.org).

AAVSB: The American Association of Veterinary State Boards recently became the owner of the Veterinary Technician National Examination (VTNE). The examination is offered during three examination periods each year. This organization helps transfer scores, offers mock examinations, lists state technician associations, and has a list of preparation reading resources for the examination (http://www.aavsb.org).

AVMA: Created in 1863, the American Veterinary Medical Association currently has 68,000 members. They have a committee that accredits veterinary technician programs around the United States and Canada (CVTEA). The AVMA acts as the collective voice for the veterinary profession. It lists state VMAs and may help you find your state VTA (http://www.avma.org).

AVTE: The Association of Veterinary Technician Educators offers a biennial symposium, continuing education, career links, recommended review materials for the VTNE, and newsletters (http://www.avte.net).

BLS.GOV: The Bureau of Labor Statistics provides information about average technician salaries, projections, and more (http://www.bls.gov).

CAAHTT: The Canadian Association of Animal Health Technologists and Technicians has resources that include a career center, VTNE study guide, list of

technician programs, and continuing education (http://www.caahtt-acttsa.ca).

CVMA: The Canadian Veterinary Medical Association has resources that include accredited programs and a career center (http://canadianveterinarians.net).

DVM360: This website offers access to a number of journals, such as *Firstline*, *Veterinary Economics*, *DVM Newsmagazine*, and *Veterinary Medicine* (http://www.dvm360.com).

FINANCIAL SIMULATOR PROGRAM: Originally created for veterinary students, this website provides access to an exceptionally valuable personal budget program. It was created by the hospital director at the University of Minnesota College of Veterinary Medicine. The various elements of this budget program can be used by technicians and students and include help to establish personal budgets, make plans to repay education and/or other loans, purchase or lease vehicles, buy homes, and plan for retirement (http://www.finsim.umn.edu).

IVNTA: The International Veterinary Nurses and Technicians Association consists of member countries that seek to foster and promote links with veterinary nursing and veterinary technician staff worldwide by communication and cooperation (http://www.ivnta.org).

MYVETERINARYCAREER: Created in 2007, this website provides personal career management and recruitment. Through their personalized approach, individual preference review, and your identified values, their team will help match you to a veterinary hospital that aligns with your personal mission, goals, and values (http://www.myveterinarycareer.com).

NAVTA: The National Association of Veterinary Technicians in America was created in 1981 to be the national voice of the veterinary technician. Currently, there are 4800 members. It is their goal to influence

Continued

BOX 3.6 Groups, Organizations, and Websites That Support the Veterinary Health Care Team—cont'd

the future of NAVTA members' professional goals, foster high standards of veterinary care, and promote the veterinary health care team. The website has resources that include a career center, continuing education, state representative contacts, specialty section, quarterly journal (TNJ), and information on student chapters (SCNAVTA) and National Veterinary Technician Week (NVTW) (http://www.navta.net).

NCVEI: Founded in 2000 by the American Veterinary Medical Association, the American Animal Hospital Association, and the American Association of Veterinary Medical Colleges and supported by corporate sponsorships, the National Commission on Veterinary Economic Issues offers benchmarking tools and other resources for veterinary practices. Recent articles include "Weathering the Economy" and "The Veterinarian's Guide to Pet Health Insurance." Technicians are greater assets to their veterinary practice if they have a basic understanding of business, profit and loss, and budgeting (http://www.ncvei.org).

NETVET: This is a veterinary resource site for veterinary professionals and animal owners (http://netvet.wustl.edu).

SAFETYVET: Created by a veterinary technician in 1998, this site has resources that include information on OSHA requirements, safety procedures, your rights as an employee, team training, controlled substance logging, radiation exposure, and pregnancy precautions (http://www.safetyvet.com).

SALARYEXPERT: This website allows for geographic research of veterinary professional salaries (http://www.salaryexpert.com).

VETMEDTEAM: Created as the first website offering continuing education to the entire health care team,

VetMedTeam offers VTNE reviews, membership polls, advanced course studies, and practice management and assistant classes (http://www.vetmedteam.com).

VETPARTNERS: VetPartners is a resource for veterinary consultants that includes veterinarians, veterinary technicians, practice managers, industry leaders, lawyers, and business associates. Review their site if you wish to become a consultant, want to network with consultants, or need to hire a consultant (http://www.vetpartners.org).

VHMA: Created in 1981, the membership of Veterinary Hospital Managers Association, currently 1500, includes a number of veterinary technicians; 25% of certified veterinary practice managers (CVPMs) are veterinary technicians. This organization offers continuing education courses, maintains certification for practice managers, conducts surveys, generates a monthly newsletter, and is growing rapidly (http://www.vhma.org).

VSPN: The Veterinary Support Personnel Network was founded in 1996 and is supported by the Veterinary Information Network (VIN). Membership is free. It offers resources that include online continuing education (since 2001), live chats, surveys, and a bookstore (http://www.vspn.org).

WHERETECHSCONNECT: The largest career center for veterinary technicians and staff, this website was created in 2001. You can post your resume, review career tips, view hospitals seeking technicians, and participate in their discussion board—all free services for veterinary technicians. Resources for continuing education are also posted (http://www.wheretechsconnect.com).

From Sirois M: Elsevier's veterinary assistant textbook, *ed 2, St Louis, 2017.*

LAWS AND ETHICS

- Ethics can be defined as the system of moral principles that determines appropriate behavior and actions within a specific group.
- Members of the medical profession are expected to adhere to the highest ethical standards.
- Professional judgment is the freedom given to all veterinarians to treat a case in a manner that they think best.
- Each state government has created laws for the veterinary profession that are written into the veterinary state practice act.
- The Board of Veterinary Medical Examiners, made up of a combination of veterinary professionals and nonveterinarians, is responsible for interpreting the law and standards of care offered to veterinary patients.
  - The board's mission is to protect the consumer and review cases brought against a licensed professional.
  - The veterinary medical board may impose penalties and fines, require further education in record keeping, send letters of guidance or admonition, and/or mandate retraining to avoid future complaints.
  - Suspension of a license to practice is the final tool that a state board uses to ensure that all individuals are practicing to a high standard.
- People who work in the veterinary profession are obligated to serve the public and in so doing, to provide medical care and treatment at a level consistent with the standards of the profession.

- The laws affecting a veterinary practice can be divided into two groups: (1) laws that ensure the quality of veterinary service to patients and (2) laws that provide a nonhostile and safe environment for employees, clients, and the public.

Laws That Ensure the Quality of Veterinary Service

Practice Acts

- The veterinary practice act of each state and province defines which persons may practice veterinary medicine and surgery in the state and under which conditions.
- Practice acts vary in different states and provinces but generally define the practice of veterinary medicine—making it illegal to practice without a license, stating the qualifications for receiving a license, stating the conditions under which a license can be revoked, and establishing penalties for violating the act.
- The practice acts generally define the practice of veterinary medicine and surgery as diagnosing, treating, prescribing, operating on, testing for the presence of animal disease, and making the public aware of your services as a licensed practitioner.
- Many of the procedures performed routinely by technicians and assistants may fall within the scope of the practice of veterinary medicine and surgery.
  - As long as the staff member is under the direction and responsible supervision of a licensed veterinarian and the staff member does not make decisions requiring a veterinary license, the licensed veterinarian, and not the staff member, is practicing veterinary medicine in such instances.
  - Whether a staff member is under the direction and responsible supervision of a licensed veterinarian is a subjective determination that considers the degree of experience and competence of the staff member, the task being performed, and the risks to the patient.

Common Law Malpractice

- When a veterinarian agrees to treat a client's animal, common law automatically imposes on that veterinarian a legal duty to provide medical or surgical care to that client's animal in accordance with that of a reasonably prudent veterinary practitioner of comparable training under the same or similar circumstances.
- A veterinarian's failure to live up to this particular duty constitutes negligence, which may also be referred to as malpractice or professional negligence.
- For malpractice to be subject to litigation, the plaintiff must prove three elements: (1) the veterinarian agreed to treat the patient; (2) the veterinarian failed to exercise the necessary legal obligation of skill and diligence in treating the patient (negligence); and (3) the negligence caused injury to the patient.

Laws That Provide a Safe Business Environment

Occupational Safety and Health Act

- Every employer with one or more employees must operate in compliance with the Occupational Safety and Health Act (OSHA).
- OSHA regulations are designed to provide a safe workplace for all persons working in any business affecting commerce.
- OSHA requires that all employers "shall furnish to each of his employees employment and a place of employment which are free from recognized hazards that are causing or are likely to cause death or serious physical harm to his employees."
- Safety Data Sheets, training, state rules and regulations, fines, and reporting information are located on the official OSHA site: http://www.osha.gov.

Common Law Ordinary Negligence

- Common law establishes for every business owner a legal duty to provide a reasonably safe work environment for employees, as well as a reasonably safe place for clients.
- Failure to provide this safe environment may constitute ordinary negligence on the part of the veterinarian or business owner.
- Ordinary negligence is distinguished from malpractice, which is negligence associated with the rendering of professional veterinary medical services.
- Ordinary negligence is not subject to legal action unless it causes injury to a client or employee.
- A veterinarian has a common law duty to supervise proper restraint of any animal under the veterinarian's control.
  - When a client's animal is being examined and the client restrains the animal, it is the veterinarian and not the client who is primarily responsible for proper restraint of that animal.
  - A veterinarian may be found guilty of ordinary negligence if she or he fails to use reasonable care to avoid foreseeable harm to the restrainer or to other people in the vicinity.

Medical Waste Management Laws

- Veterinarians who own or operate a veterinary practice may be subject to the requirements of state law governing management and disposal of medical waste.
- Local laws may impose additional restrictions on what types of waste transporters and disposal facilities may be acceptable.
- Typical waste included under these acts are discarded needles and syringes, vials containing attenuated or live vaccines, culture plates, and animal carcasses exposed to or infected with pathogens infectious to humans or euthanized with a barbiturate.

Laws That Maintain a Nonhostile Working Environment

- There is a body of federal, state, and common law that restricts a veterinarian, as the owner of a business, from engaging in hiring or firing practices that wrongfully discriminate against individuals.
- Firing an individual for discriminatory reasons constitutes a violation of the federal or state Equal Employment Opportunity (EEO) laws and may provide a basis for the terminated employee to sue the employer under common law for wrongful termination of employment.
- According to federal EEO laws, an employer of 15 or more employees may not discriminate against employees in hiring or firing practices (or in any practice, for that matter) on the basis of race, color, religion, gender, or national origin.
- Sexual harassment and discrimination on the basis of pregnancy or childbirth are forms of sex discrimination made illegal under federal law.
- Employers also cannot discriminate against individuals in hiring and firing of employees on the basis of age between 40 and 70 years or on the basis of disabilities, including AIDS and rehabilitated drug abuse.
- Common law also protects employees because it prohibits an employer from terminating that employee for discriminatory reasons or other reasons violating public policy.
- Under the common law tort of wrongful termination, an employee can sue an employer directly for firing the employee on the basis of gender, race, or religious discrimination, or on the basis that the employee is a whistleblower (i.e., has complained of sexual harassment or other violations of the law).

Laws That Govern Labor

- The Fair Labor Standard Act (FLSA) establishes minimum wage, overtime, record-keeping, and youth employment standards for employees working in the private sector and in government.
- As a veterinary practice team member, you generally fall under the nonexempt category (unless you are promoted to an administrative position).
- Nonexempt employees are entitled to paid overtime when working more than 40 hours in a work week, even those on salary.

Laws Governing Controlled Substances

- Federal and state laws have been adopted to govern the manufacture, sale, and distribution of controlled substances.
- In 1970, Congress passed the Comprehensive Drug Abuse Prevention and Control Act, regulating the manufacturing, distribution, dispensing, and delivery of certain drugs that have the potential for abuse.
- Title 2, known as the Controlled Substance Act (CSA), is the section most applicable to the veterinary community.
- The Drug Enforcement Agency (DEA) is the primary federal law enforcement agency responsible for combating the abuse of controlled drugs.
- Classifications of controlled substances are outlined in Chapter 4; carefully follow all record-keeping, storage, and ordering guidelines related to controlled substances.

RECOMMENDED READINGS

AAHA and IAAHPC End-of-Life Care Guidelines. https://www.aaha.org/globalassets/02-guidelines/end-of-life-care/2016_aaha_iaahpc_eolc_guidelines.pdf

Adler M: *How to speak, how to listen*, New York, 1997, Collier Books.

Allessandra T, Hunsaker P: *Communicating at work*, New York, 1993, Simon and Schuster.

AVMA Guidelines on Veterinary Hospice Care. https://www.avma.org/KB/Policies/Pages/Guidelines-for-Veterinary-Hospice-Care.aspx

Bacal R: *Complete idiot's guide to dealing with difficult employees*, Madison, 2000, CWL Publishing.

Bordeaux D: *12 steps to personal and professional development*, Mill Valley, 1993, Wildflower Press.

Deep S, Sussman L: *What to say to get what you want*, Reading, 1992, Addison-Wesley.

Fuller G: *The workplace survival guide*, Englewood Cliffs, 1996, Prentice Hall.

Griffin J: *How to say it at work*, ed 2, New York, 2008, Prentice Hall.

Kübler-Ross E: *On death and dying*, New York, 1969, Collier Books.

Prendergast H, editor: *Front office management for the veterinary team*, ed 2, St Louis, 2014, Saunders.

Sirois M, editor: *Principles and practice of veterinary technology*, ed 3, St Louis, 2011, Elsevier.

Pharmacology and Pharmacy

CHAPTER OUTLINE

KEY TERMS

Analgesics
Anthelmintic
Antibiotic
Anticonvulsants
Antiinflammatory drugs
Antimicrobial
Antiseptics
Bactericidal
Bacteriostatic
Bronchodilator

Continuous rate infusion
Controlled substance
Corticosteroid
Disinfection
Decongestant
Diuretic
Dose
Elixir
Emetics
Enteric-coated tablet

Expectorants
Fungicidal
Metric system
Neuroleptanalgesia
NSAIDs
Osmotic diuretic
Per os
Pharmacokinetics
Positive inotropic drugs
Prescription

Proprietary name
Residue
Sanitizers
Subcutaneous (SC) injection
Therapeutic range
Tincture
Vasodilator
Vermicide
Viricidal

LEARNING OBJECTIVES

After reviewing this chapter, the reader will be able to:

1. List the various categories of drugs and their clinical uses.
2. Identify dosage forms in which drugs are available.
3. Calculate drug dosages.
4. List and compare routes by which various types of drugs are administered.
5. Describe ways in which drugs exert their effect and affect body tissue.
6. Explain procedures used to safely store and handle drugs.
7. List the primary drugs affecting various body systems.

DRUG NAMES

- Drugs are generally referred to by three different names.
  - The chemical name, such as D-alpha-amino-*p*-hydroxybenzyl-penicillin trihydrate, describes the drug's chemical composition.
  - The nonproprietary name, sometimes called the generic name, is a more concise name given to the specific chemical compound (e.g., aspirin, acetaminophen, or amoxicillin).
  - The proprietary or trade name is a unique drug name given by a manufacturer to its particular brand of drug (e.g., Excedrin, Tylenol, or Amoxi-Tabs).
- Drug container labels must list specific items, including the generic and trade names of the medication, the drug concentration, the quantity in the drug container, the name and address of the manufacturer, the manufacturer's lot number, and the expiration date of the medication (Fig. 4.1).
  - Instructions for use must also be included, either on the label or in an insert within the package.

DOSAGE FORMS

- Drugs may be available in dosage forms that include solid, semisolid, and liquid forms (Table 4.1).

Solid and Semisolid Dosage Forms

- Solid dosage forms include tablets, which are powdered drugs compressed into pills or discs, and capsules, which are powdered drugs enclosed within gelatin capsules.
- Enteric-coated tablets have a special covering that protects the drug from the harsh acidic environment of the stomach and prevents the tablet from dissolving until it enters the intestine.
- Suppositories are inserted into the rectum, where they dissolve and release the drug to be absorbed across the membranes of the intestinal wall.
- Ointments, creams, and pastes are semisolid dosage forms that are applied to the skin (ointments, creams) or given orally (pastes).

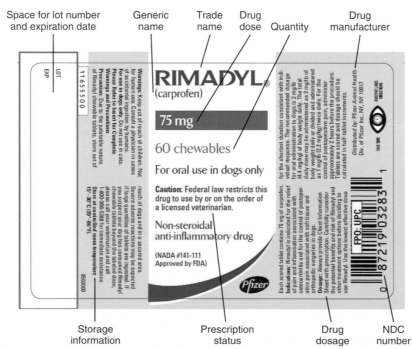

FIGURE 4.1 A label showing the components of a drug as required by the U.S. Food and Drug Administration. (From Wanamaker B, Massey M: *Applied pharmacology for veterinary technicians*, ed 5, St Louis, 2014, Saunders.)

TABLE 4.1 Dosage Forms

Solid Forms	Semisolid Forms	Liquid Forms
Tablet	Suppositories	Syrup
Capsule	Liniment	Elixir
Enteric-coated tablet	Ointment	Tincture
Sustained release	Cream	Lotion
Implant	Paste	Injectable

From Sirois M: Elsevier's veterinary assistant textbook, ed 2, St Louis, 2017, Mosby.

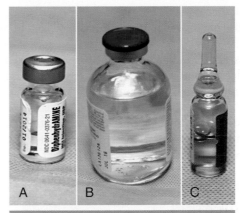

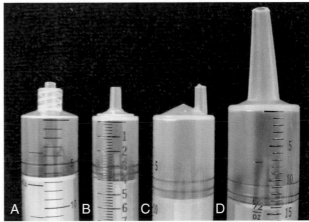

FIGURE 4.2 Parenteral medications are supplied in single-dose vials (A), multidose vials (B), ampules (C), and large-volume bottles or bags used for intravenous administration (D). (From Wanamaker B, Massey M: *Applied pharmacology for veterinary technicians*, ed 5, St Louis, 2014, Saunders.)

- Ointments and creams are designed to liquefy at body temperatures, whereas pastes tend to keep their semisolid form at body temperature.
- Implants are solid dosage forms that are injected or inserted under the skin and dissolve or release a drug over an extended period.

Liquid Dosage Forms

- A solution is a drug dissolved in a liquid vehicle that does not settle out if left standing.
- A suspension contains drug particles that are suspended, but not dissolved, in the liquid vehicle.
  - These drug particles usually settle to the bottom of the container when the container is left standing, so one must shake it back into suspension before administration to ensure consistent dosing.
- Syrups, such as cough syrups, are solutions of drugs with water and sugar (e.g., 85% sucrose).
- Elixirs are solutions of drugs dissolved in sweetened alcohol.
  - Elixirs are used for drugs that do not readily dissolve in water.
- Tinctures are alcohol solutions meant for topical application (applied onto the skin).

Injectable Drugs: Needles and Syringes

- Drugs given by injection are said to be parenterally administered, as opposed to those given enterally via the gastrointestinal (GI) tract.
- Parenteral medications may be supplied in single-dose vials, multidose vials, ampules, or large-volume bottles or bags (Fig. 4.2).
- Injectable drugs are administered via a needle and syringe.
- The most commonly used syringe sizes are 3, 6, 12, 20, 35, and 60 mL.
- Syringes may be ordered from the manufacturer with or without an attached needle.
- The tip of the syringe, where the needle attaches, can be one of four types—Luer-Lok tip (Fig. 4.3A), slip tip (see Fig. 4.3B), eccentric tip (see Fig. 4.3C), or catheter tip (see Fig. 4.3D).
- A complete syringe consists of a plunger, barrel, hub, needle, and dead space

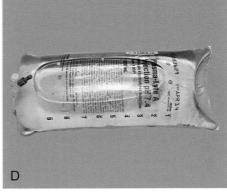

FIGURE 4.3 Syringes are available with different tips, such as a Luer-Lok tip (A), slip tip (B), eccentric tip (C), and catheter tip (D). (From Sirois M: *Elsevier's veterinary assistant textbook*, ed 2, St Louis, 2017, Mosby.)

- Tuberculin syringe: Holds up to 1 mL of medication and usually is available with a 25-gauge or smaller attached needle
- Insulin syringe: Usually is supplied with a 25-gauge needle and is divided into units instead of milliliters; it must be used only for insulin injection.

- Needles are available in various sizes and styles, but all needles have three parts: the hub, shaft, and bevel.
- Needle gauge refers to the inside diameter of the shaft; the larger the gauge number, the smaller the diameter.
- The length of the needle is measured from the tip of the hub to the end of the shaft.
- The bevel is the angle of the opening at the needle tip. Some drugs may be unstable in solution and may require reconstitution with sterile water or another diluent; these may be used immediately for injection.

PRESCRIPTIONS AND DISPENSING MEDICATION

- A prescription is an order from a licensed veterinarian directing a pharmacist to prepare a drug for use in a client's animal.
- Drugs that do not require a prescription are referred to as over-the-counter (OTC) drugs.
  - Veterinary prescription drugs must be used only by or on the order of a licensed veterinarian.
  - A valid veterinarian–client–patient relationship must exist.
  - Veterinary prescription drugs must meet proper requirements for labeling.
  - Veterinary prescription drugs should be dispensed only in a quantity necessary for the treatment of the animal(s). Unlimited refills are limited to lifelong treatments to decrease the potential of misuse of the drugs.
  - Appropriate records of all prescriptions issued must be maintained.
  - Veterinary prescription drugs must be appropriately handled and stored for safety and security.

Components of a Prescription

- Valid prescriptions must contain the following items (Fig. 4.4):
  - Name, address, and telephone number of the person who wrote the prescription

---

HOMETOWN VETERINARY ASSOCIATES

2000 West Chelsea Ave., Momack, PA
(324) 555-4313

Date: November 22, 2011

Patient: Cricket   **Species:** Canine

Owner: Lee Ann Wozniak   **Phone:** 555-0127

Address: 929 Christopher Robin Lane, Brookside, PA 13235

℞ Amoxicillin tablets 100mg #30 tabs
    Sig: 1 tab q8h POPRN until gone

                                Andrew Ryan   **D.V.M.**

FIGURE 4.4 Typical prescription for a veterinary drug. (From Sirois M: *Principles and practice of veterinary technology*, ed 3, St Louis, 2011, Mosby.)

- Date on which the prescription was written
- Owner's name, animal's name, and species of animal
- Rx symbol (abbreviation of recipe, Latin for "take thou")
- Drug name, concentration, and number of units to be dispensed
- *Sig.* (abbreviation for signa, Latin for "write" or "label"), indicating directions for the client in treating the animal
- Signature of the person who wrote the prescription
- U.S. Drug Enforcement Administration (DEA) registration number if the drug is a controlled substance

Containers for Dispensing Medication

- Many veterinary practices dispense tablets and capsules in plastic containers with a childproof lid.
- If medication is dispensed in a paper envelope and a child becomes poisoned, the veterinarian could be found negligent in dispensing the medication in a manner that placed the child at risk.
- Liquids are dispensed in individual syringes or a bottle with a syringe or dropper to draw up the amount needed at each treatment.

The Metric System

- Most of the calculations performed in veterinary practice involve units in the metric system.
- The metric system uses powers of 10 as a base for different units in the system.
- The metric system is a decimal system of notation with only three basic units for weight, volume, and length.

Measurement	Unit	Symbol
Length	Meter	m
Mass	Gram	g
Volume	Liter	l or L

- Various values can be expressed in the metric system by adding prefixes to the basic units that designate multiples or fractions of the basic units.
- The prefixes for the multiples and submultiples of basic units are provided in Table 4.2.
- Although the terms milliliter and cubic centimeter are equivalent units and are often used interchangeably, milliliter is the correct designation for use in medicine.
- As with all decimal units, any decimal number that has no whole number to the left of the decimal point should have a zero inserted as a placeholder.
- Zeroes should not be added after decimal numbers to avoid confusion in medication orders.

CALCULATING DRUG DOSES

- Common metric conversion factors used in calculating drug doses are listed in Box 4.1.
- Calculating the dose of drug to be administered involves the following steps:
  - **Step 1.** Weigh the animal and convert the weight in pounds to kilograms (if necessary).

TABLE 4.2 Prefixes for the Multiples and Submultiples of Basic Units

Power of 10	Prefix	Symbol
10^{12}	tera	T
10^{9}	giga	G
10^{6}	mega	M
10^{3}	kilo	K
10^{2}	hecto	h
10^{1}	deca or deka	da
10^{-1}	deci	d
10^{-2}	centi	c
10^{-3}	milli	m
10^{-6}	micro	mc or μ
10^{-9}	nano	n
10^{-12}	pico	p
10^{-15}	femto	f
10^{-18}	atto	a

From Hendrix CM, Sirois M: Laboratory procedures for veterinary technicians, ed 5, St Louis, 2007, Mosby Elsevier.

BOX 4.1 Metric Conversion Factors

1 kg = 1000 g = 100,000 milligrams (mg)
1 kg = 2.2 lb
1 gram = 1 gm = 1000 mg = 0.001 kg
1 gram = 1 g = 15.43 grains (gr)
1 grain = 64.8 milligrams (usually rounded to 60 or 65 mg)
1 lb = 0.454 kg = 16 ounces (oz)
1 mg = 0.001 g = 1000 micrograms (μg or mcg)
1 liter (L) = 1000 mL = 10 deciliters (dL)
1 mL = 1 cc = 1000 microliters (μL or mcL)
1 tablespoon (tbsp) = 3 teaspoons (tsp)
1 tsp = 5 mL
1 gallon (gal) = 3.786 L
1 gal = 4 quarts (qt) = 8 pints (pt) = 128 fluid ounces (fl oz)
1 pt = 2 cups (C) = 16 fl oz = 473 mL

From Sirois M: Principles and practice of veterinary technology, ed 3, St Louis, 2011, Mosby.

BOX 4.2 Simple Algebraic Calculation Used to Calculate a Drug Dose

What volume of a drug solution should we give to a 44-lb dog if the recommended dosage is 5 mg/kg and the concentration of the solution is 50 mg/mL?
Step 1: Convert pounds to kilograms.

$$X \text{ kg} = \frac{44 \text{lb}}{2.2 \dfrac{\text{lb}}{\text{kg}}} = 20 \text{ kg}$$

Step 2: Calculate the total drug dose.

$$X \text{ mg} = 5 \frac{\text{mg}}{\text{kg}} \times 20 \text{ kg} = 100 \text{ mg}$$

Step 3: Calculate the volume of solution needed.

$$X \text{ mL} = \frac{100 \text{mg}}{50 \dfrac{\text{mg}}{\text{mL}}} = 2 \text{ mL}$$

From Sirois M: Principles and practice of veterinary technology, ed 3, St Louis, 2011, Mosby.

BOX 4.3 Calculating the Number of Tablets to Dispense

How many 25-mg tablets should we dispense for a 10-lb cat if the recommended dosage is 5 mg/lb twice daily for 7 days?
Step 1: Calculate the number of tablets needed per dose.

$$10 \text{ lb} \times 5 \frac{\text{mg}}{\text{lb}} = 50 \text{ mg per dose}$$

Step 2: Calculate the number of tablets needed daily.

2 tablets per dose $\times$ twice daily = 4 tablets daily

Step 3: Calculate the number of tablets needed for 7 days.

4 tablets daily $\times$ 7 day = 28 tablets

From Sirois M: Principles and practice of veterinary technology, ed 3, St Louis, 2011, Mosby.

- **Step 2.** Set up an equation so that the units (e.g., kg, lb) are the same on the top (numerator) and bottom (denominator) on both sides of the equation; solve for X (e.g., kg of body weight) (Box 4.2).
- **Step 3.** After the total dose is determined (in mg or some other measure), calculate the volume (e.g., mL) or number of solid units (tablets, capsules) to be administered using the concentration of drug in the solution (mg of drug/mL of solution) or in each solid unit (mg of drug/tablet), solving for milliliters of liquid or number of tablets.
- When dispensing solid units (tablets, capsules), round to the nearest unit (or half- or quarter-tablet if the tablet is designed to be broken and greater accuracy is essential).
- The steps for calculating the total number of solid units required during a course of treatment are detailed in Box 4.3.

STORING AND HANDLING DRUGS IN THE PHARMACY

- Drugs that are improperly stored (e.g., exposed to extreme temperature or light) can degenerate or become inactivated.
- Drugs still on the pharmacy shelf after the listed expiration date on the container may be less effective.
- Drugs that are sensitive to light are usually kept in a dark amber container.
- Tablets and powders tend to be sensitive to moisture, and their containers usually include silica packets to absorb moisture.
- Some drugs are destroyed by physical stress such as vibrations (e.g., insulin).

STORING AND PRESCRIBING CONTROLLED SUBSTANCES

- A controlled substance is defined by law as a substance with potential for physical addiction, psychological addiction, and/or abuse.
- Controlled substances must be stored securely under lock and key to prevent access by unauthorized personnel.
- A written record must be kept describing when, for what purpose, and how much of the controlled drug was used.
  - These records must include receipts for the purchase or sale of controlled substances and must be maintained for 2 years.
- Drug manufacturers and distributors are required to identify a controlled substance on its label with an uppercase C, followed by a roman numeral, which denotes the drug's theoretical potential for abuse:
  - C-I denotes extreme potential for abuse, with no approved medicinal purpose in the United States.
    - These include such drugs as heroin, lysergic acid diethylamide (LSD), and marijuana.
  - C-II denotes a high potential for abuse.
    - Use may lead to severe physical or psychological dependence.
    - These include such drugs as opium, pentobarbital, and morphine.
  - C-III denotes some potential for abuse but less than for C-II drugs.
    - Use may lead to low-to-moderate physical dependence or high psychological dependence.
    - These include such drugs as ketamine, buprenorphine, and anabolic steroids.
  - C-IV denotes low potential for abuse.
    - Use may lead to limited physical or psychological dependence, including such drugs as phenobarbital and diazepam (Valium).
  - C-V also denotes low potential for abuse, but these drugs are subject to state and local regulation (e.g., Robitussin AC, which contains small amounts of codeine).

- For veterinarians to use, prescribe, or buy a controlled substance legally from an approved manufacturer or distributor, they must have obtained a certification number from the DEA.
- This DEA certification number must be included on all prescriptions or any order forms for Schedule (controlled) drugs.
- Even with a valid DEA number, veterinarians cannot prescribe Schedule I (C-I) drugs.
- Prescriptions for Schedule II (C-II) drugs, which have the most potential for abuse, must be in written form (many states have special forms for C-II drug prescriptions) and cannot be telephoned to a pharmacist.
  - Schedule II drug prescriptions may not be refilled; a new prescription must be written for each treatment period.

THERAPEUTIC RANGE

- The ideal range of drug concentration is referred to as the therapeutic range.
  - If an excessive dose results in accumulation of too much drug in the body, drug concentrations are said to be toxic and signs of toxicity develop.
  - If a small drug dose does not produce drug concentrations within the therapeutic range, drug concentrations are said to be at subtherapeutic levels and the drug's beneficial effect is not achieved.

DOSAGE REGIMEN

- There are three components of therapeutic administration of drugs—the dose, dosage interval, and route of administration.
- A drug's dose is the amount of drug administered at one time.
- The dose is stated in units of mass (e.g., mg, g, gr).
- Dosage interval is the time between the administration of separate drug doses.
- The dose and dosage interval together are often referred to as the dosage regimen.
- The total amount of drug delivered to the animal in 24 hours is determined by multiplying the dose by the frequency of administration.

ROUTES OF ADMINISTRATION

- The route of administration is how the drug enters the body.
- Topical administration: Drugs applied to the surface of the skin, as with lotions and liniments
- Oral administration: Drugs given by mouth, or per os (PO)
- Parenteral administration: Drugs given by injection
  - Intravenous (IV) administration involves injecting the drug directly into a vein.
    - Can be given as a single volume at one time, called a bolus

- Can be slowly injected or dripped into a vein over several seconds, minutes, or even hours as an IV infusion
  - **Continuous rate infusion** (CRI): Given over long periods of time ranging from hours to days
- Intraarterial injection: Drugs given by intraarterial injection are injected into an artery (not a vein), quickly producing high concentrations of drug in tissues supplied by that artery.
  - Inadvertent injection of drugs intraarterially can produce severe effects, such as seizures or respiratory arrest.
- Intramuscular (IM) administration involves injecting the drug into a muscle mass.
- **Subcutaneous (SC) injections** are administered deep to (beneath) the skin, into the subcutis.
- Intradermal (ID) injections are administered within (not beneath) the skin with very small needles.
  - The intradermal route is usually reserved for skin-testing procedures, such as testing for tuberculosis or reaction to allergenic substances.
- Intraperitoneal (IP) injections are administered into the abdominal body cavity and may be used when IV or IM injections are not practical, as in some laboratory animals or when large volumes of solution must be administered for rapid absorption.

Movement of Drug Molecules in the Body

- **Pharmacokinetics** describes how drugs move into, through, and out of the body and involves absorption, distribution, metabolism, and elimination.
- The movement of drug molecules from the site of administration into the systemic circulation is called absorption.
  - The length of time needed for this to occur is affected by the route of administration (Fig. 4.5).

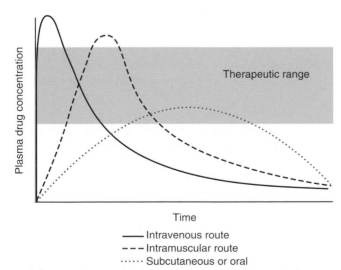

FIGURE 4.5 Plasma drug concentrations attained after intravenous, intramuscular, subcutaneous, and oral administration. (From Sirois M: *Principles and practice of veterinary technology*, ed 3, St Louis, 2011, Mosby.)

- Distribution describes the movement of a drug from the systemic circulation into tissues.
  - Drugs generally are distributed most rapidly and in greater concentrations to well-perfused (rich blood supply) tissues.
- Some drugs bind to proteins in the blood; these protein-bound drug molecules are unable to leave the systemic circulation and so are not distributed to tissues.
- Biotransformation, or drug metabolism, involves altering of a drug by the body before the drug is eliminated.
  - The altered drug molecule is referred to as a metabolite.
  - The liver is the primary organ involved in drug metabolism, or biotransformation.
  - Other tissues, such as the lung, skin, and intestinal tract, may also biotransform drug molecules.
- Removal of a drug from the body is called drug elimination or excretion.
  - The two major routes of elimination are via the kidney (into the urine) and via the liver (into the bile and subsequently into the feces).
  - Inhalant anesthetics and other volatile agents are mostly eliminated via the lungs, although some inhalant anesthetics have some hepatic biotransformation and renal excretion.
- Drug elimination is greatly affected by dehydration; kidney, liver, or heart disease; age; and other physiologic and pathologic (disease) conditions.
- For cells to respond to a drug molecule, the drug must usually combine with a specific protein molecule on or in the cell, called a receptor.

DRUGS AFFECTING THE GASTROINTESTINAL TRACT

- Drugs or functions related to the stomach (GI tract) are called gastric.
- Drugs or functions related to the duodenum, jejunum, or ileum are usually referred to as enteric.
- Drugs and functions related to the colon are referred to as colonic.

Emetics

- Drugs that induce vomiting
- Common **emetics** include apomorphine, xylazine, and hydrogen peroxide
- Most often used to induce vomiting in some cases when animals have ingested toxic substances

Antiemetics

- Antiemetics are drugs that prevent or decrease vomiting.
- Commonly used antiemetics include chlorpromazine, dimenhydrinate (Dramamine), maropitant citrate (Cerenia), and metoclopramide (Reglan).

Antidiarrheals

- Antidiarrheals are drugs used to combat various types of diarrhea.

- Narcotics commonly used to combat diarrhea include diphenoxylate (Lomotil), paregoric (tincture of opium), and loperamide (Imodium).
  - A disadvantage of narcotics when used as antidiarrheals is that their analgesic effect can mask pain that otherwise could be used to monitor progression or resolution of disease.
  - Another disadvantage is that narcotics can cause excitement in cats (so-called morphine mania).
- Bismuth subsalicylate, the active ingredient in Pepto-Bismol, breaks down in the gut to bismuth carbonate and salicylate. The bismuth tends to coat the intestinal mucosa, and the salicylate (an aspirin-like compound) decreases inflammation and blocks the formation of prostaglandins that would normally stimulate fluid secretion.

Adsorbents and Protectants

- An adsorbent causes another substance to adhere to its outer surface, thus reducing contact of that substance with the intestinal tract wall.
- Activated charcoal adsorbs enterotoxins to its surface, preventing them from contacting the bowel wall.
- Kaolin and pectin (Kaopectate) are often used together for the symptomatic relief of vomiting or diarrhea.

Laxatives, Lubricants, and Stool Softeners

- Laxatives, cathartics, and purgatives facilitate evacuation of the bowels.
- Irritant laxatives, including castor oil and phenolphthalein, work by irritating the bowel, resulting in increased peristaltic motility.
- Bulk laxatives are much gentler than irritant laxatives and work by pulling water osmotically into the bowel lumen or retaining water in the feces.
- Hydrophilic colloids or indigestible fiber (e.g., bran, methylcellulose, Metamucil) are not digested or adsorbed to any degree and therefore create an osmotic force to produce their laxative effect.
- Hypertonic salts such as magnesium (milk of magnesia, Epsom salts) and phosphate salts (Fleet Enema) are poorly absorbed and create a strong osmotic force that attracts waters into the bowel lumen.
- Lubricants (e.g., mineral oil, cod liver oil, white petrolatum, glycerin) are given to make the stool slipperier for easy passage through the bowel.
- Docusate sodium succinate (Colace) is a stool softener that acts as a wetting agent by reducing the surface tension of feces and allowing water to penetrate the dry stool.
- Lactulose is another laxative that increases osmotic pressure by drawing water into the colon, which results in fecal material containing more liquid.

Antacids

- Antacids reduce the acidity of the stomach or rumen.
- Nonsystemic antacids in liquid or tablet form are composed of calcium, magnesium, or aluminum, and they directly neutralize acid molecules in the stomach or rumen.
- OTC products such as Tums and Rolaids are nonsystemic antacids made primarily of calcium.
- Other nonsystemic antacids include magnesium products (Riopan, Carmilax), aluminum products (Amphojel), and combinations of magnesium and aluminum products (Maalox).
- Systemic antacids decrease acid production in the stomach.
- Systemic antacids include cimetidine (Tagamet), ranitidine (Zantac), and famotidine (Pepcid).

Antiulcer Drugs

- Sucralfate (Carafate) is an antiulcer drug used to treat ulcers of the stomach and upper small intestine.
- The drug forms a sticky paste and adheres to the ulcer site, protecting it from the acidic environment of the stomach.
- Omeprazole (e.g., Gastrogard, Prilosec OTC) is a gastric acid pump inhibitor that binds irreversibly to the secretory surface of cells in the stomach to decrease acid secretion (antacid) and helps support the stomach lining (antiulcer).
- Misoprostol (Cytotec) is a synthetic prostaglandin that helps decrease acid secretion in the stomach and increases production of the stomach lining (mucosa).

Appetite-Stimulating Drugs

- Cyproheptadine is a serotonin antagonist antihistamine that is mostly used as an appetite stimulant for cats.

DRUGS AFFECTING THE CARDIOVASCULAR SYSTEM

Antiarrhythmic Drugs

- Arrhythmias are divided into two general groups: arrhythmias that result in an increased heart rate (tachycardia) and those that cause a decreased heart rate (bradycardia).
  - Lidocaine, mexiletine, quinidine, and procainamide reverse arrhythmias primarily by decreasing the rate of movement of sodium into heart cells.
    - Lidocaine is available with epinephrine and is designed for use as a local anesthetic, not as an antiarrhythmic drug.
  - Procainamide and quinidine are more commonly used for their ventricular antiarrhythmic effects in dogs and cats.
  - Beta blockers: Drugs that block beta receptors are known as beta blockers and cause the heart to contract with less force.
    - Propranolol (Inderal) decreases the heart rate and prevents tachycardia in response to stress, fear, or excitement.
  - Calcium channel blockers combat arrhythmias by blocking calcium channels of cardiac muscle cells, resulting in decreased conduction of depolarization

waves and decreased automaticity of parts of the conduction system.

- Although not commonly used to treat arrhythmias in veterinary patients, verapamil and diltiazem have been used successfully for the treatment of supraventricular tachycardia, atrial fibrillation, and atrial flutter.
- A more common use of diltiazem is for cats with hypertrophic cardiomyopathy, in which the heart becomes thickened and enlarged to the point at which it cannot contract efficiently.
- Another calcium channel blocker most commonly used for hypertension in small animals is amlodipine; it dilates the peripheral arteries and thereby reduces afterload.

Positive Inotropic Agents

- Drugs that increase the strength of contraction of a weakened heart are referred to as positive inotropic drugs.
  - Digoxin exerts its effect primarily by making more calcium available for the contractile elements within cardiac muscle cells and is the drug of choice for maintaining long-term positive inotropic effects.
  - Digoxin, available as a tablet and elixir, is often used to control supraventricular tachycardia caused by atrial fibrillation.
  - Digoxin has a small therapeutic index, meaning that therapeutic concentrations are close to toxic concentrations.
  - Early signs of digoxin toxicity include anorexia, vomiting, and diarrhea.
  - Pimobendan is an inodilator because it has both inotropic and vasodilator effects and is used in conjunction with other medications in dogs to treat congestive heart failure secondary to dilated cardiomyopathy or chronic mitral valve insufficiency.
  - Dobutamine is also an inotropic agent that is generally used for the short-term management of heart failure and for shock patients when fluid therapy alone is not working.

Vasodilators

- Vasodilators open (dilate) constricted vessels, making it easier for the heart to pump blood through these vessels.
  - Hydralazine is a vasodilator that causes arteriolar smooth muscle to relax, which benefits animals with a poorly functioning left atrioventricular (mitral) valve (mitral insufficiency). Nitroglycerin relaxes the blood vessels on the venous side of the circulation; it may also help dilate coronary arterioles.
    - The drug is well absorbed through the skin and mucous membranes. The cream and nitroglycerin in patch form are applied to the skin to improve cardiac output and reduce pulmonary edema and ascites (abdominal fluid accumulation).
  - Nitroprusside acts much like nitroglycerin but is usually found only in the intensive care unit (ICU)

setting because of the necessity to monitor blood pressure constantly and the need to give the drug as a CRI.
  - Angiotensin-converting enzyme (ACE) inhibitors: Other vasodilators are enalapril (Enacard), captopril, and benazepril, which block ACE and prevent the formation of angiotensin II (a potent vasoconstrictor) and aldosterone.

Diuretics

- Diuretics are drugs that increase urine formation and promote water loss.
- In animals with congestive heart failure, sodium retention from aldosterone secretion and concomitant retention of water in the blood and body tissues lead to pulmonary edema, ascites, and an increased cardiac workload.
  - Loop diuretics such as furosemide (Lasix) produce diuresis by inhibiting sodium resorption from the loop of Henle in nephrons.
  - Because loop diuretics cause potassium to be excreted in the urine, prolonged use of loop diuretics may result in hypokalemia (low blood potassium level).

DRUGS AFFECTING THE RESPIRATORY SYSTEM

Antitussives

- Antitussives are drugs that block the cough reflex, which is coordinated by the cough center in the brainstem and are usually used in patients with nonproductive coughs.
- A productive cough refers to a cough that produces mucus and other inflammatory products that are coughed up into the oral cavity.
- A nonproductive cough is dry and hacking, and no mucus is coughed up.
- Antitussives are commonly used for treating uncomplicated tracheobronchitis (referred to as kennel cough) in dogs.
- Butorphanol (Torbutrol) is a centrally acting opioid cough suppressant that, unlike most other opioid cough suppressants, is generally not classified as a controlled substance and causes little sedation compared with stronger opioid drugs.
- Hydrocodone (Hycodan) is a C-III narcotic available only by prescription from a veterinarian with a DEA clearance for writing C-III prescriptions.
  - Sedation is often noted in treated animals, and long-term administration can result in constipation.
- Codeine is a relatively weak opioid narcotic that is a component of many cough suppressant preparations.
  - Most products containing codeine are prescription preparations with a C-V controlled substance rating.
- Dextromethorphan is a common ingredient in OTC nonprescription cough, flu, and cold preparations; its

actions are similar to those of the more potent narcotic antitussives, but it is not a controlled substance.

- Dextromethorphan is generally not as effective for controlling coughs in veterinary patients as butorphanol or other prescription antitussives.
- Although dextromethorphan in OTC products is fairly harmless, the other compounds in cold or flu preparations can cause significant harm to animals (e.g., acetaminophen can be toxic in cats).

Mucolytics, Expectorants, and Decongestants

- Mucolytic agents are designed to break up (lyse) mucus and reduce its viscosity so that the cilia can move the mucus out of the respiratory tract.
- Acetylcysteine (Mucomyst) is a mucolytic agent that decreases the viscosity of mucus.
- Expectorants are compounds that also increase the fluidity of mucus in the respiratory tract by generating liquid secretions by respiratory tract cells.
  - Guaifenesin (glyceryl guaiacolate) and saline expectorants (e.g., ammonium chloride, potassium iodide, sodium citrate) are given PO.
- Decongestants reduce congestion (vascular engorgement) of the mucous membranes.

Bronchodilators

- Drugs that inhibit bronchoconstriction are called bronchodilators.
- Terbutaline, albuterol, and clenbuterol are available in an oral dosage form and as an inhaler.
- The methylxanthines include bronchodilators such as theophylline and aminophylline.

DRUGS AFFECTING THE ENDOCRINE SYSTEM

Drugs Used to Treat Hypothyroidism

- Drugs used to treat hypothyroidism (insufficiency of thyroid hormone) include levothyroxine (T_4) and synthetic liothyronine (the L-isomer of triiodothyronine [T_3]).
- Supplementing a hypothyroid animal with T_4 provides the various organs and tissues with the appropriate amount of thyroid hormone because each organ or tissue converts T_4 to T_3.

Drugs Used to Treat Hyperthyroidism

- Hyperthyroidism (increase in thyroid hormone production) is most common in cats and is associated with a hormone-secreting thyroid tumor.
- Methimazole (Tapazole) and propylthiouracil have been used to control hyperthyroidism in cats by blocking the thyroid tumor's ability to produce T_3 and T_4.

Endocrine Pancreatic Drugs

- Lack of insulin results in diabetes mellitus, a condition characterized by high blood glucose levels (hyperglycemia) and passage of glucose in the urine (glucosuria).
- Blood glucose levels can be controlled by one or two SC insulin injections daily.
- The insulin currently approved by the Food and Drug Administration (FDA) for use in dogs and cats is porcine insulin zinc suspension (Vetsulin).
- The human recombinant protamine zinc insulin (PZI, Prozinc) is labeled as having an appropriate duration only in cats.
- Glargine (Lantus) is a long-acting insulin also used in cats.

Drugs Used to Treat Hypoadrenocorticism

- Hypoadrenocorticism (Addison disease) is characterized by a lack of glucocorticoid and/or mineralocorticoid secretion from the adrenal cortex.
- Hypoadrenocorticism is treated with corticoid supplementation.
- Mineralocorticoid supplementation is achieved with desoxycorticosterone pivalate (DOCP; Percorten-V) or fludrocortisone acetate (Florinef).
- Desoxycorticosterone is a long-acting mineralocorticoid that requires functioning kidneys to work properly.
- Fludrocortisone has mineral and glucocorticoid activity and is used in dogs and cats.
- Glucocorticoid supplementation is achieved using a number of glucocorticoid agents, including betamethasone, dexamethasone, fludrocortisone, flumethasone, hydrocortisone, methylprednisolone, prednisolone, prednisone, or triamcinolone.

Drugs Used to Treat Hyperadrenocorticism

- Hyperadrenocorticism (Cushing disease) is characterized by excess glucocorticoids in the system.
- The treatment of hyperadrenocorticism is based on suppressing the adrenal gland, either by discontinuing corticosteroid use or by surgically removing the adrenal gland.
- Mitotane (Lysodren) causes the selective necrosis of two sections of the adrenal gland, decreasing the release of corticosteroids.

DRUGS AFFECTING REPRODUCTION

- Hormone drugs, natural or synthetic, are used primarily to prevent pregnancy or alter the state of the uterus.
- Gonadotropin-releasing hormone (GnRH) drugs (e.g., Cystorelin) stimulate the release of luteinizing hormone (LH) and/or follicle-stimulating hormone (FSH) from the pituitary gland, causing the ovary to develop follicles.
- Megestrol acetate (Ovaban) is an oral progestin used for contraception in female dogs and cats.

- Mibolerone (Cheque Drops) is a testosterone analogue used as a contraceptive in female dogs.
- Estradiol cypionate (ECP) is an injectable estrogen used after mismating in dogs to prevent pregnancy.
- Oxytocin is commonly used to increase uterine contractions in animals with dystocia (difficult birth) related to a weakened or fatigued uterus.
- Anabolic steroids, such as testosterone and progesterone, have been used to increase the weight and conditioning of feedlot cattle.

DRUGS AFFECTING THE NERVOUS SYSTEM

Anesthetics

- Barbiturates are used infrequently to produce short-term anesthesia and induce general anesthesia and are frequently used to control seizures and euthanize animals.
- Thiobarbiturates contain a sulfur molecule on the barbituric acid molecule; oxybarbiturates contain an oxygen molecule.
- Thiamylal and thiopental are thiobarbiturates; methohexital, pentobarbital, and phenobarbital are oxybarbiturates.
- Thiobarbiturates have a more rapid onset but shorter duration of action than oxybarbiturates.
- Propofol is usually injected as an IV bolus and provides rapid induction of anesthesia and a short period of unconsciousness.
- Ketamine and tiletamine are short-acting injectable anesthetics that produce a rather unique form of anesthesia in which the animal feels dissociated (apart) from its body.
- The lack of muscular relaxation makes ketamine unsuitable as a sole anesthetic agent for major surgery.
- Tiletamine is included with zolazepam, a benzodiazepine tranquilizer, in a product marketed as Telazol.
- Isoflurane is an inhalant anesthetic that has gained popularity in veterinary practice because of its rapid, smooth induction of anesthesia and short recovery period.
- Other inhalant agents with properties similar to those of isoflurane include enflurane, desflurane, and sevoflurane.

Tranquilizers and Sedatives

- Acepromazine maleate is a phenothiazine tranquilizer that reduces anxiety and produces a mentally relaxed state.
- It is often used to calm animals for physical examination or transport.
- Droperidol is a butyrophenone with much more potent sedative effects than most phenothiazine tranquilizers.
- Droperidol has been combined with fentanyl, a strong narcotic analgesic with emetic activity, and marketed as a neuroleptanalgesic product called Innovar-Vet.

- Diazepam (Valium), zolazepam (contained in Telazol), midazolam, and clonazepam are benzodiazepine tranquilizers often used with other agents as part of a preanesthetic protocol for their calming and muscle relaxing effects.
- Xylazine (Rompun), dexmedetomidine (Dexdomitor), and detomidine (Dormosedan) produce a calming effect and somewhat decrease an animal's ability to respond to stimuli.

Analgesics

- Analgesics are drugs that reduce the perception of pain without loss of other sensations.
- Oxymorphone (Numorphan) and hydromorphone are commonly used for preanesthesia and anesthesia.
- Butorphanol (Torbutrol, Torbugesic) is used for cough control and GI-related pain in small animals.
- Tramadol is also used for generalized pain and cough control but has less sedating effects than butorphanol.
- Fentanyl has an analgesic effect 250 times greater than that of morphine.
- Meperidine (Demerol) is a fairly weak analgesic-sedative and is often injected SC to restrain cats.
- Pentazocine (Talwin) is a weak analgesic used for dogs recovering from painful surgery.
- Buprenorphine (Buprenex) is commonly combined with sedatives or tranquilizers (e.g., acepromazine, xylazine, detomidine).
- Butorphanol, pentazocine, and buprenorphine are sometimes used for partial reversal of some of the respiratory depression and sedation caused by stronger narcotic agents.
- Nalorphine is another reversal agent.
- Neuroleptanalgesia refers to a state of central nervous system (CNS) depression (sedation or tranquilization) and analgesia induced by a combination of a sedative (e.g., xylazine) or tranquilizer (e.g., acepromazine) and an analgesic (oxymorphone).
- Phenothiazine tranquilizers or butyrophenone tranquilizers (e.g., droperidol) calm the animal and also decrease or block the emetic (vomiting) side effect of a narcotic analgesic.

Anticonvulsants

- Drugs used to control seizures are called anticonvulsants.
- Seizures are periods of altered brain function characterized by loss of consciousness, altered muscle tone or movement, altered sensations, or other neurologic changes.
- Phenobarbital is a drug of choice for long-term control of seizures in dogs and cats.
- Diazepam (Valium) is the drug of choice for emergency treatment of convulsing animals.
- Clonazepam is occasionally used with phenobarbital in animals in which plasma concentrations of barbiturate are in the therapeutic range but the seizures are not adequately controlled.

- Potassium bromide (KBr) is the other drug of choice for long-term seizure control in dogs. It can be used alone or in conjunction with phenobarbital.
- Methocarbamol (Robaxin-V) is not an antiseizure medication, but a muscle relaxant used to help seizure-like tremoring in dogs that have metaldehyde poisoning (active ingredient in slug and snail baits).

Central Nervous System Stimulants

- CNS stimulants are primarily used to stimulate respiration in anesthetized animals or to reverse CNS depression caused by anesthetic or sedative agents.
- Doxapram (Dopram) is a CNS stimulant that increases respiration in animals with apnea (cessation of breathing) or bradypnea (slow breathing).

ANTIMICROBIALS

- Antimicrobials are drugs that kill or inhibit the growth of microorganisms or microbes, such as bacteria, protozoa, viruses, or fungi.
- The suffix -*cidal* generally describes drugs that kill the microorganism (e.g., *bactericidal*).
- The suffix -*static* usually describes drugs that inhibit replication but generally do not kill the microorganism outright (e.g., *fungistatic*).
  - Bactericidal: Kills bacteria
  - Bacteriostatic: Inhibits bacterial replication
  - Virucidal: Kills viruses
  - Protozoastatic: Inhibits protozoal replication
  - Fungicidal: Kills fungi
- Some microorganisms have developed the ability to survive in the presence of antimicrobial drugs.
- Bacteria may become resistant to certain drugs because of genetic changes inherited from previous generations of bacteria, or they may acquire resistance by spontaneous mutations of chromosomes.
- A residue is an accumulation of a drug, chemical, or its metabolites in animal tissues or food products resulting from drug administration to an animal or contamination of food products.
- Penicillins are bactericidal and can usually be recognized by their -*cillin* suffix on the drug name.
- The most frequently used penicillins in veterinary medicine include the following: the natural penicillins, penicillin G and penicillin V; the broad-spectrum aminopenicillins, ampicillin, amoxicillin, and hetacillin; the penicillinase-resistant penicillins, cloxacillin, dicloxacillin, and oxacillin; and the extended-spectrum penicillins, carbenicillin, ticarcillin, piperacillin, and others.
- Amoxicillin–clavulanate acid (Clavamox) is another bactericidal aminopenicillin with a beta-lactamase inhibitor, which expands its spectrum of coverage.
- Cephalosporins are bactericidal beta-lactam antimicrobials with a *ceph-* or *cef-* prefix in the drug name.
  - Cephalosporins are classified by generations, according to when they were first developed.

- First-generation cephalosporins are primarily effective against gram-positive bacteria (e.g., *Streptococcus*, *Staphylococcus* spp.).
- Veterinary products include cefadroxil (first generation, Cefa-Tabs), cefazolin (first generation, Ancef, Zolicef, cefazolin sodium), cephapirin (first generation, Cefa-Lak, Cefa-Dri intramammary infusions), ceftiofur (third generation, Naxcel injectable), cefovecin sodium (Convenia, 2-week injectable), and cefpodoxime proxetil (third generation, Simplicef).
- Bacitracins are a group of polypeptide antibiotics, of which bacitracin A is the major component.
  - Bacitracin is a common ingredient in topical antibiotic creams or ointments. It is often combined with polymyxin B and neomycin to provide a broad spectrum of antimicrobial activity.
- Aminoglycosides used in veterinary medicine include gentamicin, amikacin, neomycin, streptomycin, dihydrostreptomycin, apramycin, kanamycin, and tobramycin.
  - With the exception of amikacin, most aminoglycosides can be recognized by the -*micin* or -*mycin* suffix in the nonproprietary name.
  - Aminoglycosides are bactericidal and are effective against many aerobic bacteria (bacteria that require oxygen to live) but are not effective against most anaerobic bacteria (those that do not require oxygen).
- Fluoroquinolones (quinolones) are bactericidal antimicrobials used commonly for their effectiveness against a variety of pathogens.
  - Quinolones are not effective against anaerobes. Enrofloxacin (Baytril) is approved for use in dogs, cats, cattle, horses, ferrets, reptiles, birds, and rodents.
  - Ciprofloxacin (Cipro) is similar to enrofloxacin and mostly used when larger dosages are necessary.
  - Orbifloxacin (Orbax) is also similar to enrofloxacin and is approved for use against susceptible infections in dogs and cats.
  - Difloxacin (Dicural) and marbofloxacin (Zeniquin) are approved for use against susceptible infections in dogs only.
  - Ofloxacin (Ocuflox) is used as an ophthalmic medication only.
- Tetracyclines are bacteriostatic drugs with a nonproprietary name ending in -*cycline*.
  - Tetracycline and oxytetracycline have similar spectra of antibacterial activity and actions in the body.
  - Oxytetracycline is the most commonly used injectable tetracycline because of its good absorption from IM injection sites.
- Sulfonamides and potentiated sulfonamides are sometimes combined with other compounds, such as trimethoprim and ormetoprim, to potentiate (increase) their antibacterial effects.
  - Some of the more common sulfonamides used in veterinary medicine include sulfadimethoxine (combined with ormetoprim in Primor), sulfadiazine (combined with trimethoprim in Tribrissen), sulfamethoxazole

(combined with trimethoprim in Septra), and sulfasalazine (used for its antiinflammatory effect in inflammatory bowel disease).

- Lincosamide antibiotics, including lincomycin and clindamycin (Antirobe), can be bacteriostatic or bactericidal, depending on the concentration attained at the site of infection.
- Macrolide antibiotics used in dogs and cats include erythromycin and azithromycin.
  - The drugs are bacteriostatic and share similar spectra of antibacterial activity and bacterial cross-resistance.
- Metronidazole (Flagyl) is a bactericidal antimicrobial that is also effective against protozoa that cause intestinal disease, such as *Giardia* (giardiasis), *Entamoeba histolytica* (amebiasis), *Trichomonas* (trichomoniasis), and *Balantidium coli* (balantidiasis).
- The nitrofurans are a large group of antimicrobials; of these, nitrofurantoin (Furadantin) is most commonly used in veterinary medicine.
  - Nitrofurantoin is bacteriostatic or bactericidal, depending on the concentration attained at the site of infection.
- Chloramphenicol is an antimicrobial that is bacteriostatic at a low concentration but may become bactericidal when used at higher dosages.
- Florfenicol is a new drug similar to chloramphenicol but without the risk of aplastic anemia seen with chloramphenicol.
- Rifampin is a bactericidal or bacteriostatic antimicrobial belonging to the rifamycin group.
- Antifungals include amphotericin B and nystatin.
  - Amphotericin B is an antifungal that is administered IV for the treatment of deep or systemic mycotic infections.
  - Nystatin, because of its toxicity to tissues, is used only to treat *Candida* infections (candidiasis) on the skin, mucous membranes (e.g., mouth, vagina), and lining of the intestinal tract in dogs, cats, and birds.
- Flucytosine is an antifungal agent used mostly against *Cryptococcus* and *Candida*.
- Fluconazole, ketoconazole, and itraconazole are imidazole antifungals with fewer side effects than amphotericin B. Of the imidazoles, fluconazole has the fewest side effects and is apparently safe for use in multiple species.
- Griseofulvin is a fungistatic drug used primarily to treat infections with *Trichophyton, Microsporum,* and *Epidermophyton* dermatophytes (superficial fungi) in dogs and cats.

ANTIPARASITICS

- Anthelmintic is a general term used to describe compounds that kill various types of internal parasites.
  - A vermicide is an anthelmintic that kills the worm, as opposed to a vermifuge, which only paralyzes the worm and often results in the passage of live worms in the stool.

- Antinematodal compounds are used to treat infections with nematodes (roundworms). Anticestodal compounds are used to treat infections with cestodes (tapeworms or segmented flatworms).
- Antitrematodal compounds are used to treat infection with trematodes (flukes or unsegmented flatworms), including *Paragonimus, Fasciola,* and *Dicrocoelium* spp.
- Antiprotozoal compounds are used to treat infection with protozoa (single-celled organisms), including *Coccidia, Giardia,* and *Toxoplasma* spp.
- Coccidiostats are drugs that specifically inhibit the growth of coccidia.

Internal Antiparasitics

- Piperazine, a vermicide and vermifuge, is the active ingredient in most of the once-monthly dewormers sold in grocery stores and pet shops.
- The benzimidazoles include fenbendazole (Panacur), mebendazole (Telmintic), thiabendazole (Tresaderm Otic), oxibendazole (Filaribits-Plus), albendazole, oxfendazole, and cambendazole.
- Organophosphates are used as internal antiparasitics and in external antiparasitics to combat fleas, ticks, and flies.
- The organophosphates most commonly used internally are dichlorvos and trichlorfon. Ivermectin (Ivomec, Heartgard-30) is an avermectin widely used in almost every species treated by veterinarians.
- Anticestodals used in animals include praziquantel (Droncit) and epsiprantel (Cestex).
- Anthelmintics containing pyrantel (Strongid) safely remove a variety of nematodes in domestic species.
- Melarsomine dihydrochloride (Immiticide) is approved as a heartworm adulticide; it is given by IM injection.
- Milbemycin oxime, a drug similar to ivermectin, is also used as a microfilaricide.
- Many of the milbemycin products are also marketed in formulas that include spinosad, lufenuron, or praziquantel to control fleas and internal parasites (Trifexis, Sentinel, Interceptor Plus).
- Antiprotozoals are most commonly used against coccidia, *Giardia,* and other protozoa.

External Antiparasitics

- Chlorinated hydrocarbons constitute one of the oldest groups of the synthetic insecticides.
- The only chlorinated hydrocarbon currently used in veterinary medicine is lindane, which is incorporated in some dog shampoos.
- Organophosphates and carbamates are usually grouped together because of their similar mechanisms of action, effects on insects, and toxic effects.
- Unlike the chlorinated hydrocarbons, organophosphates and carbamates decompose readily in the environment and do not pose a significant threat to wildlife. Included in this group are chlorpyrifos, carbaryl, and propoxur.

- Pyrethrins and pyrethroids (synthetic pyrethrins) constitute the largest group of insecticides marketed for use against external parasites and as common household insect sprays.
- Pyrethrins and pyrethroids produce a quick knockdown effect, but the immobilized flies or fleas may recover after several minutes.
- Pyrethroids include resmethrin, allethrin, permethrin, tetramethrin, bioallethrin, and fenvalerate.
- Amitraz is a diamide insecticide that was one of the first effective agents available for the treatment of demodectic mange in dogs. The liquid form, available as a dip or sponge-on bath product (Mitaban), is used to treat demodectic mange in dogs.
- Imidacloprid (Advantage) is a chloronicotinyl nitroguanidine insecticide used topically to kill adult fleas on dogs and cats.
- Fipronil (Frontline) and selamectin (Revolution) are once-monthly flea sprays and topical applications that are similar to ivermectin in their insecticidal activity.
- Rotenone (Derris Powder) is a natural insecticide derived from derris root. It may be included with other insecticides in dips, pour-ons, and powders.
- D-Limonene, derived from citrus peel, purportedly has some slight insecticidal activity.
- Sulfur is sometimes included in tar and sulfur shampoos to help reduce skin scaling and to treat sarcoptic mange.
- Insect growth regulators are compounds that affect the immature stages of insects and prevent maturation to adults.
- Methoprene (Precor) and fenoxycarb (Insegar) were some of the first insect growth regulators incorporated into topical products or flea collars.
- Lufenuron (Program, Sentinel) is an insect development inhibitor given once monthly in tablet form for dogs and cats and as an oral liquid for cats.
- Fluralaner (Bravecto) is a systemic insecticide that kills fleas and ticks when they feed on dogs or cats and lasts up to 12 weeks per dose.
- Spinosad (Comfortis) is a neurotoxin that works on fleas only and, like lufenuron, is orally ingested and distributed throughout the animal's tissue.
- Butoxypolypropylene glycol has been incorporated into flea and tick spray products for use in dogs and cats. Diethyltoluamide (DEET) is a common ingredient in repellent products formulated for use in humans.

ANTIINFLAMMATORIES

- Drugs that relieve pain or discomfort by blocking or reducing the inflammatory process are called antiinflammatory drugs.
- There are two general classes of antiinflammatories: steroidal antiinflammatory drugs (glucocorticoids) and nonsteroidal antiinflammatory drugs (NSAIDs).

- When veterinarians use the terms cortisone or corticosteroid, they are usually referring to glucocorticoids.
- Hydrocortisone, which exerts an antiinflammatory effect for less than 12 hours, is considered a short-acting glucocorticoid.
- Intermediate-acting glucocorticoids, with activity for 12 to 36 hours, include prednisone, prednisolone, triamcinolone (Vetalog), methylprednisolone, and isoflupredone.
- Long-acting glucocorticoids, such as dexamethasone, betamethasone, and flumethasone, exert their effects for longer than 48 hours.

Nonsteroidal Antiinflammatory Drugs

- The advantage of NSAIDs over glucocorticoids is that they have fewer side effects.
- Aspirin (acetylsalicylic acid) is a fairly safe NSAID in most animal species for short-term use in low doses.
- Carprofen (Rimadyl), deracoxib (Deramaxx), etodolac (Etogesic), meloxicam (Metacam), and firocoxib (Previcox) are all cyclooxygenase (COX)-inhibiting (coxib) class, non-narcotic NSAIDs with antiinflammatory and analgesic properties.

DISINFECTANTS AND ANTISEPTICS

- Disinfection is the destruction of pathogenic microorganisms or their toxins.
- Disinfectants are chemical agents that kill or prevent the growth of microorganisms on inanimate objects (e.g., surgical equipment, floors, tabletops).
- Antiseptics are chemical agents that kill or prevent the growth of microorganisms on living tissues.
- Antiseptics and disinfectants may also be described as sanitizers or sterilizers.
- Sanitizers are chemical agents that reduce the number of microorganisms to a safe level, without completely eliminating all microorganisms.
- Sterilizers are chemicals or other agents that destroy all microorganisms completely.
- Phenols are used as scrub soaps and surface disinfectants.
- Alcohols, such as ethyl alcohol or isopropyl alcohol, are among the most common antiseptics applied to the skin.
- Solutions of 70% alcohol are used to disinfect surgical sites, injection sites, and rectal thermometers.
- Quaternary ammonium compounds are used to disinfect the surface of inanimate objects.
- One of the most commonly used quaternary ammonium compounds in veterinary medicine is benzalkonium chloride.
- Chlorine compounds, such as sodium hypochlorite (Clorox, household bleach), can kill enveloped and nonenveloped viruses and are the disinfectants of choice against parvovirus. Chlorines are also effective against fungi, algae, and vegetative forms of bacteria.
- Iodophors are used as topical antiseptics before surgical procedures or for the disinfection of tissue.

- An iodophor is a combination of iodine and a carrier molecule that releases the iodine over time, prolonging the antimicrobial activity.
- The most common iodophor is iodine combined with polyvinylpyrrolidone, more commonly known as povidone–iodine (e.g., Betadine).
- Chlorhexidine, a biguanide antiseptic, is commonly used to clean cages and to treat various superficial infections in animals.

RECOMMENDED READINGS

Bill RL: Clinical *pharmacology and therapeutics for veterinary technicians*, ed 4, St Louis, 2016, Mosby.

Plumb DC: *Veterinary drug handbook*, ed 9, Ames, 2018, Wiley-Blackwell.

Sirois M: *Principles and practice of veterinary technology*, ed 4, St Louis, 2016, Elsevier.

Wanamaker BP, Pettes CL: *Applied pharmacology for the veterinary technician*, ed 5, St Louis, 2014, Saunders.

CHAPTER OUTLINE

KEY TERMS

Aggression
Agonistic
Anthropomorphism
Behavior
Catchpole
Distraction technique
Dorsal recumbency

Elimination
Ethology
Gauntlet
Imprinting
Lateral recumbency
Muzzle
Operant conditioning

Pheromone
Punishment
Queen
Reinforcement
Selective breeding
Socialization
Sternal recumbency

Stimulus
Substrate
Veterinary behaviorist
Vital signs

LEARNING OBJECTIVES

After reviewing this chapter, the reader will be able to:

1. Describe the processes by which behaviors develop.
2. Differentiate between positive and negative reinforcement and punishment.
3. List and describe types of aggressive behavior that may be seen in dogs and cats.
4. Describe the role of veterinary professionals in preventing behavior problems.
5. List the steps in house training a puppy.
6. Describe proper litter box care.
7. List the different options cats look for in scratching posts.

8. Describe the role of veterinary professionals in managing behavior problems.
9. Describe the psychological principles underlying physical restraint techniques.
10. Explain and implement the safety precautions taken before and during physical restraint.
11. Restrain dogs and cats for routine procedures such as physical examinations, nursing care, and sample collection.
12. Give examples of behavior responses of animals to physical restraint.
13. Correctly identify and use restraint equipment.

DOG AND CAT BREEDS

- The development of different breeds of animals is primarily the result of *selective breeding*, in which humans bred specific individual animals in an effort to develop animals with certain desirable characteristics.
- Breeds of dogs have been developed for specific purposes, such as hunting and guarding.
- The development of different cat breeds was primarily the result of a desire for animals with a specific appearance.
- Some aspects of dog and cat behavior are based on instinctive behaviors common to all animals of the same species.
  - Other traits are primarily the result of selective breeding that led to the breeds of dogs and cats we now have.
- A wide variety of mixed breed dogs are also common.
  - These may also have been specifically bred from two purebred parents.

- The result of the breeding is a hybrid of the two breeds and generally has aspects of both parent breeds.
- These mixed breed dogs are sometimes referred to as "designer dogs."
- The International Cat Association (http://www.tica.org) maintains a database of recognized cat breeds.
- Common cat breeds include the domestic short hair, Abyssinian, Burmese, Persian, and Siamese.
- The American Kennel Club (AKC) (www.akc.org) maintains a database of dog breeds. Specific information on the origin of the breed, as well as the breed's physical characteristics and expected temperament, are in the database.
- The AKC organizes dogs into one of seven specific groups (Table 5.1). The groups have similar behavioral characteristics. An additional class, the miscellaneous class, contains breeds that are being developed but are not yet recognized as belonging to one of the seven groups.

TABLE 5.1 AKC-Recognized Dog Breeds

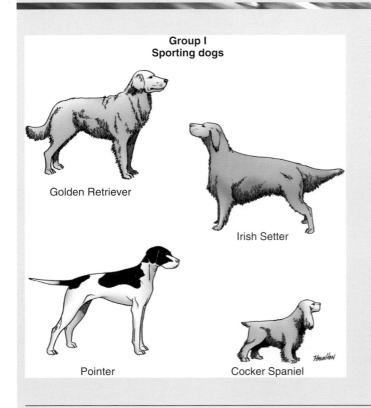

Group I
Sporting dogs

Golden Retriever

Irish Setter

Pointer

Cocker Spaniel

American Water Spaniel
Boykin Spaniel
Brittany Spaniel
Chesapeake Bay Retriever
Clumber Spaniel
Cocker Spaniel
Curly-Coated Retriever
English Cocker Spaniel
English Setter
English Springer Spaniel
Field Spaniel
Flat-Coated Retriever
German Shorthaired Pointer
German Wirehaired Pointer
Gordon Setter
Golden Retriever
Irish Red and White Setter
Irish Setter
Irish Water Spaniel
Labrador Retriever
Nova Scotia Duck Tolling Retriever
Pointer
Spinone Italiano
Sussex Spaniel
Vizsla
Weimaraner
Welsh Springer Spaniel
Wirehaired Pointing Griffon
Wirehaired Vizsla

Continued

TABLE 5.1 AKC-Recognized Dog Breeds—cont'd

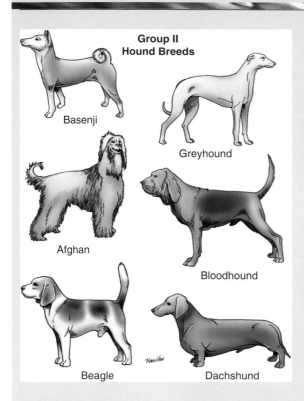

Group II
Hound Breeds

Basenji

Greyhound

Afghan

Bloodhound

Beagle

Dachshund

Afghan Hound
American English Coonhound
American Foxhound
Basenji
Basset Hound
Beagle
Black and Tan Coonhound
Bloodhound
Bluetick Coonhound
Borzoi
Cirneco dell'Etna
Dachshund
English Foxhound
Greyhound
Harrier
Ibizan Hound
Irish Wolfhound
Norwegian Elkhound
Otterhound
Petit Basset Griffon Vendeen
Pharaoh Hound
Plott
Portuguese Podeno Pequeno
Redbone Coonhound
Rhodesian Ridgeback
Saluki
Scottish Deerhound
Treeing Walker Coonhound
Whippet

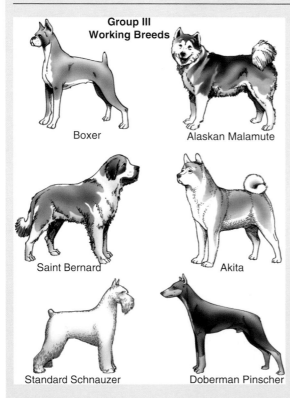

Group III
Working Breeds

Boxer

Alaskan Malamute

Saint Bernard

Akita

Standard Schnauzer

Doberman Pinscher

Akita
Alaskan Malamute
Anatolian Shepherd Dog
Bernese Mountain Dog
Black Russian Terrier
Boerboel
Boxer
Bullmastiff
Cane Corso
Doberman Pinscher
Dogue de Bordeaux
German Pinscher
Giant Schnauzer
Great Dane
Great Pyrenees
Greater Swiss Mountain Dog
Komondor
Kuvasz
Leonberger
Mastiff
Neapolitan Mastiff
Newfoundland
Portuguese Water Dog
Rottweiler
Saint Bernard
Samoyed
Siberian Husky
Standard Schnauzer
Tibetan Mastiff

TABLE 5.1 AKC-Recognized Dog Breeds—cont'd

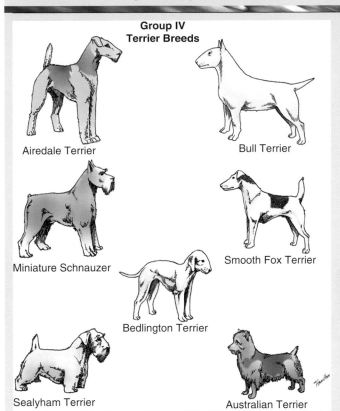

Group IV
Terrier Breeds

Airedale Terrier

Bull Terrier

Miniature Schnauzer

Smooth Fox Terrier

Bedlington Terrier

Sealyham Terrier

Australian Terrier

Airedale Terrier
American Staffordshire Terrier
Australian Terrier
Bedlington Terrier
Border Terrier
Bull Terrier
Cairn Terrier
Cesky Terrier
Dandie Dinmont Terrier
Glen of Imall Terrier
Irish Terrier
Kerry Blue Terrier
Lakeland Terrier
Manchester Terrier
Miniature Bull Terrier
Miniature Schnauzer
Norfolk Terrier
Norwich Terrier
Parson Russell Terrier
Rat Terrier
Russell Terrier
Scottish Terrier
Sealyham Terrier
Skye Terrier
Smooth Fox Terrier
Soft-Coated Wheaten Terrier
Staffordshire Bull Terrier
Welsh Terrier
West Highland White Terrier
Wire Fox Terrier

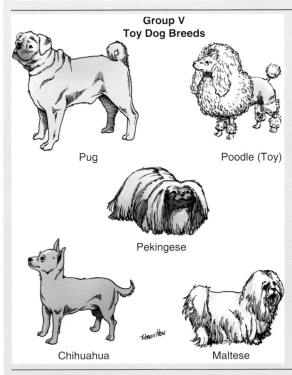

Group V
Toy Dog Breeds

Pug

Poodle (Toy)

Pekingese

Chihuahua

Maltese

Affenpinscher
Brussels Griffon
Cavalier King Charles Spaniel
Chihuahua
Chinese Crested
English Toy Spaniel
Havanese
Italian Greyhound
Japanese Chin
Maltese
Manchester Terrier (Toy)
Miniature Pinscher
Papillon
Pekingese
Pomeranian
Poodle (Toy)
Pug
Shih Tzu
Silky Terrier
Toy Fox Terrier
Yorkshire Terrier

Continued

TABLE 5.1 AKC-Recognized Dog Breeds—cont'd

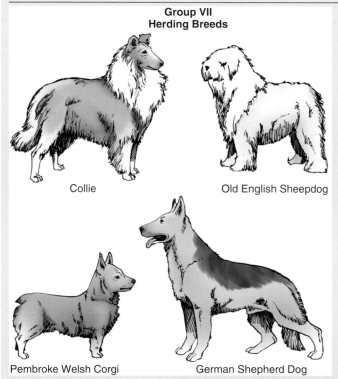

Group VI
Non-Sporting Breeds

Chow Chow

Dalmatian

English Bulldog

Schipperke

American Eskimo Dog
Bichon Frise
Boston Terrier
Bulldog
Chinese Shar-Pei
Chow-Chow
Coton de Tulear
Dalmatian
Finnish Spitz
French Bulldog
Keeshond
Lhasa Apso
Löwchen
Norwegian Lundehund
Poodle (Miniature and Standard)
Schipperke
Shiba Inu
Tibetan Spaniel
Tibetan Terrier
Xoloitzcuintli

Group VII
Herding Breeds

Collie

Old English Sheepdog

Pembroke Welsh Corgi

German Shepherd Dog

Australian Cattle Dog
Australian Shepherd
Bearded Collie
Beauceron
Belgian Malinois
Belgian Sheepdog
Belgian Tervuren
Bergamasco
Border Collie
Bouvier des Flandres
Briard
Canaan Dog
Cardigan Welsh Corgi
Collie
Entlebucher Mountain Dog
Finnish Lapphund
German Shepherd Dog
Icelandic Sheepdog
Norwegian Buhund
Old English Sheepdog
Pembroke Welsh Corgi
Polish Lowland Sheepdog
Puli
Pyrenean Shepherd
Shetland Sheepdog
Spanish Water Dog
Swedish Vallhund

Illustrations from Evans H, Lahunta A: Miller's anatomy of the dog, ed 4, St Louis, 2013, Saunders. Data from Sirois M: Elsevier's veterinary assistant textbook, ed 2, St Louis, 2017, Mosby.

WHAT IS BEHAVIOR AND WHERE DOES IT COME FROM?

- Behavior is any act done by an animal.
- For any behavior to occur, there must be a stimulus, some internal or external change that exceeds a threshold and causes stimulation of the nervous and/or endocrine systems.
- This receptor and cellular stimulation and integration of information require a number of chemical messengers in the animal's body, including epinephrine, acetylcholine, dopamine, serotonin, and many others.
  - Some problem behaviors are caused by increased or decreased amounts of these neurotransmitters.
- The study of animal behavior is referred to as ethology.
- Most ethologists agree that animal behavior is genetically programmed (instinctive) and learned (conditioned response).
- There are two general categories of conditioned responses: classical conditioning and operant conditioning.
  - Classical conditioning refers to the association of stimuli that occur at approximately the same time or in roughly the same area.
  - Operant conditioning refers to the association of a particular activity (the operant) with a punishment or reward.
- The pattern of behaviors that bonds animals to their caretakers occurs in early life and is referred to as imprinting.
- The most important period for behavior development in dogs and cats is from 3 to 12 weeks.
  - What occurs during this habituation or socialization period can affect the animal for the rest of its life.
- Operant conditioning can be used to reinforce a desired behavior or punish an undesirable one, although the latter is not recommended.
- Reinforcement refers to any stimulus that increases the likelihood of a behavior to be repeated.
- Punishment is a stimulus that decreases the likelihood of a behavior to be repeated.
- Reinforcement and punishment are referred to as positive when they involve the addition of a stimulus.
- Positive reinforcement refers to any immediate pleasant occurrence that follows a behavior.
- Withholding affection when a dog jumps up to greet you or not giving a treat when a dog is begging are examples of negative punishment.
- Box 5.1 summarizes important terms related to operant conditioning.

PREVENTING BEHAVIOR PROBLEMS IN COMPANION ANIMALS

- Most behavior problems are easier to prevent than to correct.
- Aggression is the most common problem for which owners seek guidance, but many pet owners are annoyed when their animals damage household belongings and exhibit house-soiling behavior.

> **BOX 5.1** Important Definitions for Understanding How Animals Learn
>
> **Reinforcement** is any stimulus that *increases* the chance of a behavior being repeated.
> **Positive reinforcement** involves the *presentation* of something *pleasant* (such as food) that is likely to strengthen a behavior response. (It increases the likelihood that the behavior will be repeated.)
> **Negative reinforcement** involves the *removal* of something *unpleasant* (such as escape from a fearful stimulus) that strengthens the behavior response.
> **Punishment** is any stimulus that *decreases* the chance of a behavior being repeated.
> **Positive punishment** involves the *application* of something *unpleasant or aversive*, such as a shock, verbal reprimand, squirting with water, threatening with a newspaper, etc.
> **Negative punishment** involves the *removal* of something *pleasant*, such as play or social interaction.

From Bassert JM: McCurnin's clinical textbook for veterinary technicians, ed 8, St. Louis, 2014, Saunders.

- Anthropomorphism refers to the attribution of human characteristics and emotions to animals.
  - Although many clients consider their pets to be part of the family, it is especially important that clients be provided with basic information on animal behavior to avoid the unrealistic expectations that develop when clients anthropomorphize their pets.
- Pet owners often misinterpret their pet's behavior as spite, jealousy, or guilt when the pet is in fact reacting based on learned behaviors.
- A variety of methods can be used to modify problem behaviors (Table 5.2).

House Training

- House training is one of the most important and first behaviors that young pets are expected to learn.
- Dogs and cats can be encouraged to eliminate reliably in locations that are acceptable to their human owners.
- Cats, dogs, pigs, ferrets, and rabbits can learn to use litter boxes.
- Other species of domestic companion animals are caged or kept outside because their elimination behavior is not restricted to specific locations.

Dogs

- House training requires that the dog be taken out frequently, especially when it wakes up, after it eats, and whenever it appears to be sniffing around the house.
- When a puppy cannot be monitored, it should be confined to a crate.

TABLE 5.2 Types of Behavioral Modification Programs

Method	Description	Example(s) and Possible Uses
Command–response–reward	Involves giving a command and immediately rewarding the desired response every time it is performed	Giving the command to sit and providing praise and/or treats as soon as the pet sits
Clicker training	Use of a sound to signal to the animal that it performed the right behavior and will receive a reward	Clicking when a puppy eliminates outside and immediately giving a treat
Extinction	Elimination of a problem behavior by completely removing the reinforcement for the behavior	Not providing food when a pet is begging
Aversion therapy	Associating an unpleasant stimulus with an object	Spraying an object with something that has a foul odor or taste to keep a pet from chewing it
Avoidance therapy	Associating an unpleasant stimulus with a behavior	Using a citronella collar to minimize barking behavior
Habituation	Involves surrounding the animal with the stimulus at low levels until the animal becomes acclimated to the stimulus and is no longer afraid of it	Playing recordings of thunderstorms or vacuum cleaners to a litter of puppies so that they become accustomed to the sound
Counterconditioning	Replacing an undesirable behavior with a desirable one	Using rewards to teach a pet to pull a bell on a string rather than scratching at the door to be let inside
Desensitization	Often used in combination with counterconditioning; involves diminishing a particular behavior by gradually exposing the animal to the stimulus that produces the inappropriate response	Exposing a pet that is afraid of children to children using longer periods of time and decreasing distance
Environmental modification	Changing one or more environmental parameters	Placing pet in crate when unsupervised; changing the location of a litter box
Surgery	Anatomic alteration	Castration of male pets to decrease aggressiveness and territorial urine marking
Medication	Sedatives, hormonal agents, herbal remedies	Canine cognitive dysfunction; as an adjunct to other behavioral therapies in aggressive or extremely fearful animals

From Sirois M: Principles and practice of veterinary technology, ed 3, St Louis, 2011, Mosby.

- Crate training is also useful for preventing destructive behaviors such as chewing.
- The use of the crate should not be excessive because 8-week-old puppies cannot hold their bowels longer than 4 to 6 hours.
- For young puppies, bladder control can be as little as 1 hour or sometimes as long as 2 or 3 hours at a time.
- The dog must be actively taught, by reinforcing correct behavior, the desired location for elimination.
- Owners should reward elimination outside with verbal praise and petting, and possibly a special tidbit.
- To reinforce the elimination behavior, the owner must go outside with the puppy and provide reinforcement immediately following elimination at the location where it occurs.
- Clicker training may also be useful for house training of puppies.
- Use of physical punishment in regard to house training is never appropriate.

Cats
- The process of encouraging cats to use litter boxes consistently is based on different developmental events than house training dogs.
- It is normal instinctual behavior for kittens and cats to use a substrate for elimination.
- Kittens do not need to observe the queen eliminating or have the owner demonstrate part of the process by raking the cat's paws in the litter.
- Providing a clean, easily accessible litter box with an acceptable substrate is sufficient.
- The major complaint of cat owners is that their cats stop or inconsistently use the litter box and choose to eliminate somewhere else in the house.

- Because there are many reasons for a cat to stop using its litter box, a detailed history is needed to determine the cause.
- Because kittens are physically and behaviorally immature, a litter box should be within easy access at all times.
  - This may mean providing several litter boxes at strategic locations in the house or initially limiting the cat's access to only portions of the house.
- The litter box should be easily accessible but also should afford some privacy.
- Proximity to appliances that make unexpected startling noises, such as the washer, furnace, or hot water heater, should also be avoided.
- Cats may avoid litter that is consistently dirty, too deep, or scented.
- General guidelines are to keep the litter depth at no more than 2 inches, remove feces and urine clumps daily, change the litter frequently enough to prevent odors from developing, and ensure that most of the litter is always dry.
- Advise owners to provide one litter box per cat, plus one extra, and to keep the boxes in different locations so that a single cat cannot block another cat's access to the litter box area.

Preventing Destructive Behavior By Cats

- Scratching objects should be provided in locations in which the behavior is likely to be triggered.
- The scratching objects must match the cat's preferences for desirable locations and with regard to height, orientation, and texture.
- Many scratching posts available commercially do not permit the cat to reach vertically to its full height to scratch, as many cats like to do.
- Some cats may prefer to stretch their legs out in front and rake backward in a horizontal motion.
  - If this is the case, the cat may be more likely to use a flat horizontal object (Fig. 5.1) than a vertical post.
- Texture: As with other aspects of the behavioral pattern of scratching, cats vary in the textures that they prefer.
- Cats that like to rake their claws in long vertical motions may be more likely to use an object with a texture that permits this.
- Other cats use more of a picking motion and may prefer items covered with sisal, wrapped horizontally.
- The scratching object should be placed in a location where the cat is likely to be motivated to scratch or adjacent to an unacceptable item that the cat is already using.
- To encourage the cat to use the desirable object, it can be scented with catnip or a commercial pheromone (Feliway, CEVA Animal Health, St Louis), or a toy can be attached to the top to entice the cat to reach high up the post.

Preventing Destructive Behavior By Dogs

- Destructive behavior is a classification of behavior based more on the owner's view of the result (destruction) than on the actual behavior that caused it.

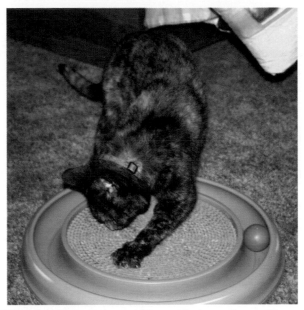

FIGURE 5.1 Horizontal scratching objects such as this pad scented with catnip may be preferred over vertical objects. (From Sirois M: *Principles and practice of veterinary technology*, ed 3, St Louis, 2011, Mosby. Courtesy Donna Harris.)

- Digging, chewing, tearing, scratching, moving objects from one place to another, and removing the contents from the trash are all considered destructive behavior and are self-rewarding.
- Destructive behavior that is the symptomatic manifestation of other problems, such as separation anxiety or noise phobias, can be treated but may not be prevented.
- Destructive behavior that occurs as the result of a normal developmental process, such as teething, play, and investigative behavior, can often be prevented or at least minimized.
- Toys should be available for chewing and tearing, as well as for carrying and chasing, if the dog displays both patterns of play behavior.
- If the dog is caught chewing an unacceptable item, the item should be taken away and replaced with one that is acceptable.
- Dogs that insist on digging outside can be provided with their own area in which to do so. This area should consist of loose soil or sand to facilitate digging.
  - Owners can bury enticing items shallowly in this area to attract the dog.

Preventing Aggressive Behavior Problems

- Aggression is the most common type of behavior problem reported in dogs and occurs in cats as well.
- Aggressive behavior is normal behavior for most species of animals, including companion animals.
- Aggression, defined as behavior that is intended to harm another individual, is an aspect of agonistic behavior.
- Agonistic behaviors are behaviors that animals show in situations involving social conflict. Submission, avoidance,

TABLE 5.3 Common Types of Aggressive Behavior in Dogs and Cats

Type of Aggression	Comments
Conflict related	Result of unpredictable environment or inconsistent or inappropriate use of punishment
Fear induced	Fearful situations (e.g., noises, being in the veterinary office)
Predatory	Instinctual stalking and pouncing with no warning growl
Pain induced	Protective instinct
Intermale	Natural instinct usually eliminated by castration
Territorial	Dogs—usually directed toward humans that are not members of their household Cats—usually directed toward other cats
Maternal	Normal protective instinct

From Sirois M: Principles and practice of veterinary technology, ed 3, St Louis, 2011, Mosby.

escaping, offensive and defensive threats, and offensive and defensive aggression are all part of the agonistic behavior system.
- Many different types of aggression are displayed by dogs and cats (Table 5.3).
- The most common complaint from dog owners is aggression toward people, whereas the most common complaint from cat owners is aggression toward other cats.
- Castrating male animals clearly reduces some forms of aggressive behavior in many species, including dogs, cats, and horses.
  - In addition to aggression, castration prevents other potential problems such as roaming, urine marking, and prostate problems.

Socialization

- Many species of mammals and birds have sensitive periods of development of normal species-typical social behavior. This sensitive period has been well studied in dogs and to a lesser degree in cats and horses.
- The sensitive socialization period usually occurs fairly early in life; in dogs, it is from 3 to 12 weeks of age and in cats, from 2 to 7 weeks.
- Companion animals must have a variety of pleasant experiences with different types of people, other animals, and environments during these sensitive periods so that they are able to accept humans as their social peers later in life.
- It is also important to habituate the puppy and kitten to a variety of environmental situations.

- Fear of people or specific situations can sometimes develop into defensive aggression problems.

Fear-Free Handling

- Prevention of problem behaviors includes use of techniques both in the home and in the veterinary clinic that are designed to reduce fear, stress, and anxiety in pets.
- Although it is not possible to only use fear-free techniques with every animal that is presented to the veterinary practice, use of these techniques should be the first choice with all pets.
- Veterinary staff members and practice teams can become certified in fear-free techniques. Visit https://fearfreepets.com/ for more information on fear-free techniques and certification.
- The fear-free approach involves a variety of techniques that are used both at home by the client and in the veterinary practice by the veterinary health care team.
- Educate new pet owners about methods that can be used to keep their pet calm when preparing for and traveling to the veterinary practice.
- Cats should be allowed daily access to their carrier so that they become acclimated to it and it becomes a comfortable resting spot.
- Allow pets to become accustomed to car rides as a positive experience.
- Consider the use of calming pheromones before car rides and veterinary visits.
- Have the client withhold food the day of the veterinary visit so that treat rewards used by the veterinary practice team will be more effective.
- Pheromones can be used in the examination room to help the patient remain calm.
- Allow the patient to approach staff members on its own.
  - Stand sideways rather than directly in front of the patient and toss some small treats to entice the patient to approach you.
- Common signs of fear in dogs include panting, pacing, licking the lips, furrowed brows, and yawning.
- Fearful cats will often try to hide and may exhibit signs of agitation or aggression such as dilated pupils, piloerection, and hissing.
- When preparing to restrain for specific procedures, work with the pet to find a position in which they are comfortable while still secure enough to safely perform the procedure.
- If signs of fear become evident, stop the procedure and consider sedation.

PATIENT HISTORY AND CLIENT INTERACTION

- Astute observations from the veterinarian and the veterinary staff are crucial when performing the physical examination.

- The interviewer must be able to ask questions that are easily understood and are geared toward the animal's owner.
- If necessary, slang words describing certain conditions may be used to facilitate communication and avoid misunderstanding.
- Determine the primary medical problem (presenting or chief complaint), as well as how the specific signs of illness are observed by the client.
- An important interviewing technique uses reflective listening methods that incorporate active listening, infrequent interruption, limited speaking, and asking for clarification when needed.
- Once the client has reported the facts, repeat important information, indicating that you have heard him or her and understand the concern.
- If the history given is vague, use direct questioning; asking how, where, and when is generally more effective than asking why.

Obtaining a History

- Open the interview by introducing yourself and explaining what you will be doing.
- You can then validate the preliminary data, if needed, and go on to obtain the history for the presenting complaint.

Patient Characteristics

- The interviewer should verify that the patient's age, breed, gender, and reproductive status have been correctly recorded and note any changes since the patient's last visit (e.g., if the patient has been spayed or castrated).
- Congenital and infectious diseases, parasitism, ingestion of foreign bodies, and intussusceptions are usually predominant in young animals.
- Degenerative diseases and neoplasia are more common in adult animals.
- Certain species or breeds are predisposed to particular problems.
- The patient's gender and reproductive status are important because certain conditions are gender-specific and determine which areas should be given special attention in the patient evaluation.
- The incidence of some diseases decreases markedly as a result of ovariohysterectomy (spay) or castration.

Origin, Prior Ownership, and Current Environment

- Questions concerning geographic origin and prior ownership may indicate exposure to infectious or parasitic diseases.
- Information on the pet's current environment, including information about the patient's diet, is also needed to help identify risk factors for specific diseases.

Past Medical History

- Past medical history provides information about the patient's health before the current illness. Carefully inquire about and record the dates of previous illnesses and treatment, hospitalization, and surgeries, followed by a brief description of each problem, how it was managed, and how the patient responded to treatment.
- Ask the client to describe any allergies (e.g., environmental, ingestible, drug related) and how these were diagnosed.
- Note any medications that the patient is currently receiving and whether the client is giving medications as prescribed.
- Question the client about the patient's vaccination status, when any vaccinations were given, and when diagnostic tests (e.g., heartworm infection test) were performed.

Presenting Complaint

- The presenting complaint is why the client has sought veterinary care for the animal.
- The presenting complaint is what the client perceives the patient's problem to be.
- It is important to determine whether the client understands the meaning of the medical terms that he or she uses to describe the problem.
- Record the clinical signs observed and not the client's presumptive diagnosis.
- Once the presenting complaint is listed, record the information gathered in chronologic order to clarify areas of possible confusion.
- Separate the client's observations from his or her conclusions and amplify certain portions of the complaint that may be important.
- The history of the presenting complaint is best recorded by chronology (i.e., in the order in which events occurred).

Physical Examination

- The physical examination assesses the animal's current state of health and is generally performed by the veterinary technician or veterinarian, with the veterinary assistant providing restraint and record-keeping support.
- Patients are evaluated using a combination of methods: inspection, palpation, auscultation, and percussion.
- Vital signs include the body temperature, respiratory rate and effort, heart rate and rhythm, and indications of perfusion (Table 5.4).

RESTRAINT AND HANDLING OF DOGS

- Most dogs brought to veterinary facilities are friendly and require minimal restraint. However, it is best to be cautious with every dog.
- All animals can become startled or anxious in a medical facility.
- The proper way to approach an unknown dog is to extend your hand palm down, with fingers bent slightly, allowing the dog to sniff the back of your hand.

TABLE 5.4 Normal Ranges of Heart Rate, Respiratory Rate, and Rectal Temperature in Adults of Some Domestic Species

Animal	Heart Rate (beats/min)	Respiratory Rate (breaths/min)	Rectal Temperature
Dog	70–60	8–20	99.5°–102.2°F (37.5°–39°C)
Cat	150–210	8–30	100.4°–102.2°F (38°–39°C)
Hamster	250–500	35–135	98.6°–100.4°F (37°–38°C)
Guinea pig	230–280	42–104	99°–103.1°F (37.2°–39.5°C)
Rabbit	130–325	30–60	101.3°–104°F (38.5°–40°C)

Adapted from Sirois M: Principles and practice of veterinary technology, ed 3, St Louis, 2011, Mosby.

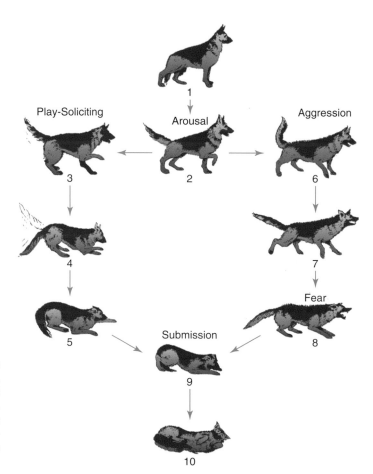

FIGURE 5.2 General body postures of dogs. Dog 1 shows a relaxed dog. Dog 2 is alert. Dog 3 shows playful behavior. Dogs 4 and 5 show increasing fear and submission. Dog 6 displays offensive aggression. Dog 7 shows mixed motivations of offensive and defensive aggression. Dog 8 shows defensive aggression. Dogs 9 and 10 show fear and/or submission. (From Millis D, Levine, D: *Canine rehabilitation and physical therapy*, ed 2, St Louis, 2014, Saunders.)

Canine Body Language

- Dogs exhibit a number of personalities that can be identified by their body language (Fig. 5.2).
- Happy dogs greet you with a wagging tail and a slightly lowered and cocked head and initiate affection.
- Nervous or fearful dogs have their ears drawn down and back, showing white around the pupils of their eyes, not making any eye contact, and cowering.
  - If cornered, they feel threatened and often bite.
- Aggressive dogs hold their head lowered between the shoulders, have a level stare with the tail straight out (possibly wagging), and perhaps a grimace or growl (Fig 5.3).
  - These dogs take offense at anyone's improper body language, such as a direct look into their eyes or a frontal approach.
- Aggressive dogs and nervous or fearful dogs should be handled with the knowledge that they will bite, and appropriate steps, such as a muzzle and sedation, should be considered before working with this type of dog.

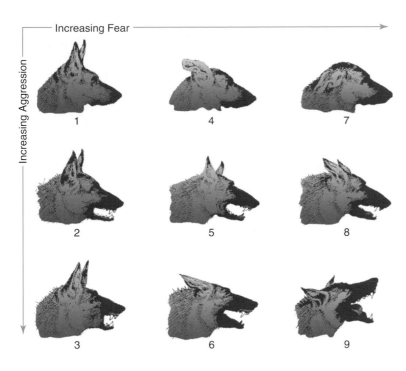

FIGURE 5.3 Facial postures of dogs. Figures from left to right show increasing fear. Figures from top to bottom show increasing aggressive motivation. Dog 1 is an alert dog. Dog 3 is offensively aggressive. Dog 7 is fearful and/or submissive. Dog 9 is defensively aggressive. All others are intermediate in fear and/or aggression. (From Millis D, Levine, D: *Canine rehabilitation and physical therapy*, ed 2, St Louis, 2014, Saunders.)

- Regardless of personality, if a dog is curling its lips, showing its teeth, growling, or raising its hackles, it is imperative to control its muzzle to avoid being bitten.

Restraint Devices

Mechanical Devices

- Leash: The rope leash can be made of a rolled or flat nylon rope with a handle at one end and a slip ring to form a sliding loop at the other.
- Gauntlets: Gauntlets are heavy leather gloves designed to protect the hands and forearms when working with fractious dogs, cats, and birds.
  - Even though they are made of thick leather, most dogs, cats, and birds can pinch or actually bite through them.
- Muzzle: Many types of commercially manufactured muzzles are available and should be fitted to the dog by the owner.
- Catchpole: Many types of catchpoles are available commercially and are used to move an aggressive or fearful dog to or from a run or cage.
  - The loop at the end of the pole is placed around the dog's neck and tightened (Fig. 5.4).
- Voice: Dogs often respond to voice commands and tones.
  - When using it to direct an animal, make the tone of your voice deep and commanding.

Mobility-Limiting Devices

- Movement-limiting devices are designed to prevent a dog from chewing on itself or its bandages, or generally to restrict movement.

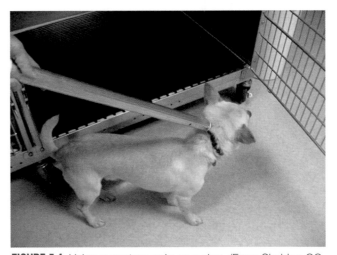

FIGURE 5.4 Using a capture pole on a dog. (From Sheldon CC, Sonsthagen T, Topel JA: *Animal restraint for veterinary professionals*, St Louis, 2006, Mosby.)

- Elizabethan collars are cone-shaped collars that fit around a dog's neck.
  - They can be attached to the dog's collar or secured around its neck.
  - The collar should extend past the end of the nose and be snug but not constrictive around the neck.
- No-bite collars are designed to fit snugly around the dog's neck, much like a cervical collar for humans.

Special Handling

- Puppies must be watched constantly; never place them on an examination table or countertop without making sure that your hand is always in contact with them.

- In the advanced stages of pregnancy, applying excessive pressure on the dog's abdominal organs during restraint can have severe repercussions.
- When restraining a pregnant bitch, always be aware of where your hands are and how much pressure you are applying to the dog's abdomen.
- Old dogs can be arthritic and should not be maneuvered into awkward positions.
- Nervous dogs must be handled with great caution because they can be easily provoked to bite.
- Aggressive dogs: Signs of impending aggression include a head held low, either below or level with the dog's shoulders, a gaze that is averted to the side, raised hair along the back, ears down and tail straight out, and an ominous growl or snarl.
  - Dogs showing any of these signs should be handled with extreme caution and must always be considered dangerous.
  - Avoid looking directly at an aggressive dog and stand sideways instead of facing the dog straight on.
- Injured dogs must always be treated with extreme caution and care.
  - An injured dog should be muzzled before being moved or handled.
  - The exception to this rule is if the dog has an injury to the head or is vomiting.
  - The best way to transport an injured animal is on a stretcher or flat board.

Restraint Techniques

Removing Dogs from Cages or Runs
- Make certain that all escape routes are closed before opening any kennel door.

Nonaggressive, Nonfearful Dogs
- Small dogs usually can be grasped gently and lifted out of the cage with one hand around and under the dog's thorax.
- Hold its body snugly, close to yours, or place a leash around its neck and place the dog on the floor.
- Medium-sized to large dogs are usually led out with a leash from a floor-level cage.

Fearful and Aggressive Dogs
- Ideally, dogs that are likely to bite should be muzzled, sedated, or both before placed in a cage or run.
- With a dog in a run or floor-level cage, open the door narrowly, stepping behind the door to allow the dog to exit.
- As the dog's head comes through the doorway, quickly flip a leash over its head and move out with it.
- If a dog is attacking the leash or the front of the kennel, the use of a capture pole is warranted, regardless of whether the dog is small, medium, or large.

Lifting a Dog
- Small dogs are draped over a forearm, with the other hand holding onto the head just below the mandible.

- Medium-sized dogs are held around the neck with one arm and around its rear end or under the abdomen with the other.
- Large dogs should be lifted by two people: one with an arm around the neck and thorax and the other with an arm around the abdomen and rear quarters.
- Procedures should be done on the floor when the pet is nervous.

Standing Restraint
- This hold is used for physical examinations, including tests of temperature, pulse, and respiration.
  - You can also use this hold when subcutaneous (SC) and intramuscular (IM) injections must be administered, as well as to express anal glands, administer enemas, and examine the animal's limbs.
- Wrap one arm around the dog's neck to control its head and keep it pressed close to your shoulder; place the other arm under its abdomen to maintain the dog in a standing position and close to your body (Fig. 5.5).
- If you have a very small dog, lift it into your arms and snug it close.

Sitting or Sternal Recumbency
- Sternal recumbency is usually used on the examination table and sometimes on the floor with large dogs.
- This technique is useful for blood collection from the cephalic or jugular vein, intravenous (IV) injection, nail trimming, oral and ophthalmic examination or medication, and some radiographs.

Lateral Recumbency
- Lateral recumbency is usually used on the examination table but also can be used on the floor.

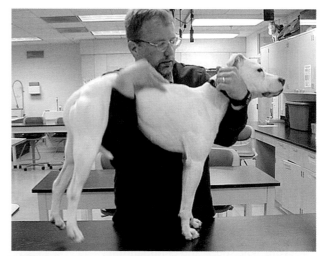

FIGURE 5.5 Wrap one arm around the dog's neck to control its head and keep it pressed close to your shoulder. Place your other arm under its abdomen to maintain the dog in a standing position and close to your body. (From Sheldon CC, Sonsthagen T, Topel JA: *Animal restraint for veterinary professionals*, St Louis, 2006, Mosby.)

- It is useful for urinary catheterization, radiographs, suture removal, electrocardiography, access to the lateral saphenous vein, nail trims, and other short procedures.

Dorsal Recumbency

- **Dorsal recumbency** is used for procedures such as radiography, cystocentesis, and blood collection from the jugular vein.
- Place the dog in lateral recumbency and then roll it onto its back.
- If it is a very deep-chested dog, a V trough or foam wedges may be necessary to keep the dog from rolling.
- The forepaws are stretched cranially and the back paws are stretched caudally, exposing the thorax and abdomen.

RESTRAINT AND HANDLING OF CATS

- Rough handling, extreme physical restraint, and a hot temper are counterproductive and have no place in cat restraint.
- Relax the cat by petting it, speaking to it gently, and finding its favorite spot where it likes to be scratched.
- When restraining a cat, start with a minimum amount of restraint and perform the procedure as quickly as possible.
- Many procedures can be accomplished by barely holding on, but you need to be ready to tighten the hold as necessary.
- If the cat begins to resist, tighten your grip so no one gets hurt; if the cat vigorously resists the restraint, release it and consider using a chemical restraint after it has calmed down.

Mechanical Devices

Towel and Blanket

- A large towel can be used to wrap the cat's body snugly, thus controlling the feet and body.
- A front or back leg can be pulled out for a cephalic or femoral vein exposure or for an IM injection, the cat can be rolled onto its back for a jugular venipuncture, and oral or ophthalmic medicines can be given without fear of being scratched.
- Covering the head with a towel often calms the cat down.

Feline Restraint Bags

- Manufactured nylon or canvas bags can be used to secure a cat's legs and body and have a number of strategically placed zippered openings.
- Choose a properly sized bag and ensure that it is clean and has no residual odor of another animal.

Muzzles

- Muzzles must be wide enough to cover the cat's entire face, including the eyes, but have an opening positioned so that the cat can still breathe through its nose.

- It may be difficult to secure them behind the cat's ears because its head is so rounded and there is not much ledge there to keep the strap from moving forward.
- The restrainer may inadvertently pull the muzzle off if the cat moves its head or body violently.
- Secure the muzzle tabs behind the ears as low and tight as they will go.
- Check that the muzzle does not cover the cat's nares.

Distraction Techniques

- Methods to get the cat to concentrate on what you are doing and ignore the procedure being performed.

Caveman Pats

- Caveman pats are exaggerated, heavy but gentle pats or rubbing on the head.
- They can be rapid or slow and steady.
- Varying the pressure and stroke is usually more successful than a continuous pattern.

Puffs of Air

- Blowing or puffing air into a cat's face is another way to redirect its interest.
- Vary the speed and force of the puff of air to obtain better results.

Restraint Techniques

Removal from a Carrier

- Most cats will not willingly walk out of a carrier on demand.
- Open the carrier door as soon as the client is escorted into the examination room; the cat may decide to walk out and explore.
- If the cat is friendly, reach in, gently grasp the scruff, and bring it forward until you can get a hand around its midsection.
- If the cat resists, elevate the rear of the carrier and allow the cat to slide out.
- You can also dismantle most carriers quickly.

Removal from a Cage

- If the cat is friendly, reach in across its shoulders, grasp the front feet, quickly lift it out of the cage, and hold its body snugly against yours.
- If the cat is upset, throwing a large beach towel or small blanket over the cat and then scooping it up works well to get it out of the cage.
- It is recommended that you wear gauntlets while getting it out of the cage.
- If the cat is terribly upset, use a device designed to trap and/or pin it to the floor of a cage or inside a device so a sedative can be administered (Fig. 5.6).
- A dose of ketamine can be given by squirting it into the cat's eyes or open mouth if it is hissing. It is absorbed through the mucous membranes, and the cat will quickly become sedated.

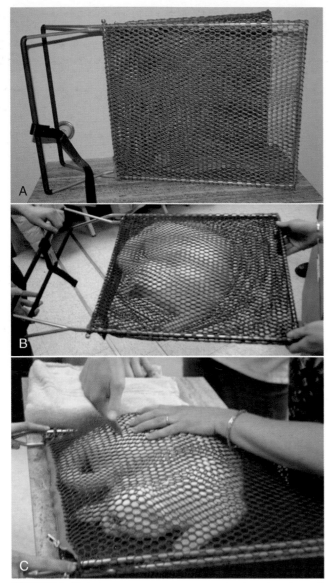

FIGURE 5.6 (A) A device such as the easy nabber tool works well in subduing an aggressive cat. (B) You can transport the cat to an examination table or wherever you need to take it. (C) The cat is encircled inside the nabber and cannot move much, so IM or SC injections can be given through the netting. (From Sheldon CC, Sonsthagen T, Topel JA: *Animal restraint for veterinary professionals*, St Louis, 2006, Mosby.)

Sitting or Sternal Recumbency

- This procedure can be used for physical examinations, oral and ophthalmic examinations and medications, and cephalic or jugular venipuncture.
- For a routine physical examination, have the cat sit and place one hand in front of its chest while the other hand steadies its back.
- When it is time to examine the head or perform a more invasive procedure, encircle the neck, holding its mandibles with one hand; with the other hand, reach across the back and grasp its front feet. Hold the cat snugly up against your body.

Restraint for Cephalic Venipunctures

- Cephalic venipuncture requires the cat to be in sternal recumbency.
- Grasp the cat with your right hand, with your thumb pointing toward the cat's back end.
- Slide the cat to the edge of the table and then bring your left hand around the side of the cat's body and hold it snugly against your body.
- Turn the cat's head away from your partner and toward your body.
- With your left hand cradling the cat's left elbow, wrap your thumb across the proximal part of the forearm as you extend its left leg forward, toward your partner.
- To occlude the vessel, keep your thumb in place but roll it laterally so that it ends up perpendicular to the vessel.

Applying a Tourniquet for Cephalic Venipuncture

- Place the cat in sternal recumbency using the same technique as you would for a cephalic venipuncture.
- The restrainer extends the limb to be used by cradling the elbow in the palm of the left hand without laying the thumb across the vessel.
- The phlebotomist slips the tourniquet over the paw.
- The tourniquet goes proximal to the cat's elbow, and the tails and clip are on the caudolateral aspect of the elbow.
- To release the tourniquet, grab both sides (top and bottom) of the clip and pull it away from the base as you pull the entire locking mechanism away from the leg.

Restraint for Jugular Venipuncture

- There are two holds to use for jugular venipuncture.
- The first method involves starting just as you would for the cephalic hold.
  - Once to the edge of the table, shift your left hand to a cupping technique with your fingers under the mandible and the thumb on top of the cat's head.
  - Gently move your right hand under the cat and grasp both front legs above the elbows, with your finger in between the legs for added gripping power.
  - Extend its head upward while extending its legs down so that you can see the jugular vessel.
- The second method is to hold the cat on its back.
  - It is easier to do this if the cat is wrapped in a towel or placed in a cat bag. Once the cat is wrapped up in the towel, roll it over so that it is lying on its back.
  - The restrainer uses one hand to grasp the head from the back and holds the cat's front feet under the towel and down toward its chest.
  - When ready, the phlebotomist takes the cat's head and the restrainer occludes the vessels.

Lateral Recumbency

- Cats can be restrained in lateral recumbency; however, they are agile and can often maneuver their heads around and bite.

- This method should be reserved for very placid cats and noninvasive procedures.
- A fetal hold or scruffing technique is more useful for giving subcutaneous or intramuscular injections or placing a rectal thermometer.
- Do not use this on cats weighing more than 7 pounds because it can cause damage to tissues and vertebrae.

Dorsal Recumbency
- This technique is used for blood collection from the jugular vein, radiography, and cystocentesis.

Chemical Restraint
- An inhalation chamber is a great tool that can be used for cats that will not surrender, no matter what you do.
- Another chemical restraint technique is to squirt ketamine into the cat's mouth. It is absorbed by the mucous membranes and the cat is sedated.
- Load a dose of ketamine into a syringe with a Tom Cat catheter attached and, as the cat hisses, squirt it into the cat's mouth.

Cat Lasso
- The cat lasso is really a tool of last resort. The pole has a noose at one end that draws tight when placed around the cat's body.
- If the noose can be placed around the cat's shoulders, you avoid choking it.
- If you capture it around the neck, the cat will often react violently because it feels threatened by this hold.

ADMINISTERING MEDICATIONS

Topical Administration
- Medication applied to the skin provides a local effect and may also be absorbed through the skin into the circulation.
- Shaving and cleaning the area or parting the hair before application facilitates absorption of the medication.
- Wear examination gloves and/or plastic aprons when giving a medicated bath or applying topical medication.
- Topical medications include medicated shampoos for skin diseases, fentanyl transdermal patches for analgesia, spot-on flea and tick control, topical anesthetics, nitroglycerin ointment for cardiac disease, and other various antibiotic and cortisone creams and ointments.

Oral Administration
- Oral administration is the route most commonly used to administer medications.
- Medications given orally are metabolized slowly.
- The patient must be able to swallow and have normal digestive function if medication is given by mouth (PO).

- If necessary, tablets can be crushed or capsule contents dissolved in water and given with a syringe or feeding tube.
- If the patient has a good appetite, the medication may be placed in a meatball of canned food; however, this does not work well with sick cats.
- If the oral cavity is damaged, the medication can be given directly into the gastrointestinal (GI) tract via nasogastric or gastrostomy tube after mixing with water for easy tube passage.
- A pilling device can be used to avoid being bitten (Fig. 5.7).
- Place small patients at waist level and large dogs on the floor.
- Medicate cats by grasping the upper jaw over the top of the head and tipping the head back.
- Place the pill in the center groove of the tongue, at the back of the throat.
- In dogs, grasp the muzzle using the fingers and thumb to press the skin against the teeth.
- Slip the thumb of the left hand into the mouth and press up on the hard palate, keeping the lips against the teeth.
- Place the pill on the base of the tongue at the back of the throat.
- Keep the head slightly elevated, close the mouth, and hold it shut while rubbing the throat until the patient swallows.
- To administer liquid medication in a syringe, tilt the head back slightly and pull the lips outward slightly to form a pocket.
- Place the syringe between the lips and back teeth so that the liquid flows between the molars and into the throat.
- Administer slowly in small boluses to allow the patient to swallow and not aspirate.
- Buccal or transmucosal administration of medications can also be effectively achieved in the feline patient.

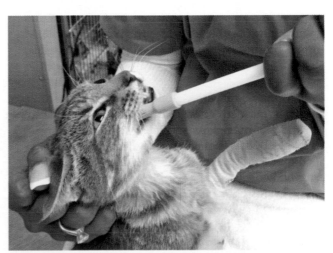

FIGURE 5.7 A pill gun is useful for administering medications to the difficult patient. (From Sirois M: *Principles and practice of veterinary technology*, ed 3, St Louis, 2011, Mosby.)

RECOMMENDED READINGS

Beaver BV: *Canine behavior: Insights and answers*, ed 2, St Louis, 2009, Saunders.

Beaver BV: *Feline behavior: A guide for veterinarians*, ed 2, St Louis, 2003, Saunders.

Horwitz D, Neilson J: *Blackwell's five-minute veterinary consult clinical companion: Canine and feline behavior*, Indianapolis, 2007, Wiley-Blackwell.

Landsberg G, Hunthausen W, Ackerman L: *The handbook of behavior problems in the dog and cat*, ed 2, Philadelphia, 2003, Saunders.

Miklosi A: *Dog behaviour, evolution, and cognition*, Oxford, England, 2009, Oxford University Press.

Shaw J: *Companion animal behavior for veterinary technicians and nurses*, Indianapolis, 2014, Wiley-Blackwell.

Sheldon CC, Sonsthagen T, Topel JA: *Animal restraint for veterinary professionals*, ed 2, St Louis, 2016, Mosby.

Sirois M: *Principles and practice of veterinary technology*, ed 4, St Louis, 2019, Elsevier.

Tully T, Mitchell M: *A technician's guide to exotic animal care*, Lakewood, 2001, AAHA Press.

Turner D, Bateson P: *The domestic cat: The biology of its behaviour*, ed 2, Cambridge, England, 2000, Cambridge University Press.

Yin S: *Low stress handling*, Davis, 2009, Cattle Dog Publications.

Small Animal Nursing

KEY TERMS

Ad libitum	Erythema	Nonessential amino acids	Vaccine
Body condition scoring	Essential amino acids	Nutrient	Virus
Capsid	Etiology	Pathology	Vitamins
Concussion	Fibrosis	Penrose drain	Wound
Contusion	Granulation tissue	Public health	Zoonoses
Débridement	Laceration	Pyrogen	
Decubital ulcers	Lavage	Reservoir	
Edema	Necropsy	Sanitizer	

LEARNING OBJECTIVES

After reviewing this chapter, the reader will be able to:

1. Describe techniques used in the general nursing care of dogs and cats.
2. Describe procedures used in grooming and skin, nail, and ear care.
3. List basic energy-producing and non–energy-producing nutrients.
4. Describe considerations for feeding young and adult dogs.
5. Describe considerations for feeding young and adult cats.
6. Discuss the fundamentals of exotic pet diet considerations.
7. List and describe common diseases and ways in which they can affect people.

8. Discuss methods used to control the spread of zoonotic diseases.
9. Explain the general principles underlying disease prevention.
10. Discuss features of appropriate housing and nutrition for animals.
11. List and discuss types of vaccinations and schedules of vaccinations for domestic animal species.
12. Describe factors that predispose to disease.
13. Explain the principles of first aid treatment of wounds.
14. Explain the principles of wound closure.
15. Give examples of the types and applications of bandages.

GROOMING AND SKIN CARE

Bathing

- The basic technique for bathing dogs and cats is to wet the coat thoroughly and then apply small amounts of shampoo, starting at the head and working back to the tail.
- Rubbing the shampoo into the coat until a lather is produced, again starting from the head and working back to the tail, is a generally accepted bathing method.
- The eyes should be protected from chemical injury by instilling a drop of mineral oil or a small amount of boric acid ophthalmic ointment in each eye before the bath.
- Care should be taken to prevent water from entering the external ear canal; this can be accomplished by placing a small piece of cotton in each ear.
- Thermal injury from excessively hot water can be prevented by monitoring the water temperature constantly.
- Thorough rinsing with clean water prevents irritation of the skin from residual shampoo.
- The axillary and scrotal regions of long-haired dogs are particularly vulnerable to residual shampoo irritation.
- Shampoos containing insecticides should be used only with the approval of the attending veterinarian because of the possibility of cumulative toxicity or drug interactions with medications or other topically applied insecticides.
- If a complete immersion bath is contraindicated, localized soiling of the animal may be handled with a sponge bath.
- Orthopedic or neurologic patients may not be able to stand steady in the bathtub; therefore a rubber mat should be placed in the tub to help reduce the risk of injury.
- Cover any clean and dry bandages with plastic to reduce the need for bandaging after the bath.
- When a patient is admitted and its condition has been stabilized, any vomit, diarrhea, urine, or blood should be removed from the skin to prevent secondary infections.
- Skin care of the hospitalized patient involves bathing to remove body fluids, skin oil, or exudates; brushing to prevent mat formation; padding to prevent decubital ulcer (pressure sore) formation; and medicating affected areas of skin.

- Surgical patients with diarrhea should be cleaned frequently to prevent incisional infections.
  - Any long hair should be trimmed to prevent moisture from being trapped and causing a secondary infection.
  - Carefully shave the hair around the perianal and inguinal areas for ease of cleaning.
  - Apply a light tail wrap on long-haired patients with diarrhea to help keep the tail clean and prevent scalding.
  - Wrap the tail loosely and incorporate some of the hair to keep the wrap in place.
- Before placing the patient back in the cage, make sure that the patient is completely dry and all irritated areas on the skin are examined, shaved if necessary, cleaned, and treated appropriately.
- Ointments, creams, lotions, drying solutions, or powders can be reapplied at this time.
- For recumbent patients, place clean towels or padding between the patient's legs to aerate the skin, make the patient more comfortable, and prevent scrotal edema.
- Roll a stockinette into a donut shape to pad any decubital ulcers, which typically form on bony prominences such as the scapula or femur (Fig. 6.1).

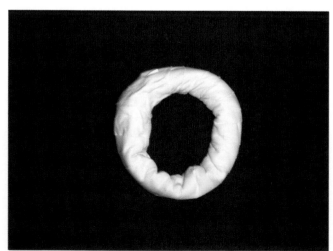

FIGURE 6.1 A donut-shaped pad used to help treat decubital ulcers. (From Sirois M: *Principles and practice of veterinary technology*, ed 3, St Louis, 2011, Mosby.)

Nail Trimming

- Nail trimming (pedicure) is an important general care technique.
- Excessive nail length results in altered gait and the potential accentuation of lameness problems.
  - Excessively long nails are more likely to split or to be traumatically avulsed.
  - Untrimmed nails can become ingrown (usually into the footpads), resulting in cellulite or abscess formation.
- Two common types of nail trimmers are available (Whites, Resco).
- To avoid cutting pigmented (black) nails too short in the dog, the cutting surface of the nail trimmer should be held parallel to the palmar or plantar surface of the digital footpads and the nail cut in this plane.
- In cats, the nails can be exposed by grasping the paw between the thumb and index finger and sliding the skin on the dorsum of the paw away from the nails.
- Nails that have not been trimmed regularly have a quick, or nail vein, that extends farther out into the claw than that of regularly trimmed nails.
  - The center of the nail takes on a fleshy, shining appearance in the region next to the quick. This is an indicator to trim no farther.
- The nail should be cut cleanly, with no frayed edges; smooth off any rough edges with nail file or Dremel tool.
- If the quick is accidentally cut, apply pressure with a cotton ball or gauze sponge directly on the quick to stop the bleeding gradually, or apply a cauterizing agent, such as silver nitrate applicators or Quick Stop powder.

Anal Sac Care

- The anal sacs are paired sacs located beneath the skin on either side of the anus at the 4 and 8 o'clock positions, each with a duct opening directly into the terminal rectum.
- The anal sacs normally empty their malodorous secretions during defecation.
- Occasionally, animals (rarely, cats) may not be able to empty their anal sacs naturally and develop painful distention or impaction of the anal sacs.
- Signs include scooting on the hindquarters and licking of the anal area.
- The anal sacs are emptied with the dog restrained in the standing position.
- Anal sac expression may cause discomfort, and a muzzle may be necessary.
- The veterinarian or veterinary technician performs internal anal sac expression by first donning examination gloves that are well lubricated with a water-soluble lubricant or 2% lidocaine jelly.
- With the veterinary assistant holding the tail dorsally or laterally, the veterinarian or veterinary technician inserts the first joint of the index finger into the rectum and gently palpates the anal sac between the thumb (externally) and forefinger.
- Gentle massage with light to moderate pressure milks the secretions medially into the anal opening.
- External expression of the anal sacs is a technique that requires squeezing of the anal glands from the external anal sphincter.
- This technique is not recommended because of the frequent occluding of the ducts, inability to empty the sacs completely, and excessive pain that it may cause the patient.

Ear Care

- Before cleaning ears, visually examine the external ear canal and tympanic membrane for any irregularity.
- Look for any redness, discharge, ulceration, excessive tissue formation, narrowing (stenosis) of the canal, abnormal odor, or debris in the outer ear and on the pinna.
- Evaluate the patient for signs of pain during the aural examination; these could indicate a bacterial or yeast infection, ear mite infestation, or tumors.
  - Thickening of the pinna could indicate an aural hematoma.
- Signs of ear disease include excessive shaking of the head, scratching at the ears, head tilt, nystagmus, and ataxia.
- Occasionally, the ear canal is occluded with debris and must be cleaned and flushed with saline to visualize the tympanic membrane.
- If cultures or cytologic samples are required, obtain the samples before cleaning the ears.
- Some dog breeds, such as poodles, have hair growth in the ear canal that traps moisture and debris and increases the likelihood of infection.
- Hair in the ear canal should be plucked out with a hemostat or the fingertips a few strands at a time.
  - This procedure may be painful, so appropriate restraint of the head is necessary.
  - Sedation or tranquilization may be necessary.
- Ensure that the tympanic membrane is intact before any cleaning.
- Most cleaning solutions are ototoxic if the tympanic membrane is not intact.
- If the membrane is not intact, use a saline solution to clean the ears.
- Various ceruminolytics are available for breaking up debris and cleansing.
- Cleansing products with a drying agent are good for cleaning the ears of dogs with long droopy ears, such as poodles and cocker spaniels.
- It is good public relations to have the patient looking better (as well as feeling better) on discharge than when it was admitted. Examine every patient before discharge to ensure that all extraneous bandages are removed. Ensure that the patient is bathed, groomed, dematted, and smelling good and that the nails are trimmed, ears cleaned, and anal sacs expressed. Brush one last time and spray with a lightly scented spray.

Preventive Medicine

- A great deal of nursing care involves preventive medicine.
- Preventive medicine is the science of preventing disease in animals.
- The three major components of a preventive medicine program include husbandry, vaccination or prevention through medication, and sanitation.
  - Husbandry involves the housing, diet, and environment of animals.
  - Vaccination involves the use of vaccines or bacterins to prevent diseases such as rabies or canine distemper; medication can be given regularly to prevent diseases such as heartworm infections or flea infestations.
  - Sanitation focuses on cleanliness and the use of disinfectants to prevent infection or disease transmission.
- The goal of any preventive medicine program is the lowest possible incidence of disease in animals under the care of the veterinary practice.

ANIMAL NUTRITION

- Animals must have free access to fresh potable water and be fed a wholesome, palatable diet on a regular schedule and in sufficient quantity.
- The diet fed should be formulated for that species.
- The quality of a pet's life can be dramatically influenced by the intake of nutrients balanced to its lifestyle and state of health.
- A nutrient is any constituent of food that is ingested to support life.
- The six basic nutrients are proteins, fats, carbohydrates, water, vitamins, and minerals. Energy-producing nutrients have a hydrocarbon structure that produces energy through digestion, metabolism, or transformation.
- Non–energy-producing nutrients play an important role throughout the body system and are often called the gatekeepers of metabolism.

Energy-Producing Nutrients
Proteins
- Dietary protein is used to build body tissues.
- Amino acids, the building blocks of protein, are categorized as either essential or nonessential.
- Essential amino acids cannot be synthesized in the body and so must be supplied by the diet (Box 6.1).
- Nonessential amino acids are synthesized in the body.
- The proportion of essential and nonessential amino acids largely determines the quality, or biologic value, of a particular protein source.
- A protein's biologic value represents the amount that is retained by the body after ingestion.

Fats
- Vegetable and animal fats, oils, and lipids are composed of fatty acids and contain more energy per unit of weight than any other nutrient.

BOX 6.1 Essential Amino Acids

- Arginine
- Histidine
- Isoleucine
- Leucine
- Lysine
- Methionine
- Phenylalanine
- Threonine
- Tryptophan
- Valine
- Taurine

From Sirois M: Principles and practice of veterinary technology, ed 3, St Louis, 2011, Mosby.

BOX 6.2 Essential Fatty Acids

Dogs
- Linolenic
- Linoleic

Cats
- Linolenic
- Linoleic
- Arachidonic

From Sirois M: Principles and practice of veterinary technology, ed 3, St Louis, 2011, Mosby.

- There is a direct correlation between fat content and caloric density in a diet; the more fat there is in a diet, the more calories it contains.
- Cats require three essential fatty acids in their diet, whereas only two are essential in dogs (Box 6.2).

Carbohydrates
- Carbohydrates are classified as soluble or insoluble, based on their digestibility.
- Mammals cannot digest insoluble carbohydrates, such as fiber, although bacteria can degrade fiber in the stomach of herbivores.
- Fiber decreases a diet's digestibility and caloric density.
- Soluble carbohydrates, such as sugar and starches, can be readily digested and are metabolized for energy needs.

Non–Energy-Producing Nutrients
Water
- Water provides the foundation for the metabolism of all nutrients in the body.
- Minor alterations in the body's water content and distribution can result in dramatic alterations in nutritional requirements.

- Water balance in the system affects the ability to excrete waste into the urine by the kidneys. Water is also essential for absorption and metabolism of water-soluble vitamins B and C.

Vitamins

- Vitamins play a very important role in maintaining normal physiologic functions.
- These organic molecules are required only in minute amounts to exert their function as coenzymes, enzymes, or precursors in metabolism.
- Water-soluble vitamins are passively absorbed from the small intestine, and excess amounts are excreted in the urine.
- Fat-soluble vitamins are metabolized in a manner similar to that of fats and stored in the liver. Because of this storage mechanism, toxicity from excessive intake of fat-soluble vitamins can occur.
- A deficiency of fat-soluble vitamins is not as common as with water-soluble vitamins (Box 6.3).

Minerals

- Within the body, minerals are often distributed in ionized form as a cation or anion electrolyte.
- In ionic form, they are involved with acid–base balance, clotting factors, osmolality, nerve conduction, muscle contraction, and other cellular activities.
- Deficiencies or excesses in mineral intake can lead to problems through imbalances.
- Minerals are closely interrelated, and an imbalance in one mineral can affect several others.
- Dietary minerals include calcium, phosphorus, potassium, sodium, chloride, magnesium, iron, zinc, copper, manganese, selenium, iodine, and boron.

BOX 6.3 Vitamins

Water-Soluble
- Thiamin
- Riboflavin
- Niacin
- Pyridoxine
- Pantothenic acid
- Folic acid
- Cobalamin
- Vitamin C
- Choline
- L-Carnitine

Fat-Soluble
- A
- D
- E
- K

From Sirois M: Principles and practice of veterinary technology, ed 3, St Louis, 2011, Mosby.

Feeding Methods

Portion Control

- After determining the animal's nutritional requirements, the daily portion is offered to the animal in a single feeding or divided into several portions offered several times per day.
- The animal is then allowed to consume the food throughout the day or during 5 to 10 minutes for each divided portion.

Free Choice

- In free-choice feeding, also referred to as **ad libitum** (ad lib), the animal is allowed access to food 24 hours per day.
- Free-choice feeding is not recommended for puppies and obese dogs, but it works well for cats.

Time Control

- In time-controlled feeding, a portion of food is offered and the animal is allowed access for only 5 to 10 minutes.
- Puppies are commonly fed in this manner.
- A review of nutritional considerations for different life stages in the cat and dog can be found in Table 6.1.

Feeding Considerations for Dogs

- Contrary to popular belief, frequent changes in diet have few positive effects, encourage finicky eating, and can cause digestive disorders.
- Weight loss or gain indicates a need to reevaluate the amount being fed or diet selection. **Body condition scoring** is a valuable way to assess the appropriate amount of food.

Feeding the Gestating or Lactating Dog

- The daily energy requirement during gestation in the bitch increases during the length of the pregnancy.
- The goal is to increase food intake gradually, assessing weight gain carefully during the pregnancy.
- Excessive weight gain in the gestating bitch can make parturition more difficult and affect the overall health of the dog.
- In the lactation phase, many dogs will require free feeding because they will need to eat smaller meals more frequently to reduce their absence from the puppies during this critical growth phase.

Feeding Puppies

- With puppies born by cesarean section, or if the bitch has no milk, the veterinary staff must intervene and provide nutritional support to neonatal puppies.
- Puppies can be raised successfully on canine milk replacer; cow's milk is not an acceptable substitute because it contains inappropriate levels of protein and lactose.
- It may be necessary to use orogastric intubation or a feeding syringe and then gradually adopt a regular small animal feeding bottle as the puppies begin to thrive.
- Daily or twice-daily weighing and physical examination of the puppies help identify problems early enough to

TABLE 6.1 Nutrient Considerations for Different Life Stages in Cats and Dogs

Life Stage	Food Characteristics	Comments
Cats Kittens 8 wk–1 yr; gestation, lactation	Metabolizable energy, 4.5 kcal/g dry matter Digestibility ≤80% Protein, 35%–50% Fat, 17%–30% Fiber ≥5% Calcium-to-phosphorus ratio, 1.0–1.8 to 0.8–1.5 Magnesium ≤20 mg/100 kcal	Transition queen to growth diet at 3 wk of gestation.
Adult cat	Metabolizable energy, 3.75 kcal/g dry matter Digestibility >78% Protein, 0%–45% Fat, 9%–25% Magnesium <20 mg/100 kcal	Ad lib feeding acceptable to kittens and queens. Free-feeding adults may result in overnutrition.
Obese-prone cat	Metabolizable energy, 3.50–3.75 kcal/g dry matter Digestibility >75% Protein, 30%–45% Fiber, 7%–12% Fat, 9%25% Magnesium <20 mg/100 kcal	Feed multiple (three or four) times daily. Fiber provides satiety and decreased caloric density.
Geriatric cat	Metabolizable energy, 3.75 kcal/g dry matter Digestibility >80% Protein, 35%–45% Fiber, 7%–12% Fat, 9%–25% Magnesium <20 mg/100 kcal	Watch excess sodium and energy intake. Increased palatability may be needed.
Dogs Puppies; gestation, lactation	Metabolizable energy >3.9 kcal/g of diet Digestibility >80% Protein, 27%–30% Fiber <4% Fat, 8%–20% Calcium-to-phosphorus ratio, 1.0–1.8 to 0.8–1.6	Avoid excessive weight during pregnancy. Puppies reach skeletal maturity at approximately 12 mo of age.
Adult dog	Metabolizable energy >3.5 kcal/g of diet Digestibility >75% Protein, 15%–25% Fiber ≥5% Fat, 7%–15%	Food and feeding consistency encouraged.
Obesity-prone dog	Metabolizable energy <3.5 kcal/g of diet Digestibility >80% Protein, 15%–25% Fiber >5% Fat, 6%–10%	Free feeding can contribute to obesity.
Increased activity or stressed dog	Metabolizable energy >4.2 kcal/g of diet Digestibility >82% Protein, 25%–32% Fiber <4% Fat, 23%–27%	
Geriatric dog	Metabolizable energy = 3.75 kcal/g of diet Digestibility >80% Protein, 14%–21% Fiber >4% Fat, 10%–12% Control sodium	The average small-to-medium breed dog is considered geriatric after 7 yr. Giant and large breeds are geriatric at 5 yr of age.

From Sirois M: Principles and practice of veterinary technology, ed 3, St Louis, 2011, Mosby.

adjust feeding protocols or begin other therapeutic measures to avoid mortality.

- Puppies typically gain 2 to 4 g/kg of anticipated adult weight each day.
- Some neonatal puppies fail to gain weight when nursing the bitch because they cannot compete with siblings for a nipple.
- Puppies in this situation tend to be restless and whimper excessively.
- Normal weight can be restored by allowing these puppies to nurse the bitch without competition three to four times daily.
- Weaning begins at approximately 3 to 4 weeks of age in large-breed puppies and at 4 to 5 weeks of age in smaller breeds.
- To facilitate the transition to solid foods, begin by making a gruel or slurry of a growth type of diet.
- Gruel is created by mixing equal parts of food and water together to form a homogeneous consistency.
- Gruel should be offered three to four times daily during the weaning process.
- Feed the puppy with increasing amounts until the puppy can be maintained without nursing, at 5 to 7 weeks in large-breed puppies and 6 to 7 weeks in smaller breeds.
- Once weaning is complete, decrease the volume of water added to the mixture until the puppy is eating the desired diet and drinking water voluntarily.

Feeding Adult Dogs

- As a dog matures, be sure to monitor activity level and predisposition to obesity to preserve a neutral energy equilibrium.
- Reassess feeding methods because inappropriate techniques commonly result in excessive nutrient intake and obesity.

Feeding Active Dogs

- Active dogs require energy to sustain hunting, obedience trials, or other activities.
- The diets for active dogs must have enhanced levels of fat, the most energy-dense nutrient, as well as increased total digestibility.
- Any increase in food portions to condition a dog for work should be gradually instituted over a 7- to 10-day period.
- Hunting dogs should be fed just before a period of increased activity to avoid hypoglycemia.

Feeding Geriatric Dogs

- Older dogs are less able to adjust to prolonged periods of poor nutrition.
- Dietary protein should be of high biologic value to reduce the level of metabolites that must be excreted through the kidneys.
- Dietary fats must be sufficiently digestible to provide adequate levels of essential fatty acids without an excess that could lead to obesity.

- Because of its detrimental effects on the kidneys, dietary phosphorus should be limited. Increased levels of zinc; copper; and vitamins A, B complex, and E may be required in the diet of older dogs.

Feeding Considerations for Cats
Feeding Kittens

- Kittens that are orphaned or born to queens unable to nurse must be hand fed.
- Weaning should not commence until 7 weeks of age.
- Kittens can be gradually introduced to a diet by first offering a slurry of canned food mixed with kitten milk replacer.

Feeding Adult Cats

- Adult cats typically eat several small meals throughout a 24-hour period.
- Overfeeding can be prevented by offering limited amounts of food throughout the day.

Feeding Cats With Lower Urinary Tract Disease

- Feline urinary tract disease is a complex disease characterized by bouts of frequent painful urination, bloody urine, and, in males, possible urethral obstruction.
- It tends to occur more often in obese, sedentary cats.
- Factors other than diet are involved in lower urinary tract disease, but careful attention to the diet of affected cats can help prevent future episodes.
- Depending on the type of uroliths (small stones composed of cellular debris and mineral crystals) present in the urinary tract (struvite or calcium oxalate), prevention involves manipulation of dietary mineral, fiber, and water intake.
- Special commercial diets are available for the dietary management of feline urinary tract disease.

Feeding Geriatric Cats

- Because aging can diminish the senses of smell and taste, it is sometimes necessary to enhance the aroma and taste of foods to improve their palatability for aged cats.
- Successful techniques include warming canned food to body temperature in the microwave to improve the aroma, applying garlic powder to canned food before it is warmed, and adding aromatic foodstuffs, such as clam juice or bits of canned fish.

Feeding the Gestating and Lactating Cat

- Food intake for the gestating queen is not as dramatic as that found in the canine.
- Allow the queen to have free access to food during the last 30 days of gestation.
- Free food should be available to the queen throughout lactation to ensure ample milk availability to the kittens.

Pet Food Considerations

- To evaluate commercial diets for dogs and cats accurately, it is necessary to obtain accurate information about the common pet foods that clients consider feeding and that are recommended by the veterinary practice.

- Assessing pet food begins with making an overview of general considerations and then progressing to more specific evaluations as the diet continues to meet nutritional expectations.
- A review of information available on a pet food label is shown in Fig. 6.2.
- Occasionally, clients inquire regarding their potential to produce a homemade diet.
  - Most homemade diet recipes have not been analyzed for adequacy, possess ingredients that are often hard to come by, and are hard to reproduce consistently.
- Pet foods should also be tested by the Association of American Feed Control Officials (AAFCO; http://www.aafco.org).
  - AAFCO provides a resource to formulate uniform and equitable regulations and policies. These guidelines apply to ingredient definitions, labeling, and feeding trials.
  - Diets to be considered for veterinary clinic recommendation should be tested by AAFCO with approved feeding trials to substantiate adequacy regarding actual application of the diet to a particular species and life stage as it is intended to be fed.
- Decisions on feeding for pets must be based on activity level, breed, age, health status, and reproductive condition (spayed or neutered).
- A dry food may be a better choice than canned when there are concerns regarding dental health.
  - Some pets that are finicky may find canned food to be their preference over dry food.

Nutritional Support
For Ill or Debilitated Patients

- Sick or injured patients need good nutritional support to counteract the immunosuppressive effects of sepsis, neoplasia, chemotherapy, anesthesia, and surgery.
- Nutritional support enhances wound healing and minimizes the length of hospitalization without significant weight loss and muscle atrophy.
- Initiation of nutritional support early in the course of hospitalization is crucial for a successful outcome.
- Nutritional status should be assessed when the patient is admitted to the hospital and daily during hospitalization.
- Cats, especially overweight cats, can only go a few days without nutritional support before ill effects develop, such as hepatic lipidosis.
- During the physical examination, the patient's weight is recorded and compared with that of previous visits.
- During hospitalization, the patient is a candidate for nutritional support if the following occurs:
  1. The patient loses more than 10% of body weight.
  2. The patient has a decreased appetite or anorexia.
  3. The patient loses body condition from vomiting, diarrhea, trauma, or wounds.
  4. The patient has increased needs because of fever, sepsis, wounds, surgery, low serum albumin level, organ dysfunction, or chronic disease.
- The goal of nutritional support is to provide the patient's nutritional requirements while it is recovering from its disease process and/or anorexia, trauma, or surgery until the patient is able to eat enough on a regular basis to accommodate any ongoing losses.

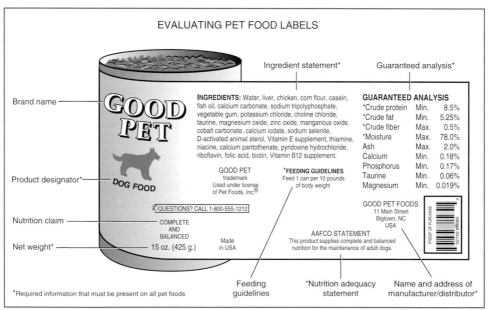

FIGURE 6.2 A pet food label is the contract between the manufacturer and consumer. A label provides information required by law and may have optional information, such as a statement of calorie content, the universal product code, batch information, and/or a freshness date.

- The route of nutritional support administration can be enteral, parenteral, or a combination of both.
  - Enteral feeding may be accomplished with orogastric, nasogastric, nasoesophageal, pharyngostomy, gastrostomy, and jejunostomy tubes.
  - Parenteral nutrition is administered via a catheter placed in the cranial or caudal vena cava.
- The route selected depends on factors such as function of the gastrointestinal (GI) tract, disease process, duration of support, equipment and personnel available to provide the necessary support, and cost of the chosen method.
- Enteral support is chosen most often because it is physiologically sound, easy, relatively free of complications, and inexpensive.
  - If the GI tract is functional and the patient can swallow, use as much as possible.
- Parenteral support should be used if the patient has a medical or surgical condition that prevents ingestion or digestion of nutrients (e.g., vomiting, diarrhea, ileus, pancreatitis, malabsorption, reconstructive surgery, coma) and as adjunctive therapy for patients with organ failure or when malnutrition is severe.

Enteral Nutritional Support

- Hand feeding favorite foods and tempting with warm, odoriferous foods in multiple small meals can be used in conjunction with other methods of nutritional support.
- Forced feeding can be stressful to the patient and may deliver only a portion of the nutrition required for recovery.
- Orogastric intubation is excellent for rapid administration but can cause aspiration and trauma and is stressful for patients other than neonates. This method is for short-term use only.
- Placement of a nasoesophageal or nasogastric tube is an easy, simple, and relatively inexpensive procedure that allows liquid nutritional support for an extended time.
- A nasoesophageal or nasogastric tube is placed through the nasal cavity into the distal esophagus or stomach to bypass the oral cavity (Fig. 6.3).
  - Placement is contraindicated in patients with nasal masses, esophageal disorders (e.g., megaesophagus), or no gag reflex.
  - It is tolerated by most patients and used when the animal is anorexic, too stressed for forced feeding, and not receiving enough nutrition through hand feeding.
  - The tube can remain in place for 1 week or longer until the patient's appetite increases or the oral cavity can be used again.
  - Common problems with nasoesophageal or nasogastric tubes include epistaxis (nosebleed) when the tube is first placed, accidental placement in the trachea, patient intolerance of the tube, and tube obstruction by medications or diet.
- Soft, flexible pediatric feeding tubes; red rubber tubes; and seamless polyurethane tubes in a variety of lengths and diameters are used for cats and dogs.

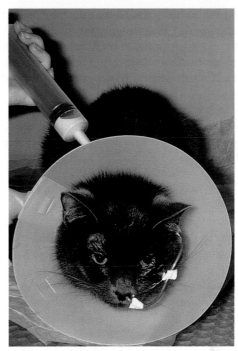

FIGURE 6.3 Nasoesophageal tube in place in a cat being fed a liquid enteral diet. (From Nelson RW, Couto G: *Small animal internal medicine*, ed 4, St Louis, 2009, Mosby.)

- Animals weighing less than 5 kg require a 5-Fr feeding tube, whereas some cats and all dogs weighing 5 to 15 kg can accept an 8-Fr tube.
- For nasoesophageal placement with the tube tip at the level of the midthoracic esophagus, measure from the tip of the nose to the eighth or ninth rib.
- For nasogastric placement, measure from the tip of the nose to the 13th rib to ensure safety in its position.
- Before each feeding, also assess tube location by injecting 3 mL of sterile water through the tube and listening for coughing or gagging.
- A pharyngostomy tube is placed through the wall of the pharynx into the esophagus or stomach, bypassing the oral cavity.
  - Placement requires general anesthesia and surgery.
  - The many possible complications (e.g., esophagitis, pharyngitis, laryngitis, vomiting, regurgitation, aspiration pneumonia) and the difficulty of pharyngostomy tube placement outweigh the benefits.
- A jejunostomy tube is a feeding tube surgically placed in the mid-to-distal duodenum or proximal jejunum, bypassing the stomach.
- Continuous feeding of easily digestible diets through the jejunostomy tube requires prolonged hospitalization, without the benefits of home care.
  - This procedure is rarely used because of the cost of placement and maintenance and possible complications.
- A gastrostomy or percutaneous endoscopic gastrostomy (PEG) tube is placed through the body wall into the lumen of the stomach, bypassing the mouth and esophagus.

- A gastrostomy tube is used for patients requiring long-term nutritional supplementation because of orofacial neoplasia, surgery or trauma, esophageal disorders, or liver disease.
- The tube's bulb or mushroom tip helps retain the tube in the desired location.
- Gastrostomy tubes can be placed with the use of endoscopic equipment (e.g., percutaneous endoscopic gastrostomy) or without endoscopic equipment (e.g., blind percutaneous gastrostomy).

Enteral Nutrition Daily Caloric Requirements

- Diet selection is based on caloric density, diameter of the feeding tube, and daily caloric needs of the patient.
- Each illness is assigned a factor to increase the calculated estimate of the patient's basal energy requirements by 25% to 75%.
- The volume and consistency of the diet are limited by the size of the animal's stomach and diameter of the feeding tube, but total caloric requirements can usually be delivered when using a calorically dense diet.
- Stomach volume is approximately 20 mL/kg body weight; daily water requirement is 12 mL/kg body weight.
- Patients with a nasoesophageal or nasogastric tube require a liquid diet because of the small tube diameter.
- Liquid veterinary products are available; canned diets, such as Hill's a/d and Eukanuba Nutritional Recovery Formula, can also be delivered through a feeding tube as small as 8-Fr.
- Select the appropriate diet of canned food and calculate the caloric density (kcal/mL) of the diet based on information on the label or supplied by the manufacturer.
- The total volume (mL) to be delivered daily is calculated by using the maintenance energy requirement (MER) and caloric density (Box 6.4).
- For anorexic patients, after placement of the tube, the volume fed is gradually increased over 3 days, with 5 mL of water administered through the tube every 2 hours for 12 hours.
  - Change to the selected diet and double the volume to 10 mL every 2 hours for 12 to 24 hours.
  - Gradually increase the volume to achieve full caloric intake, divided into four to six feedings daily, by the third day.
- Animals with feeding tubes in place should be offered fresh food before each feeding once the oral cavity and esophagus can be used.
  - Most animals begin to eat with the feeding tube still in place.
- When the animal begins voluntarily to eat at least half of its MER daily, the amount of food given through the feeding tube can be decreased until the patient is consuming its full caloric intake by mouth (PO).
- The change from enteral feedings to the normal diet should be gradual, over 3 to 5 days, if the patient's normal diet is not used for enteral feedings.

BOX 6.4 Enteral Feeding Calculation

- Calculate resting energy requirement (RER):

$$RER = 70 \times BW \text{ (body weight in kg)}$$

- Calculate illness/infection/injury energy requirements (IER):

$$Factor = 1.2 - 1.5$$

- Multiply chosen factor by RER to equal IER.
- Choose a veterinary-specific critical care formula.
- Calculate the volume of diet required and identify amount of kcal/mL:

$$\frac{IER}{\frac{kcal}{mL}} = mL \text{ of diet/day}$$

- Calculate the number and volume of feedings:

(mL of diet/day) /(number of feedings/day) = mL diet / feeding

From Sirois M: Principles and practice of veterinary technology, ed 3, St Louis, 2011, Mosby.

Parenteral Nutritional Support

- Patients that cannot receive enteral nutrients must be supported by total parenteral nutrition (TPN), which involves intravenous (IV) infusion of nutrient solutions.
- Carbohydrates are administered in the form of dextrose.
  - The most common concentration used is 50% dextrose, which provides 1.7 kcal/mL.
- Gradual introduction of dextrose is necessary to avoid hyperglycemia.
- Lipids, including essential fatty acids, provide the fat required by the patient.
  - These are available in 10% and 20% solutions, with 20% used more commonly.
- Proteins are supplied in the form of crystalline amino acids, made of essential and nonessential amino acids, available in a variety of concentrations, with or without electrolytes.
  - The most common concentration used is 8.5% with electrolytes.
- If TPN is to be continued for longer than 1 week, supplementation of taurine is essential in cats.
  - Electrolytes can be included in the amino acid solutions.
- Hypokalemia is the most common electrolyte abnormality.
  - For patients with ongoing potassium losses (e.g., because of vomiting), additional supplementation may be necessary.
- Vitamins are administered as a multivitamin supplement.
  - B complex vitamins should be added daily to the feeding solution.

- Vitamin K is incompatible with parenteral solutions and should be administered by subcutaneous or intramuscular injection only if parenteral nutrition is continued longer than 1 week.
- Trace elements only need to be supplemented if long-term (>1 week) parenteral nutritional support is needed.
  - Zinc may need to be supplemented after 1 week in patients with GI disease.
  - Phosphorus may be added for diabetics.
- The total daily fluid volume for maintenance TPN is 30 mL/lb of body weight.
- If the total volume of TPN is less than the calculated required amount, add an additional amount of balanced electrolyte solution or sterile water to equal the calculated fluid requirements.
- If the patient is experiencing ongoing fluid losses, a second catheter, or an additional lumen on a central catheter, can be used to deliver the fluids.
  - When mixing the appropriate solutions, strict asepsis is essential.
  - Add the dextrose and amino acids before the lipids to prevent lipid destabilization. Add the water or electrolyte solutions next, and any vitamins last.
- Parenteral nutrition is administered via a catheter in the cranial or caudal vena cava.
- A double-lumen catheter is of benefit if additional medication, fluids, blood products, or blood sampling is needed.

- Administration by a fluid pump is the most accurate method of delivering parenteral nutrition.
- Many complications of parenteral nutrition involve problems with the catheter.
  - Sepsis is another complication of parenteral nutrition.
  - Nutrient solutions are an excellent growth medium for bacteria.
  - Contamination of the solutions, lines, or catheters can cause fever, depression, and pain or swelling at the catheter insertion site.
  - Administering TPN through a dedicated IV line can decrease the likelihood of sepsis.
  - The catheter should be used for parenteral nutrition only and not for blood sampling, medication administration, or central venous pressure (CVP) monitoring.
- All administration lines should be changed every 48 hours when the bag is changed. The catheter bandage should be replaced whenever it is soiled, as well as every 48 hours, when the administration lines are changed.
- Gradual tapering of TPN can prevent hypoglycemia.
  - If TPN must be discontinued abruptly, use a 5% dextrose solution to maintain blood glucose levels.
- Patients on TPN longer than 1 week may develop intestinal villous atrophy.
- Table 6.2 summarizes the nutritional requirements of pets with various diseases.

TABLE 6.2 Summary of Small Animal Clinical Nutrition*

Objectives	Considerations	Product†	Comments
Allergy, Food			
Dogs			
Reduce antigen ingestion.	Novel highly digestible protein source or protein hydrolysate. Reduce total protein content Simplify food. Distilled H_2O	Hill's Prescription Diet—Canine d/d or Canine z/d	8- to 10-wk trial period Avoid treats, snacks, access to other food sources, chewable medications, supplements.
Cats			
Reduce antigen ingestion.	Same as dog except control Mg^{2+} intake. Provide taurine. Control urine pH.	Hill's Prescription Diet—Feline d/d or Feline z/d	
Anemia			
Support RBC production.	↑ Iron, cobalt, and copper ↑ B complex vitamins ↑ Protein	Hill's Prescription Diet—Canine p/d Feline p/d	
Anorexia			
Prevent protein and caloric malnutrition. Stimulate appetite.	Establish fluid–electrolyte balance and acid–base balance. ↑ Protein and fat ↑ Micronutrients	Hill's Prescription Diet—Feline, Canine a/d, Canine p/d, Feline p/d	Cat foods are suitable for dogs in acute care settings.

Continued

TABLE 6.2 Summary of Small Animal Clinical Nutrition*—cont'd

Objectives	Considerations	Product†	Comments
Ascites Reduce fluid retention.	Restrict sodium chloride. Maintain hydration.	Hill's Prescription Diet—Canine h/d, k/d; Feline h/d, k/d	h/d = marked salt restriction k/d = moderate salt restriction
Bone Loss and Fracture Healing Correct deficiency of energy and protein.	↑ Protein ↑ Energy Avoid supplementation.	Hill's Prescription Diet—Canine p/d, Feline p/d	Extra dietary calcium does not increase rate of fracture healing.
Cancer Increase longevity and quality of life.	↓ Soluble carbohydrate ↑ Fat and n-3 fatty acids ↑ Arginine	Hill's Prescription Diet—Canine n/d, Canine/Feline a/d	Use in conjunction with chemotherapy or other forms of cancer therapy.
Colitis Normalize gastrointestinal motility. Rebalance microflora. Provide local healing factors.	Feed small meals three to six times/day. Control dietary antigens. Vary levels of dietary fiber.	Hill's Prescription Diet—Canine w/d, i/d, d/d; Feline w/d, d/d	
Constipation Normalize gastrointestinal motility. Maintain stool water. Maintain stool bulk.	>10% fiber	Hill's Prescription Diet—Canine w/d, Feline w/d	No table scraps or bones Increase exercise. Encourage water intake. Cats: keep litter box clean.
Copper Storage Disease Restrict copper intake.	<1.2 mg copper/100 g dry diet	Hill's Prescription Diet—Canine l/d	No table scraps or treats
Debilitation Restore tissue, plasma, and nutrients.	↑ Protein ↑ Fat ↑ Macronutrients and micronutrients	Hill's Prescription Diet—Canine a/d, Feline a/d	Assist feed if needed.
Developmental Orthopedic Disease Reduce rapid growth.	↓ Fat and energy density ↓ Calcium	Hill's Prescription Diet—Canine p/d, large breed	Avoid calcium–phosphorus supplements.
Diabetes Mellitus Even rate of glucose absorption. Provide consistent caloric intake.	>10% fiber ↓ Soluble carbohydrates	Hill's Prescription Diet—Canine w/d, Feline w/d	Weigh animal frequently and note in medical record.
Diarrhea, Acute Normalize GI tract motility and secretion.	Withhold food for 1–2 days. Feed small amounts three to six times/day. ↓ Fiber ↓ Sugar ↑ Digestibility	Hill's Prescription Diet—Canine i/d Feline i/d	Electrolyte disturbances and dehydration are common.
Eclampsia Provide Ca and P in correct quantity and ratio prepartum.	High digestibility of diet Balanced minerals, vitamins	Hill's Prescription Diet—Canine p/d Feline p/d	Avoid supplementation.
Flatulence Decrease aerophagia. Avoid food fermentation.	Avoid milk or milk products. Feed small meals three to six times/day. ↑ Caloric density	Hill's Prescription Diet—Canine i/d, Feline i/d	Feed in a flat, open dish. Avoid vitamin or fatty acid supplementation. Separate competitive eaters.

TABLE 6.2 Summary of Small Animal Clinical Nutrition*—cont'd

Objectives	Considerations	Product†	Comments
Gastric Dilation and Bloat (Postoperative)			
Prevent gastric distention.	Avoid exercise before and after feeding. ↑ Digestibility of diet Small frequent feedings	Hill's Prescription Diet—Canine i/d	Diet form or type is *not* related to risk of occurrence or recurrence.
Heart Failure *Dogs*			
Control Na⁺ retention.	↓ Na⁺ intake Maintain energy and protein intake. ↑ B-complex vitamins ↓ Na⁺ intake	Hill's Prescription Diet—Canine h/d, Canine k/d	Hill's Prescription Diet—k/d has moderate Na⁺ restriction.
Cats			
Control Na⁺ retention.	↑ Taurine Control Mg²⁺ levels.	Hill's Prescription Diet—Feline h/d, Feline k/d	Avoid high-Na⁺ treats and water.
Hyperlipidemia			
Control fat intake.	↑ Fiber intake ↓ Fat intake	Hill's Prescription Diet—Canine w/d, Feline w/d	Common in schnauzers Consider fat in treats, table foods, and supplements.
Hyperthyroidism (Cats)			
Support increased energy need.	↑ Energy intake ↑ Vitamins and minerals ↑ Protein	Hill's Prescription Diet—Feline a/d	Monitor for evidence of concurrent renal disease.
Liver Disease (Fat-Tolerant)			
Reduce protein metabolism. Maintain liver glycogen. Prevent ammonia toxicity.	↑ Digestible energy Protein restriction High–biologic value proteins Control Na⁺ intake.	Hill's Prescription Diet—Canine l/d, Feline l/d	May feed small meals (four to six times/day)
Lymphangiectasia			
Decrease dietary fat.	↓ Intake of long-chain triglycerides Control protein levels. Consider medium-chain triglycerides.	Hill's Prescription Diet—Canine w/d or r/d	Medium-chain triglyceride oils and powder can increase caloric density.
Obesity			
Maintain intake of all nutrients except energy.	↓ Energy digestibility Replace digestible calories with indigestible fiber. Increase bulk to control hunger. Add carnitine.	Hill's Prescription Diet—Canine r/d, Feline r/d	Requires professional advice and teamwork with veterinary technician and client.
Oral Disease: Gingivitis (Gum Inflammation), Periodontitis (Loss of Tooth Attachment)			
Control accumulation of plaque, stains, and calculus. Maintain gingival health.	Provide food that promotes chewing and mechanical cleansing of teeth.	Hill's Prescription Diet—Canine t/d, Feline t/d	Many treats make dental claims but are not effective.
Pancreatitis, Acute (Recovery Phase)			
Control pancreatic secretions.	↓ Fat ↑ Digestibility Feed small meals three to six times/day	Hill's Prescription Diet—Canine i/d, Feline i/d	Frequent, small meals

Continued

TABLE 6.2 Summary of Small Animal Clinical Nutrition*—cont'd

Objectives	Considerations	Product†	Comments
Pancreatic Exocrine Insufficiency			
Reduce requirements for digestive enzymes.	↓ Fiber ↓ Fat Highly digestible carbohydrates ↑ Caloric density	Hill's Prescription Diet—Canine i/d, Feline i/d	Pancreatic enzymes complement highly digestible food.
Renal Failure			
Reduce signs of uremia. Slow progression of disease.	↓ Protein (↑ biologic value of protein) ↑ Nonprotein calories ↓ Phosphorus and sodium ↑ B complex vitamins	Hill's Prescription Diet—Canine k/d, Canine g/d, Canine u/d Hill's Prescription Diet—Feline k/d, Feline g/d	Small meals four to six times/day. Conversion to a protein-restricted diet may take 7–10 days. Water available at all times.
Canine Urolithiasis (Struvite)			
Treatment			
Increase water intake. Restrict Mg^{2+}, NH_4^+, and PO_4.	↓ Protein ↓ PO_4, Mg^{2+} ↑ Na^+ ↓ Urine pH (5.9–6.1)	Hill's Prescription Diet—Canine s/d	Evaluate and treat urinary tract infection. Average duration of stone dissolution is 36 days; follow up via radiography.
Prevention			
Maintain physiologic level of urinary solutes and urine pH.	Control protein excess. ↓ Ca^{2+}, P, Ma^{2+} ↓ Sodium mildly ↓ Urine pH (6.2–6.4)	Hill's Prescription Diet—Canine c/d	Monitor urine sediment for crystalluria and infection.
Canine Urolithiasis (Ammonium Urate)			
Prevention			
	↓ Protein ↑ Nonprotein calories ↓ Nucleic acids ↓ Ca^{2+}, P, Mg^{2+}, Na^+ Urine pH (6.7–7.0)	Hill's Prescription Diet—Canine u/d	Drugs plus diet may be successful treatment. Monitor urinary crystalluria. Prevention may require long-term drug treatment.
Canine Urolithiasis (Calcium Oxalate and Cystine)			
Prevention			
↓ Urinary concentration of calcium oxalate or cystine	↓ Protein ↑ Nonprotein calories ↓ Ca^{2+}, P, Na^+, Mg^{2+} ↑ Urine pH (6.1–7.0)	Hill's Prescription Diet—Canine u/d	Treat by surgical removal. Prevent by dietary management ± drugs.
Feline Urolithiasis (Struvite)			
Treatment			
↑ Urine volume ↓ Urine pH (5.9–6.1) Restrict Mg^{2+}, Ca^{2+}, and PO_4.	↑ Caloric density ↓ P and Ca^{2+} Mg^{2+} >20 mg/100 kcal ↑ Na^+ Urine pH (6.2–6.4)	Hill's Prescription Diet—Feline s/d	Dissolution is complete 1 mo after negative x-rays. Recurrence is high if prevention is not implemented.
Prevention			
Maintain physiologic levels of urinary solutes and urine pH.	Mg^{2+} >20 mg/100 kcal (0.1% DMB) ↓ P ↑ Caloric density Urine pH (6.2–6.4)	Hill's Prescription Diet—Feline c/d-s	For obesity, use calorie-restricted diets that maintain urine pH at 6.2–6.4 (Hill's Prescription Diet w/d is suggested).

TABLE 6.2 Summary of Small Animal Clinical Nutrition*—cont'd

Objectives	Considerations	Product†	Comments
Feline Urolithiasis (Calcium Oxalate)			
Prevention			
↑ Urine volume ↓ Urinary Ca^{2+}, oxalate ↑ Urine pH	↓ Protein ↑ Nonprotein calories ↓ P, Ca^{2+}, Na$^+$ Mg^{2+} <20 mg/100 kcal	Hill's Prescription Diet—Feline c/d-oxl	Monitor urinary crystalluria.
Vomiting			
Minimize gastric secretion. Provide GI rest.	↑ Digestibility ↑ Caloric density	Hill's Prescription Diet—Canine i/d, Feline i/d	Frequent, small meals

From Sirois M: Principles and practice of veterinary technology, ed 3, St Louis, 2011, Mosby.
Ca, Calcium; DMB, dry matter basis; Mg, magnesium; Na, sodium; NH4, ammonium; P, phosphorus; PO4, phosphate; RBC, red blood cells.
*Nutrients in table are expressed on a dry weight basis.
†Other North American therapeutic brands with wide distribution include the following: CNM (Purina), Eukanuba Veterinary Diets (Iams), and Waltham Veterinary Diets (Mars).

FLUID THERAPY

- Fluid therapy is one of the most commonly used supportive measures in veterinary medicine and is an important aspect of almost every critical care case.
  - It is primarily used to correct fluid deficits, electrolyte disturbances, and acid–base imbalances.
- The veterinarian will determine the need for fluid administration based on assessment of the patient's state of hydration and estimation of fluid deficits through subjective patient evaluation.
- Formulation of a fluid therapy regimen is based on information gathered from an accurate history, thorough physical examination, and laboratory tests.
- An appropriate route through which fluid solutions can be administered is chosen after careful evaluation of a number of factors.
  - These factors will be influenced by the cause and severity of the condition and include the following:
    - Volume of fluid loss
    - Rate of fluid loss (acute virtually chronic)
    - Fluid solution selected for administration
    - Volume and rate of infusion
    - Patient status
- In small animal medicine, medical, practical, and economic considerations may affect the fluid solution chosen and administration route used.
- The IV route of fluid administration is preferable when treating animals that are critically ill, severely dehydrated, hypovolemic, or experiencing some electrolyte or metabolic disorder.
- Many factors influence the rate of fluid administration (e.g., disease process, rate of fluid loss, severity of clinical signs, fluid composition and delivery route, cardiac and renal function).
- Regular monitoring of fluid therapy patients is needed to detect overhydration or underhydration.

- The patient's weight, body temperature, mucous membrane color, capillary refill time, heart and respiratory rate, respiratory rhythm, pulse rate and quality, and urine output are recorded at regular intervals for the duration of fluid therapy.
- The catheter and IV fluid line are also checked regularly for signs that might indicate that the catheter has become dislodged or contaminated.
- Edema (swelling) around the catheter site often indicates that the catheter is no longer in the vein and must be replaced.
- Any redness or excessive warmth around the catheter site also signifies problems that must be addressed.

COMMON DISEASES

- Disease is any alteration from the normal state of health.
- A pathologist is one who studies diseases and often is responsible for accurate diagnosis, as well as determining the cause of those diseases.
- Pathologists are trained in different areas of expertise, including anatomic pathology or clinical pathology.
- The primary responsibility of a veterinary anatomic pathologist is the prosection (dissection) of cadavers (carcasses) presented for necropsy, which is analogous to an autopsy in humans.
  - During necropsy, the pathologist collects tissue sections from lesions, which are grossly observable diseased tissues, and examines them with a microscope.
- Evaluating tissues with a microscope is termed histopathology.
- The study of causes of disease, or sometimes the causes themselves, is referred to as the etiology.
- Prognosis is the expected outcome of the patient affected by the disease and is usually stated as good, guarded, or poor.

- Veterinary clinical pathologists evaluate components of the blood as well as types of body fluids, such as transudates and exudates.

Terminology

- Pathologists use specific terms to describe the lesions observed at necropsy and with the microscope.
- Gross lesions are described by stating the location, color, size, texture, and appearance of the altered tissue.
- The diagnosis may be a morphologic (anatomic) diagnosis or an etiologic (causative) diagnosis.

Fever, Inflammation, and Response to Injury

- Fever and inflammation are protective responses of the animal's body to fight infection resulting from pathogens (disease-causing agents).
- Pathogens include viruses, bacteria, parasites, fungi, and molds. Pathogens are described in more detail later in the chapter.
- Fever, also called pyrexia, is an abnormal increase in body temperature caused by the release of agents, called pyrogens, within the body.
- Pyrogens can be thought of as substances that cause the body to adjust its biologic thermostat to a higher setting.
  - This differs from hyperthermia, in which the body temperature increases above the body's thermostat setting because of such things as drugs, toxins, or external temperatures, as in heat stroke.
- Many pyrogens are released by the body's own immune cells when they encounter pathogens; however, some pathogens also produce substances that act as pyrogens.

Signs of Inflammation

- The five cardinal signs of inflammation are heat, redness, swelling, pain, and loss of function (Box 6.5).
- The cells involved in the inflammatory process are the leukocytes (white blood cells).
- The first response of the blood vessel to vascular injury is dilation, which means the diameter of the blood vessel increases, allowing more blood to flow into the affected area.
- Next, there is increased vascular permeability, which means that the blood vessels become slightly leaky.
- Immediately after vascular permeability increases, the process of exudation allows an influx of leukocytes and red blood cells to the inflammatory site.

BOX 6.5 Signs of Inflammation

Heat
Swelling
Pain
Redness
Loss of function

- Congestion of the blood vessels occurs in the next step, which means stasis or sludging of blood flow in the vessels from fluid loss through exudation.

Healing and Repair of Damaged Tissues

- In almost every organ system, the end result of tissue repair is fibrosis, or scarring. Repair can take place by first- or second-intention healing of a wound.
- A wound is an injury caused by physical means, with disruption of normal structures.
- First-intention healing occurs when the edges of the wound surfaces close together with no discernible scarring.
  - This type of healing generally occurs when the edges of a fresh wound are evenly opposed with the aid of a bandage, sutures, or skin staples.
- Second-intention healing repairs wounds involving much greater tissue damage. Second-intention healing produces much more granulation tissue.
  - Granulation tissue is a highly vascularized connective tissue that is only produced after extensive tissue damage.

Pathogens

- Pathogens are infectious organisms that can cause disease in a host.
- Pathogenic agents include multicelled and single-celled parasites, protozoans, bacteria, fungi, rickettsiae, mycoplasmas, chlamydiae, and viruses.

Parasites

- Parasites are organisms that have adapted to live on or within a host organism, deriving all their nutrients from that host, ideally without killing the host.
- We generally use the word parasite only in conjunction with multicelled organisms such as worms, flukes, and arthropods or single-celled protozoans; we tend to classify bacteria, fungi, rickettsiae, mycoplasmas, chlamydiae, and viruses separately.

Bacteria

- Bacteria are single-celled organisms referred to as prokaryotes because they lack a nucleus and organelles and their DNA consists of one double-stranded chromosome.
- Most bacteria have a cell wall outside their cell membrane, as do plant and fungal eukaryotic cells, although composed of different materials.
- Bacteria are classified as gram positive or gram negative, depending on the staining characteristics of their cell walls with Gram stain.
  - Gram-positive organisms stain purple, and gram-negative organisms stain red.

Viruses

- Viruses are extremely small infectious agents that can cause disease in a wide variety of animals.

- For viruses to cause disease, they must enter the animal's body, bind to the surface of a host cell, enter the cell, and destroy it.
- Viruses are technically nonliving agents, which consist of genetic material in the form of DNA or RNA surrounded by a protein coat, called a capsid.
- After the virus enters a host cell, it uses the host cell's machinery to transcribe, translate, and replicate the viral genetic material, thereby creating new viral proteins and new viruses.
- Viruses can destroy the cells by suppressing the cells' metabolic activity or causing them to lyse, releasing the newly formed viruses.

Nonpathogens

- Nonpathogenic causes of disease include trauma associated with mechanical, sonic, thermal, and electrical injuries, temperature extremes, and irradiation.
- Trauma is a physical wound or injury.
  - The primary effects of trauma, regardless of the initiating cause, are tissue necrosis and hemorrhage.
- An abrasion is an injury whereby the epithelium is removed from the tissue surface.
- A contusion is a bruise or injury with no break in the surface of the tissue.
- A laceration is a tear or jagged wound.
- A concussion is a violent shock or jarring of the tissue, a common injury to the brain after blunt trauma to the head.

Immune Response

- The immune system is a highly complex and complicated system that has many components that, along with the inflammatory process, prevent pathogens from causing disease.

- The immune system consists of nonspecific and specific defenses.
- Nonspecific defenses include the body's defenses against pathogens in general, regardless of pathogen type.
  - These include mechanical barriers to infection such as skin and mucous membranes, chemical barriers such as lysozymes in tears, salt in sweat, antiviral substances such as interferon in blood, and acid in the stomach.
  - Fever and inflammation, discussed earlier, are also part of the nonspecific defenses.
- Specific defenses comprise what is normally thought of as immunity, the body's protection against specific pathogens.
  - Specific defenses include antibodies and a number of other cells and biochemicals that work together to protect an animal from disease.

Zoonotic Diseases

- Zoonoses are the major area of involvement for veterinarians in public health.
- Zoonoses are diseases transmitted between animals and people; some diseases are indirect zoonoses and can be transmitted to animals and humans, and between species, by arthropods such as ticks or mosquitoes.
- Other infectious diseases are common to but not transmitted between animals and people; these can be caused by similar exposures to the same infectious organism.
- More than 150 zoonoses have been reported, and diseases not previously thought to be zoonotic are frequently added to the list.
- Zoonoses are a significant cause of human disability, hospitalization, death, and high economic cost in the United States and underdeveloped countries.
- Table 6.3 lists the causative organism, hosts, and mode of transmission for some common zoonoses.

TABLE 6.3 Causative Organisms, Animal Hosts, and Modes of Transmission for Selected Common Zoonoses

Disease	Causative Organism	HOSTS Small Animals	Wildlife	Modes of Transmission
Viral Diseases				
Rabies	Rhabdovirus	Most	Most	Animal bite
Encephalitis (eastern equine encephalitis [EEE], western equine encephalitis [WEE])	Togavirus		Birds, rodents	Mosquito bite
Lymphocytic choriomeningitis	Arenavirus	Mice		Varied
Contagious ecthyma (orf)	Poxvirus	Sometimes dogs		Contact
Simian herpes (B virus)	*Herpesvirus simiae*		Primates	Animal bite, direct contact

Continued

TABLE 6.3 Causative Organisms, Animal Hosts, and Modes of Transmission for Selected Common Zoonoses—cont'd

| | | HOSTS | | |
Disease	Causative Organism	Small Animals	Wildlife	Modes of Transmission
Newcastle disease	Paramyxovirus	Domestic birds	Wild fowl	Contact, inhalation
Yellow fever	Togavirus		Primates	Mosquito bite
Hantavirus infection	Hantavirus		Rodents	Contact
Rickettsial Diseases Q fever	*Coxiella burnetii*		Birds, rabbits, rodents	Inhalation, milk ingestion, contact
Rocky Mountain spotted fever	*Rickettsia rickettsii*	Dogs	Rodents, rabbits	Tick bite
Psittacosis	*Chlamydia psittaci*	Psittacine birds	Birds	Inhalation
Mycoses Ringworm	*Trichophyton* spp., *Microsporum* spp.	Cats, dogs	Rodents	Contact
Parasitic Diseases Trichinosis	*Trichinella spiralis*		Rats, bears, carnivores	Ingestion
Scabies	*Sarcoptes scabiei*	Dogs, rodents, cats	Primates	Contact
Taeniasis, cysticercosis	*Taenia* spp., *Cysticercus*		Boars	Ingestion
Hydatid disease	*Echinococcus* spp.	Dogs	Wolves	Ingestion
Schistosomiasis	*Schistosoma* spp.	Dogs, cats	Rodents	Contact
Larva migrans	*Toxocara, Ancylostoma, Strongyloides*	Dogs, cats	Raccoons	Ingestion
Bacterial Diseases Anthrax	*Bacillus anthracis*	Dogs	Most, except primates	Contact
Brucellosis	*Brucella* spp.	Dogs	All, except primates	Contact, inhalation, ingestion
Plague	*Yersinia pestis*	Cats	Rodents, rabbits	Flea bite
Campylobacteriosis	*Campylobacter fetus*	Dogs, cats	Rodents, birds	Ingestion, contact
Cat scratch disease	*Bartonella henselae*	Cats	Cats	Cat bite, scratch
Leptospirosis	*Leptospira* spp.	All, especially dogs	Rats, raccoons	Contact with urine
Salmonellosis	*Salmonella* spp.	All, especially dogs, cats	Rodents, reptiles	Ingestion
Tuberculosis	*Mycobacteria* spp.	Dogs, cats	All except rodents, monkeys	Ingestion, inhalation
Tularemia	*Francisella tularensis*	All	Rodents, rabbits	Tick bites, contact with tissue
Erysipelas	*Erysipelothrix rhusiopathiae*		Rodents	Contact
Tetanus	*Clostridium tetani*		Reptiles	Wound
Lyme disease	*Borrelia burgdorferi*	Dogs, cats	Deer, birds, rodents	Tick bite
Protozoal Diseases Cryptosporidiosis	*Cryptosporidium* spp.	Most	Birds	Ingestion

TABLE 6.3 Causative Organisms, Animal Hosts, and Modes of Transmission for Selected Common Zoonoses—cont'd

| | | HOSTS | | |
Disease	Causative Organism	Small Animals	Wildlife	Modes of Transmission
Toxoplasmosis	*Toxoplasma gondii*	Cats, rabbits, guinea pigs	Cats	Ingestion
Balantidiasis	*Balantidium coli*		Rats, primates	Ingestion
Sarcocystosis	*Sarcocystis* spp.	Dogs, cats		Ingestion
Giardiasis	*Giardia lamblia*	Dogs, cats	Beavers, zoo monkeys	Ingestion

From Sirois M: Principles and practice of veterinary technology, ed 3, St Louis, 2011, Mosby.

Disease Transmission

- For an infectious disease to survive in a population, the agent causing the disease must be transmitted.
- The mode of transmission is an important epidemiologic clue for understanding the disease.
- Reservoirs and hosts of a specific disease are important to identify because these are essential for the transmission of a disease and its maintenance in the population.
- Control programs for a disease are often aimed at the reservoirs, or hosts of the disease.
- Reservoirs can be inanimate (e.g., soil) or animate (e.g., animals, people, birds).
- Hosts are living beings that offer an environment for maintenance of the organism, but they are not necessary for the organism's survival.
- Direct transmission of disease requires close association or contact between a reservoir of the disease and a susceptible host.
- Contact with infected skin, mucous membranes, or droplets from an infected human or animal can cause disease.
- Animal bites can be a source of infections, trauma, and even zoonotic disease.
  - *Pasteurella* is responsible for 50% of dog bite infections and 90% of cat bite infections.
  - Cat bites are 10 times more likely to become infected than dog bites.
- Soil or vegetation contaminated with parasites, bacteria, or spores may be another source of direct transmission.
- Visceral larval migrans is transmitted when children eat soil or vegetables that have been contaminated with feces that contain *Toxocara canis* or *T. cati* (roundworm) eggs.
  - A similar disease occurs with *Ancylostoma* spp. (hookworm). The signs of cutaneous larval migrans are those of dermatitis, which is caused by the hookworm larvae migrating in the skin.
- Indirect transmission of disease is more complicated and involves intermediaries that carry the agent of disease from one source to another.

- The intermediary may be airborne, vector-borne (an arthropod), or vehicle-borne through water, food, blood, or an inanimate object.
- A vector is a living organism that transports the infectious agent.
- A vehicle is simply the mode of transmission of an infectious agent from the reservoir to the host.
- Indirect airborne transmission involves spread of the agent through tiny dust or droplet particles over long distances.
- Droplet spread is differentiated from airborne transmission by the fact that the droplets travel only a short distance (i.e., a few feet) and involve larger particles that often are removed by mechanisms in the upper respiratory passages.
- Various types of arthropods may serve as vectors of disease; these may include mosquitoes, ticks, and fleas.
  - Food and water are also vehicles of indirect transmission of disease.
- Foodborne intoxications are caused by toxins produced by certain bacteria that may contaminate food, such as *Staphylococcus aureus*.
- The toxins may be present in the food or may be formed in the intestinal tract after the contaminated food is eaten.
- Foodborne infections are caused by bacterial or viral organisms that cause infection.
- Parasitic diseases are also transmitted through food and water.
- Nematode and trematode infections are usually transmitted through the ingestion of eggs or undercooked meat that contains cysts.
  - *Giardia* is a protozoan that causes gastrointestinal disease in people; giardiasis can be serious in immunosuppressed individuals.
- Animals admitted to the veterinary clinic for hospitalization and treatment of any disease caused by a transmissible pathogen must be kept in isolation to avoid infecting other animals in the clinic.
- Personnel working with these animals must take appropriate protective measures, such as wearing disposable gowns and gloves, while treating these patients.

Control of Zoonotic Diseases

- Because of their regular contact with animals, animal tissues, animal environments, and pet owners, veterinarians and veterinary staff members are often the first to notice a zoonotic disease or the potential for one.
- It is important to determine which diseases are most common in certain animal species so that the risk of contracting a particular disease can be estimated.
- Children and older adults are more susceptible to zoonotic diseases and suffer more serious effects because their immune systems function at a lower level than those of normal healthy adults.
- Control of zoonotic diseases is aimed at the reservoir of disease or the intermediaries that transmit the disease.
- Control measures include spraying for mosquitoes, use of tick repellent, pasteurization of milk, adequate water filtration, and proper cooking and handling of food.
- Control programs also include the treatment of infected animals in the reservoir population and decreased contact with infected animals in the reservoir to prevent further transmission.
- Prevention programs require a thorough knowledge of the disease and how it is maintained and transmitted to help break the cycle of disease in the population and/or prevent disease transmission.
- Prevention programs include vaccination of animals in the reservoir population, potential hosts, and people, if vaccines against that disease are available.
- Prevention of human infection is possible by the treatment of infected animals that may transmit the disease to humans.

Vaccination and Preventive Medications

- There are two basic ways that an animal can acquire the immunity that it needs: passively and actively.
- Passive immunity occurs when the animal acquires preformed antibodies to various pathogens.
  - This can take place naturally, such as when maternal antibodies cross the placenta into the fetus or neonates ingest the dam's colostrum.
- Active immunity is when an animal develops its own antibodies to pathogens.
  - This can also occur naturally, through infection or exposure to the pathogen, or artificially through vaccination.
- Animals can be vaccinated against a wide variety of diseases.
- The vaccine does not cause disease but stimulates the cells of the immune system to develop antibodies against the portion of the pathogen that is antigenic.
  - On the next exposure to the pathogen, a vaccinated animal will not become infected because it has been immunized.
- A vaccine consists of a particular antigen unique to a pathogen, such as the cell wall of the causative bacterium or a small unit of the virus.

- The pathogen can be in several forms, including modified live, inactivated, or recombinant.
  - A modified live vaccine consists of a weakened version of the pathogen, which will induce an immune response but is attenuated enough so that it will not cause disease.
  - An inactivated or noninfectious vaccine consists of whole killed pathogens or selected antigenic subunits, enough to induce immunity.
  - A recombinant vaccine consists of a live nonpathogenic virus into which the gene for a pathogen-related antigen has been inserted.
- When the virus is injected into the animal, viral genes, including the inserted gene for the antigen of interest, will be expressed.
  - This will cause the animal to produce antibodies to the antigen without ever having been exposed to the pathogen.
- Serious diseases such as parvovirus infection and distemper in dogs and panleukopenia and feline leukemia virus infection in cats can be prevented by vaccination.
- The decision as to whether to vaccinate an animal is influenced by the risk of contracting the disease, effects of the disease, and benefits and cost of vaccination.
- Vaccination may not be warranted if the disease is unlikely to develop or causes only mild illness.
- A growing number of practitioners are concerned about the apparent association between vaccines and a particular type of cancer (sarcoma) at the injection site in cats.
  - The American Association of Feline Practitioners (AAFP) currently recommends using different vaccines at different locations on the body.
  - It is recommended that feline leukemia virus (FeLV) vaccine be given in the left rear limb as distally as possible and rabies vaccine be given in the right rear limb as distally as possible.
- Many products are available with multiple combinations of pathogens to accommodate different animal needs based on their lifestyles.
- Core vaccines are recommended for all dogs, whereas noncore vaccines are recommended based on a dog's lifestyle.

Vaccination
Vaccination of Dogs

- The following vaccines are available for dogs:
  - Rabies
  - Distemper
  - Parvovirus
  - Coronavirus
  - Canine adenovirus (CAV-1 or CAV-2)
  - Canine influenza
  - *Bordetella bronchiseptica*
  - Parainfluenza
  - Leptospirosis
  - *Borrelia burgdorferi*

- Puppies are usually immunized with one to three doses in the first few months of life and then annually as adults.
- The American Animal Hospital Association (AAHA) vaccination guidelines for dogs offer specific recommendations about which vaccines are core and noncore and when vaccinations should be administered.
- A less common vaccine available for dogs is the *Crotalus atrox* toxoid, which protects against rattlesnake venom. The vaccine is only administered to dogs with a defined risk for exposure.

Vaccination of Cats
- The following vaccines are available for cats:
  - Rabies
  - Panleukopenia (feline distemper)
  - Feline herpesvirus 1
  - *Chlamydophila felis*
  - FeLV
  - Rhinotracheitis
  - Calicivirus
  - Feline immunodeficiency virus (FIV)
  - *B. bronchiseptica*
- Most cats begin receiving vaccines as kittens, usually at approximately 6 weeks of age. Kittens require boosters after an original series of vaccines.
- Adult cats may require annual boosters against each of these diseases.
- The AAFP vaccination guidelines for cats offer specific recommendations about which vaccines are core and noncore and when vaccinations should be administered.

Antibody Titers Instead of Vaccination
- Although mostly safe, annual vaccinations are a source of controversy because of risks that may be associated with vaccine use.

- Reactions to vaccine administration ranging from localized swelling to anaphylaxis and sarcoma formation (especially in cats) have been reported.
- Although there are recommendations for appropriate vaccination protocols, optimal intervals have not been established for many vaccines.
- It is likely that the vaccinations currently in use provide long-term immunity; however, some patients at risk for contracting common diseases may still need vaccination.
- Some veterinarians are now recommending the measurement of antibody titers to diseases normally vaccinated against as an alternative to routine annual vaccination.
- An antibody titer may help determine whether a patient is likely to need booster vaccinations.
- There is disagreement and inconsistency about the level of antibodies that constitutes protection against a disease if the animal were infected or challenged with the pathogen.

Use of Preventive Medication
- Certain diseases can be prevented by the regular administration of preventive medication.
- This is best exemplified by the use of anthelmintics and other parasiticides to prevent heartworm infection and control internal and external parasites in dogs and cats.

Factors Predisposing to Disease
- Although some factors that predispose to disease are beyond our control, we can often establish conditions so that even uncontrollable factors have only minimal impact on our animals.
- Table 6.4 lists some common diseases of dogs and cats. Animals are predisposed to disease by genetic, dietary, environmental, and metabolic factors.

TABLE 6.4 Common Diseases of Dogs and Cats

Disease	Cause(s)	Common Signs and Symptoms
Anal sacculitis	Impaction, inflammation, or infection of anal glands	Scooting, tail chewing, malodorous perianal discharge
Anemia	Hemorrhage, iron deficiency, toxins, immune disorders	Anorexia, weakness, depression, tachycardia, tachypnea, pale mucous membranes
Arthritis	Acute—sepsis, trauma, immune-mediated	Lameness, swelling, crepitus
	Osteoarthritis—progressive degeneration of hyaline cartilage	
Asthma (feline)	Inflammation of airways, bronchoconstriction	Dyspnea (acute onset), coughing, lethargy
Atopy	Allergic reaction to inhaled substances	Pruritus, alopecia, dermatitis
Aural hematoma	Trauma causing buildup of blood beneath skin surface	Head shaking, scratching at ear
Brachycephalic respiratory distress syndrome	Congenital airway obstruction	Coughing, exercise intolerance, cyanosis, dyspnea

Continued

TABLE 6.4 Common Diseases of Dogs and Cats—cont'd

Disease	Cause(s)	Common Signs and Symptoms
Calicivirus (feline)	Viral infection of upper respiratory tract	Anorexia, lethargy, fever ulcerative stomatitis, nasal discharge
Cataracts	Inherited or secondary to diabetes and other diseases	Opaque pupillary opening, progressive vision loss
Congestive heart failure	Valvular insufficiency, myocarditis, hypertension, dilated cardiomyopathy	Anorexia, syncope, pulmonary edema
Coronavirus	Viral infection of GI system	Asymptomatic or anorexia, dehydration, V, D
Cushing disease	Hyperadrenocorticism	Bilateral, symmetrical alopecia
Cystitis	Inflammation or bacterial infection of urinary bladder	Hematuria, dysuria, inappropriate urination, pollakiuria, polyuria
Demodex	Infestation of hair follicles with *Demodex* mites	Alopecia, erythema, secondary pyoderma, pruritus
Dermatophytosis	*Microsporum canis, M. gypseum,* or *Trichophyton mentagrophytes* infection	Circular area of alopecia; lesion may be raised, red, crusty
Diabetes mellitus	Deficient or defective production of insulin	PU, PD, weight loss, polyphagia
Dilated cardiomyopathy	Dilation of all chambers of the heart	Ascites, hepatomegaly, weight loss, abdominal distension, dyspnea
Distemper (canine)	Paramyxoviral infection	Fever, cough, mucopurulent ocular and nasal discharge, V, D, hyperkeratosis of foot pads, ataxia
Dystocia	Primary uterine inertia, fetal obstruction	Active prolonged straining with no fetus produced; green, purulent, or hemorrhagic vaginal discharge; pain
Feline fibrosarcoma	Vaccine-induced	Swelling and rapidly growing firm mass at site of recent vaccination
Flea allergy dermatitis	Hypersensitivity to *Ctenocephalides* infestation	Pruritus, licking, chewing, erythema, alopecia
Fungal infection (systemic)	*Blastomyces dermatitidis*	Anorexia, depression, fever, dyspnea
	Coccidioides immitis	Cough, fever, anorexia, weight loss
	Histoplasma capsulatum	Weight loss, fever, anorexia
Geriatric vestibular syndrome	Otitis media	Head tilt, circling, disorientation, ataxia, nystagmus
Glaucoma	Increased intraocular fluid production	Ocular pain, corneal edema, buphthalmos, blindness
Heartworm disease	*Dirofilaria immitis* parasite	Exercise intolerance (dogs), dyspnea, coughing, ascites (dogs), vomiting (cats)
Hemobartonellosis	Mycoplasma, rickettsial infection	Pale or icteric mucous membranes, fever, tachypnea, tachycardia
Hip dysplasia	Laxity and subluxation of the hip joint	Lameness, gait abnormality, muscle atrophy
Histiocytoma	Benign skin tumor	Fast-growing dome or button-like nodules; may be ulcerated
Hyperthyroidism	Overproduction of thyroid hormone	Weight loss, polyphagia, vomiting, enlarged thyroid
Hypothyroidism	Underproduction of thyroid hormone	Weight gain, bilateral, symmetrical alopecia, cold intolerance

TABLE 6.4 Common Diseases of Dogs and Cats—cont'd

Disease	Cause(s)	Common Signs and Symptoms
Hepatic lipidosis	Accumulation of triglycerides in liver	Prolonged anorexia, V, D, lethargy
Immune-mediated hemolytic anemia	Accelerated red blood cell destruction	Anorexia, depression, tachycardia, tachypnea, pale mucous membranes
Immunodeficiency virus (feline)	Lentivirus infection	Chronic infections (e.g., of oral cavity, skin, respiratory tract); chronic fever, cachexia
Infectious canine tracheobronchitis (kennel cough)	Bacterial and viral infection of lower respiratory tract (e.g., *Bordetella bronchiseptica,* canine adenovirus)	Dry, hacking, paroxysmal cough
Inflammatory bowel disease	Inflammation of intestinal mucosa	Diarrhea, increased frequency and volume of defecation
Intestinal parasitism	Infection with parasites including nematodes (e.g., ascarids, hookworms, whipworms), coccidia, protozoa (e.g., *Giardia*), cestodes	Depending on species of parasite; diarrhea, weight loss, anemia, unthriftiness
Lipoma	Benign fatty tumor	Soft, round or oval subcuticular mass
Liver disease	Drugs, toxins, bile duct inflammation	Anorexia, V, D, PU, PD, jaundice
Lyme disease	*Borrelia burgdorferi*	Fever, anorexia, lameness, lymphadenopathy
Sarcoptic mange	*Sarcoptes scabiei canis* mite infestation	Red, crusty lesions, intense pruritus
Osteochondrosis dissecans	Degeneration and reossification of bone and cartilage	
Otitis externa	Primary or secondary parasitic, bacterial or yeast infection of the soft tissues of the ear	Head shaking, head tilt, pain, foul odor
Panleukopenia (feline)	Parvoviral infection	Anorexia, fever, V, D, abdominal pain
Panosteitis	Possible viral infection, metabolic disease, allergic reaction, hormonal excesses	Intermittent lameness, anorexia, fever, weight loss
Pancreatitis	Inflammation of the pancreas caused by obesity, overingestion of fats, other diseases	Depression, anorexia, V, D, dehydration
Parvovirus (canine)	Viral infection of GI tract	Bloody diarrhea, lethargy, vomiting, dehydration, fever
Patella luxation	Genetic predisposition, trauma	Abnormal gait with rotation of limbs
Periodontal disease	Bacterial infection of tissues surrounding teeth that leads to plaque accumulation and causes calculus buildup	Increased depth of periodontal pockets, increased tooth mobility, foul oral odor, pain
Peritonitis	Inflammatory process	Abdominal pain, reluctance to move, tachycardia, tachypnea, fever, V, D, dehydration
Pyoderma (deep)	Bacterial infection of the skin usually caused by *Staphylococcus intermedius*	Papules, pustules, draining fistulous tracts
Pyometra	Bacterial infection (e.g., *Escherichia coli, Staphylococcus, Pasteurella*)	Vulvar discharge, abdominal enlargement, PU, PD, dehydration
Renal failure	Damage to nephron causing reduction in glomerular filtration	Oliguria, polyuria, V, D, anorexia, dehydration
Skin tumors (sebaceous cysts, adenoma, adenocarcinoma, melanoma)	Unknown; possible genetic causes	Usually round masses, may be encapsulated or ulcerated
Thrombocytopenia	Numerous viral, bacterial, immune-mediated, and other noninfectious causes	Petechial hemorrhage, ecchymosis, epistaxis, lethargy

Continued

TABLE 6.4 Common Diseases of Dogs and Cats—cont'd

Disease	Cause(s)	Common Signs and Symptoms
Tick-borne rickettsial disease	*Rickettsia rickettsii* (Rocky Mountain spotted fever)	Fever, anorexia, mucopurulent ocular discharge, coughing, tachypnea, V, D
	Ehrlichia canis, E. ewingi, E. equi (ehrlichiosis)	Lymphadenopathy, anemia, depression, anorexia, fever lethargy, lameness, muscular stiffness
Ulcerative keratitis (corneal ulcers)	Trauma, bacterial infection, feline herpesvirus	Ocular pain, corneal edema, photophobia
Urolithiasis	Precipitation of mineral substances in urine	Dysuria, hematuria
Viral rhinotracheitis (feline)	Herpesvirus infection	Acute onset of sneezing, conjunctivitis, purulent rhinitis, fever
Von Willebrand disease	Decreased or deficient production of von Willebrand factor	Purpura, prolonged bleeding from venipuncture or surgical sites
Viral enteritis	Parvovirus, coronavirus, rotavirus	Bloody diarrhea, lethargy, vomiting, dehydration, fever

D, Diarrhea; PD, polydipsia; PU, polyuria; V, vomiting.
From Sirois M: Principles and practice of veterinary technology, ed 3, St Louis, 2011, Mosby.

Genetic Factors

- Genetic factors are largely not controllable, although their effects can be reduced to some extent by selective breeding.
  - These include, for example, gender predisposition, inherited mutations, immunodeficiencies, and the effect of inbreeding.
  - Immunodeficiencies may be noted by an increased incidence of infections.
  - Inbreeding can lead to physical abnormalities or diminished mental (intellectual) capacities.

Environmental Factors

- Environmental factors, such as climatic extremes or sudden climatic changes, can clearly cause distress or even death.
- Additional bedding improves the insulation around animals housed in extremely cold conditions.
- Overhead cover is needed to prevent sunburn and heat prostration and shield animals from precipitation.
- Inadequate ventilation increases the incidence of respiratory diseases through increased ammonia levels and large numbers of microorganisms in the air.
- Inadequate ventilation also impairs cooling in animals that use respiration to regulate body temperature (e.g., dogs) and prevents radiation of body heat.
- Inadequate ventilation inhibits the drying of bedding, favoring proliferation of bacteria or parasites.
- Excessive ventilation is also stressful; drafts or excessive ventilation can cause chilling, dehydration, or inflamed ocular tissues.

Metabolic Factors

- Metabolic factors beyond our control include the age of the animal and reproductive status, concurrent disease, and nonspecific stressors.
- Young, old, pregnant, and lactating animals have different physiologic needs than other animals.
  - These needs may require alteration of the animal's diet and housing.
- A common metabolic problem that influences the health of many companion animals, and that can be effectively managed by the animal owner, is obesity from overfeeding and lack of exercise.

WOUND CARE AND BANDAGING

- A wound is a disruption of cellular and anatomic functional continuity.
- Acute wounds are those induced by surgery or trauma that heal normally, with healing time determined by the depth and size of the lesion.
- Examples of acute wounds include surgical incisions, blunt trauma, bite wounds, burns, gunshots, and avulsion injuries.
- Chronic wounds have various causes and, as determined by their underlying pathology, may take months or years to heal completely.
- Decubital ulcers, diabetic ulcers, and vascular ulcers are examples of chronic wounds.

Wound Contamination and Infection

- Wound contamination is not the same as wound infection.

- Microorganisms in the environment contaminate all wounds, even those created during surgery using strict aseptic technique.
- Initially, these organisms are loosely attached to tissues and do not invade adjacent tissue; there is no host immune response to these organisms.
- Over time, these microorganisms multiply.
- Infection is the process whereby organisms bind to tissue, multiply, and then invade viable tissue, eliciting an immune response.
- Tissue infection depends on the number and pathogenicity (or virulence) of the microorganisms.
- In general, a wound is infected when the number of microorganisms reaches 100,000/g of tissue or milliliter of fluid.
- If the patient presents for treatment more than 12 hours after injury, any wounds should be considered infected.
- Infection is characterized by erythema (reddening of the skin), edema, pus, fever, elevated neutrophil count, pain, change in color of exudate, and/or uncharacteristic odor.
- Contaminated wounds may become infected under the following circumstances:
  - Foreign bodies are present (e.g., organic material, bone fragments, suture material, glove powder, bone plates, screws).
  - Excessive necrotic tissue is left in the wound.
  - Excessive bleeding results in higher levels of ferric ion (necessary for bacterial replication).
  - Local tissue defenses are impeded (e.g., excessive hemoglobin level in burn patients or patients receiving immunosuppressive drugs).
  - The vascular supply is altered.
  - Dirt and debris are present.
- Appropriate treatment soon after injury is important to avoid infection.

Wound Categories

- Open traumatic wounds can be categorized according to the degree of contamination present (Box 6.6).
- Management of these wounds varies according to the severity of the injury and the patient's condition.
- Until contamination and infection can be eliminated, open wound management is necessary.
- Dead and dying tissues must be excised (débrided) to minimize the potential for bacterial infection and create a viable wound bed.
- Traumatic wounds, as opposed to clean surgical wounds, may contain devitalized tissue and/or foreign material and are contaminated by microorganisms.
- Chronic (long-standing) wounds offer an ideal environment for bacterial proliferation, with copious wound fluid, necrotic tissue, and deep cracks and crevices on the wound surface.
- In these cases, antibacterials with a broad spectrum of antimicrobial activity are given systemically.
- Generally, water-soluble antibacterial products tend to impede wound healing more than ointments or creams.

BOX 6.6 Categories of Wounds

Clean
- Surgical wounds
- Elective incisions
- Highly vascular tissues not predisposed to infection

Clean-Contaminated
- Minor contamination evident
- Surgical wounds with minor break in aseptic technique
- Elective surgery in tissues with normal resident bacterial flora (e.g., gastrointestinal, respiratory, genitourinary tract)
- No spillage of organ contents

Contaminated
- Moderate contamination evident
- Fresh traumatic injuries, open fractures, penetrating wounds
- Surgery with gross spillage of organ contents
- Presence of bile or infected urine
- Surgical wounds with major break in aseptic technique

Dirty
- Grossly contaminated or infected
- Contaminated traumatic wounds more than 4 hr old
- Perforated viscera, abscess, necrotic tissue, foreign material

Adapted from Sirois M: Principles and practice of veterinary technology, ed 3, St Louis, 2011, Mosby.

- Solutions tend to evaporate, contributing to drying of the wound surface.
- Ointments and creams remain in contact with the wound longer than solutions, preventing drying of the wound surface but also trapping bacteria in the wound and allowing for infection.

First Aid

- In the field and/or before transport to a treatment facility, the wound should be protected with an occlusive bandage.
- An occlusive bandage controls hemorrhage, prevents additional contamination, and provides immobilization of the extremity.
- Open fractures should be splinted.
- In open or compound fractures, exposed bone should not be forced into position below the skin.
- The wound should be protected during preparation of the surrounding area (e.g., clipping, scrubbing).
- Wound assessment includes evaluation of the wound's location, size, and depth; exudate (drainage); tissue in the wound bed; and any signs of infection.

- Wound management revolves around three considerations—cleansing, closing, and covering.
- Control of hemorrhage is usually the first step in wound management.

Clipping

- In initial wound treatment, the wound must be protected while areas around the wound are clipped and cleaned.
- Before the area around the wound is clipped and cleaned, cover the wound with a water-soluble sterile ointment (e.g., K-Y Lubricating Jelly, Johnson & Johnson, New Brunswick, NJ) or moistened sterile gauze sponges.
- This helps prevent loose hairs from contaminating the wound further.
- Before clipping and shaving areas around head or face wounds, an ophthalmic ointment should be instilled in the conjunctival sac to protect the cornea and conjunctiva.
- If the patient is covered with dirt and debris and is not in critical condition, it should be bathed before clipping.
- Hair at wound edges may be trimmed with scissors or a handheld no. 10 scalpel blade dipped in mineral oil, K-Y jelly, or water so that the hair sticks to the blade and does not enter the wound.

Scrubbing

- After the area around the wound has been clipped, place gauze sponges or gel over the wound.
- Gently scrub the surrounding intact skin, not the wound itself.
- The most commonly used surgical scrubs for skin preparation contain an antimicrobial agent plus a detergent-surfactant, such as chlorhexidine or povidone-iodine (Betadine).

Lavage

- Cleansing of the wound (lavage) and débridement begin after the surrounding area has been cleaned.
- Obvious foreign bodies and gross contamination must be removed.
- Lavaging with a sterile solution and gentle scrubbing are the primary methods used for cleaning the wound.
- Take care not to use forceful lavage or scrub too vigorously; this may force bacteria into the wound and spread contamination.
- Lavage solutions are most effective when delivered to the wound with a fluid jet with a pressure of at least 7 pounds per square inch (psi).
- Isotonic (normal) saline, lactated Ringer's solution, or plain Ringer's solution may be used for lavage.
- Dilutions of povidone-iodine in the range of 1% to 2% are commonly used to lavage wounds because of its broad antimicrobial spectrum.
- Povidone-iodine is inactivated by blood, exudate, and organic soil, reducing the period of residual action.

- The detergent form of povidone-iodine (scrub) is deleterious to wound tissues, causing irritation and potentiation of wound infection.
- Chlorhexidine diacetate solution has a broad antimicrobial spectrum and is commonly used on small animals.
- In dogs it is more effective against *S. aureus* than povidone-iodine.
- Currently, 0.05% chlorhexidine solutions are recommended for use in wound lavage.
- Hydrogen peroxide is commonly used as a foaming wound irrigant.
- In concentrations of 3% and higher, hydrogen peroxide is damaging to tissues.
- It also causes thrombosis in the microvasculature adjacent to the wound margins, impairing proliferation of blood vessels.

Débridement

- Débridement is the removal of devitalized or necrotic tissue.
- Débridement removes sources of contamination, infection, and mechanical obstructions to healing.
- Débridement is complete when the wound bed consists of only healthy tissue, commonly referred to as a clean wound.
- Acute traumatic wounds are usually débrided to facilitate surgical closure, whereas chronic wounds are usually débrided to reduce the risk of infection and facilitate second-intention healing.
- Wounds are generally débrided by mechanical means, such as with surgical instruments, irrigation, and dry-to-dry or wet-to-dry dressings.

Drainage

- Drains implanted in a wound provide an escape path for unwanted air and/or wound fluids, thus preventing or reducing seroma or hematoma formation in tissue pockets or dead space.
- Drains are indicated when wounds produce fluids and exudates for several days after initial treatment as follows:
  - For treatment of an abscess cavity
  - When foreign material and nonviable tissue are present and cannot be excised
  - When contamination is inevitable (e.g., wounds near the anal area)
  - To obliterate dead space
  - As prophylaxis against anticipated fluid or air collection after a surgical procedure
- Penrose drains are made of soft latex rubber and range from ¼ to 1 inch in diameter and 12 to 18 inches long.
- Fluid flows through the drain's lumen and around the tube and is related to the surface area of the tubing.
- Penrose drains should not be left in place for more than 3 to 5 days because most gravitational drainage has subsided by that time.

- **Closed-suction drains** provide drainage with a vacuum applied to the drain lumen, with no air vent.
- Closed-suction drains allow wounds and dressings to stay dry, prevent bacterial movement through and around the drain, afford continuous drainage, and eliminate the need for irrigation.

WOUND CLOSURE

- The patient's ability to tolerate anesthesia influences initial wound management.
- It is usually best to close fresh wounds as quickly as possible, when the risk of infection and complication is low.
- Wounds with minor contamination may be cleaned, débrided, and closed.
- Wounds that require optimal wound drainage because of gross contamination, tissue necrosis, and/or infection are managed as open wounds until they can be closed at a later time.
- Table 6.5 summarizes the types of closure used with different types of wounds.

Covering Wounds

- Nature provides natural bandages as a part of normal healing.
- A partial-thickness wound that forms a blister rarely becomes infected and heals more rapidly if the blister is not broken.
- The scab of a full-thickness wound and the eschar (necrotic layer that sloughs off) of a burn also serve as natural bandages.

Principles of Bandage Application

- In veterinary application, bandages have the following functions:
  - Protect wounds.
  - Hold clean or sterile dressings in place.
  - Absorb exudate and débride a wound.
  - Serve as a vehicle for therapeutic agents.
  - Serve as an indicator of wound secretions.
  - Pack the wound.
  - Provide support for bony anatomic structures.
  - Support and stabilize soft tissue.

TABLE 6.5 Types of Wound Closures

Type of Closure	Type of Wound Healing	Conditions of Use
Primary closure	First-intention healing	Wound closed with sutures or staples Full-thickness apposition of wound edges Tissues in direct apposition Minimal edema No local infection No serous discharge Minimal scar formation Rapid healing
Nonclosure	Second-intention healing	Wound left open because of infection, extensive trauma, tissue loss, or incorrect apposition of tissues Healing by contraction and epithelialization from inner layers to outer surface Contraction starts after ≈72 hr; stops when wound edges meet or tension exceeds strength of contraction Epithelialization starts within 24 hr after injury; requires a moist, oxygen-rich environment Delayed by healing
Delayed primary closure	Form of third-intention healing	Closure 3–5 days after cleaning and débridement, but before granulation tissue forms Wound strength and rate of healing not affected by delaying primary closure
Secondary closure	Form of third-intention healing	Closure after >3–5 days after granulation tissue has formed in the wound bed
	Third-intention healing	Safe method for repair of dirty, contaminated, or infected wounds with extensive tissue damage Allows for management of infection or necrosis before closure Surgeon débrides damaged tissue; wound closed, with accurate apposition of tissues
Adnexal reepithelialization	Second-intention healing	Partial-thickness skin loss with epithelialization primarily from compound hair follicles (so-called road burns)

Adapted from Sirois M: Principles and practice of veterinary technology, ed 3, St Louis, 2011, Mosby.

- Secure splints.
- Prevent weight bearing.
- Provide compression to control hemorrhage, dead space, and tissue edema.
- Discourage self-grooming.
- Restrict motion to eliminate stress of the wound edges.
- Provide patient comfort.
- Provide an aesthetic appearance.
- The basic principles of bandage application are as follows:
  - Properly prepare the area before application of a bandage. This may require clipping the hair, wound débridement, and/or cleaning of surrounding skin.
  - Use porous materials when possible. This allows circulation of air and escape of excessive moisture.
  - Use absorbent materials when exudates may be a problem. Change absorbent dressings when they become saturated and before saturation is evident externally.
  - Use appropriate materials of adequate width to avoid producing a tourniquet effect.
  - Apply bandage materials as smoothly as possible. Ridges and lumps lead to skin irritation and necrosis.
  - Secure protective wound pads to the skin so that they do not shift from the site.
  - Check bandages frequently to determine whether there is persistent swelling, skin discoloration, or coolness. A bandage applied too tightly can impair circulation, resulting in serious damage to soft tissues.
  - Instruct clients on basic care of bandages and signs of bandage failure. This includes the physical appearance of the bandage, as well as behavior of the patient.
  - Ideally, materials used for bandaging should have the following properties:
    - Permeable to oxygen and other gases
    - Conform to body contours
    - Acceptable appearance
    - Inert
    - Long storage life
    - Inexpensive
    - Easily sterilized
    - Unaffected by disinfecting and cleaning solutions
    - Nonflammable
    - Will not shred (so particles do not contaminate the wound)
    - Compatible with topical therapeutic agents
    - Will not adhere to the wound but can remove exudate and debris from the wound
    - Maintains a moist wound surface that is free from exudate

Bandage Components

- In most situations, bandages are generally composed of three layers, each with its own properties and function.
- The primary layer rests on the wound and may or may not be adherent.

- The secondary layer provides absorbency and padding.
- The tertiary layer is the outer layer that holds the underlying layers in place.

Primary Layer
- When débridement is the goal, an adherent layer is used for the primary bandage.
- Once the wound is in the proliferation phase and granulation tissue has formed, use a nonadherent dressing to avoid disruption of the new tissue.
- The primary layer should be sterile and comfortable, allow fluids to pass to the secondary layer, protect the wound from exogenous contamination, and be nontoxic and nonirritating to tissue.
- Adherent bandaging material, such as sterile gauze sponges with wide mesh openings and noncotton filler, can be used to provide débridement during the early stage of wound healing.
- This layer removes devitalized tissue and wound exudate when it is taken off during a bandage change.
- Adherent dressings may be wet or dry, depending on the nature of the wound.
- If loose necrotic tissue or foreign material is present on the surface of the wound, a dry-to-dry dressing may be the best type to use.
- Dry gauze with a large mesh is placed directly on the wound.
- An absorbent layer is placed over this primary layer and fluid is absorbed from the wound and allowed to dry.
- If the exudate is especially viscous or dried foreign matter must be removed, a wet-to-dry dressing may be appropriate.
- The bandage is applied wet, which dilutes the exudate for absorption.
- As the bandage dries, the foreign material adheres to the bandage and is later removed with the bandage.
- Solutions used to wet the primary layer include physiologic (0.9%) saline or a water-soluble bacteriostatic or bactericidal compound, such as 0.05% chlorhexidine diacetate solution.
- For wounds with copious exudate or transudate, a wet-to-wet dressing may be best.
- Wet dressings absorb fluid more rapidly than dry dressings.
- The primary layer is applied wet and kept wet after the secondary and tertiary layers have been applied.
- Wet-to-wet dressings cause less pain than dry dressings when removed; by using a warm solution, patient comfort is increased.
- A nonadherent primary layer is indicated during the reparative stage of wound healing, with the formation of granulation tissue and production of a more serosanguineous exudate.
- Nonadherent dressings are used to cover lacerations, skin graft donor sites, minor burns, abrasions, and surgical incisions.
- The main goal is to minimize tissue injury on removal.

Secondary Layer

- The secondary (intermediate) layer provides support and moves exudate or transudate away from the wound.
- Materials used in this layer include gauze bandaging material, cast padding, and bandaging cotton.
- The secondary layer should be thick enough to absorb moisture, pad the wound from trauma, and inhibit wound movement.

Tertiary Layer

- The tertiary (outer) layer holds the underlying bandage layers in place.
- Materials used in this layer include adhesive tapes, elastic bandages, and conforming stretch gauze.
- This layer should be applied carefully to provide support without constricting.
- If using Vet Wrap, it is best to unroll the wrap and then loosely reroll it before placing.
- Porous adhesive tape allows evaporation of fluid from the bandage.
- Waterproof adhesive tape repels water but also prevents evaporation.

OCCUPATIONAL HEALTH AND SAFETY IN VETERINARY PRACTICE

- Veterinary health care team members may be exposed to many hazards in their daily routine and in the performance of nonroutine functions.
- Hazards can include exposure to pathogenic microorganisms, chemicals, or radiation in addition to the obvious physical dangers.
- The veterinary hospital must offer training specific to the exposure in the workplace.
- In every state, an employee can be legally disciplined, including being terminated, for failure to follow safety rules for the workplace.

Safety in the Workplace

- Machinery and moving parts: Equipment such as fans, chutes, and dryers have moving parts that can cause severe injury.
  - Long hair should be tied back to prevent it from getting caught in fans or other moving objects.
  - Avoid wearing excessive jewelry, very loose-fitting clothing, or open-toed shoes.
- Slips and falls: You can reduce the chance of personal injury from slips and falls by wearing slip-proof shoes and using nonslip mats or strips in wet areas.
- Lifting: When lifting patients, supplies, or equipment, remember to keep your back straight and lift with your legs.
  - Recruit help when lifting patients weighing more than 40 pounds.
- Storing supplies: Store heavy supplies or equipment on the lower shelves to prevent unnecessary strains.
  - Store chemicals on shelves at or below eye level.

- Never climb on cabinets, shelves, chairs, buckets, or comparable items to reach high locations; use an appropriate ladder or stepstool.
- Toxic substances: Eat or drink only in areas free of toxic and biologically harmful substances as outlined in the employee handbook.
  - Store food, drinks, condiments, and snacks in a refrigerator free from biologic or chemical hazards; vaccines, drugs, and laboratory samples are all potential contamination sources.
  - It is best to have a minimum of two refrigerators, one for biologic substances and one for employees' food.
- Heating devices: Learn the rules for safe operation of any heating devices.
  - Burns, especially from steam, are painful and serious and can almost always be prevented.
  - When opening an autoclave, first release the pressure with the vent device and let the steam rise completely before opening the door fully.
  - Always assume that cautery devices and branding irons are hot, and use the insulated handle whenever you handle them.
- Eye safety: Familiarize yourself with the locations and use of eye wash stations.
  - Always use safety glasses and other personal protective equipment (PPE) when required.
  - If you splash a chemical in your eyes, call for help.
  - With a coworker's assistance, go to the eye wash station and flush both eyes, even if only one eye is affected.
  - Contact lenses should not be worn when working with chemicals because the contact lens will impair the ability of the eye wash to remove any splashed chemicals.

Hazards of Animal Handling

- Stay alert when working with and around animals.
- Sudden noises, movements, or even light can cause an animal to react.

Protective Gear

- Your employer is obligated to provide you with PPE.
- Some hazards that you may be exposed to when working in a veterinary hospital and the required PPE are listed in Table 6.6.
- Make use of any available capture or restraint equipment, such as cages, snares, cat bags, and poles, when appropriate.
- Wear examination gloves and a surgical mask when handling a stray, wild, or unvaccinated animal.
- Maintain an appropriate distance from the work area or animal; for example, do not place your face close to the mouth of the animal.
- Wear protective leather gloves when handling a fractious animal.
- Long-term exposure to excess noise levels can contribute to hearing loss.

TABLE 6.6 Hazards and Personal Protective Equipment

Potential Hazards	Protective Equipment
Radiation exposure while taking x-rays	Lead aprons, gloves, thyroid collars
Bites and scratches	Leashes, muzzles, bags, towels
Bacterial exposure	Safety glasses, eye shields
Exposure to hazardous chemical fumes	Masks
Exposure to hazardous, caustic solutions	Examination gloves, rubber gloves
Loud noises	Ear plugs
Burns	Oven mitts and hot pads

- Short-time exposure, such as going into the kennel to retrieve a patient, poses no serious damage to your hearing.
- When working in noisy areas for extended periods (e.g., when cleaning cages), always wear personal hearing protectors rated to filter the noise by at least 20 dB. (The package label indicates the rating.)

Hazards of Bathing and Dipping

Ventilation
- Always use the ventilation fan when bathing or dipping patients.
- Be sure to wear appropriate protective gear that includes safety glasses, gloves, and apron.

Chemical Storage
- Chemicals used for bathing and dipping animals can be harmful and must be stored properly. Bottles of dips, shampoos, and parasiticides should be stored in a cabinet at or below eye level. The bottle should be properly labeled, including contents and any appropriate hazard warning.

Zoonotic Hazards
- When handling specimens such as fecal samples, laboratory samples, or wound exudates, wear protective gloves and always wash your hands immediately after completing the procedure. Contamination with these types of materials can usually be cleaned up with paper towels soaked in an appropriate disinfecting solution.
- Disposable gloves should be worn and then discarded with the cleaned-up materials.
- When treating patients with diseases that are infectious to people or other animals (zoonotic hazards), wear a protective apron, examination gloves, face mask, and eye

protection. Thoroughly wash your hands with a disinfecting agent, such as chlorhexidine or povidone-iodine scrub, at the completion of treatment. Any clothing that has been contaminated should be changed immediately.

Radiation Hazards
- Infrequent exposure to small amounts of radiation, such as routine thoracic or dental x-rays, poses little threat to your overall health.
  - Long-term exposure to small doses of radiation has been linked to genetic, cutaneous, glandular, and other disorders.
  - Exposure to large doses of radiation can cause skin changes, cell damage, and gastrointestinal and bone marrow disorders that can be fatal.

Radiation Safety
- When using radiographic equipment, never place any part of your body in the primary beam, even a hand wearing a lead-lined glove.
- Always wear the appropriate protective equipment, such as lead-lined aprons, thyroid collar, and lead gloves.
- Lead-impregnated glasses are also recommended.
- Always use the collimator to restrict the primary beam to an area smaller than the size of the cassette, creating a clear border around all four sides of the film.
- Digital radiographs add safety protection in that fewer x-rays are taken because the film can be digitally enhanced or altered.
- Proper exposure techniques are still necessary to provide diagnostic-quality images and reduce exposure to radiation.
- Portable x-ray machines, such as those used for dental radiography and in mobile practices, can be particularly dangerous because the primary beam of these machines can be aimed in any direction.
- When using a portable machine, always be sure that there is no human body part in the path of the primary beam, even at a distance.
- Never hold a cassette during the radiograph procedure, whether wearing lead-lined gloves or not; always use a cassette-holding device.
- Everyone involved with radiography must wear a dosimetry badge to measure any radiation that you may receive during the procedure.

Anesthetic Hazards
- Long-term exposure to waste anesthetic gases has been linked to congenital abnormalities in children, spontaneous abortions, and liver and kidney damage.
- The Occupational Safety and Health Administration (OSHA) has set the safe exposure limit for halogenated anesthetic agents (e.g., isoflurane) at 2 parts per million (ppm).
- Always check for leaks in the hoses and anesthetic machine before use.

- Use hoses and rebreathing bags that are the correct size and consider inflating the endotracheal tube cuff before connecting the patient to the machine.
- Have anesthetic machines professionally serviced on an annual basis.
- A well-designed scavenging system captures excess gases directly at the source and transports them to a safe exhaust port, usually outside the building.
- When refilling the anesthetic machine vaporizer, move the machine to a well-ventilated area and use a pouring funnel; avoid overfilling the vaporizer or spilling the liquid anesthetic.

Hazards of Compressed Gases

- Store cylinders of compressed gas (e.g., oxygen) in a dry, cool place, away from potential heat sources such as furnaces, water heaters, and direct sunlight.
- Always secure the tanks in an upright position by means of a chain or strap, including small tanks.

Hazards of Sharp Objects

- The most serious hazard of sharp objects (termed sharps) in a veterinary environment is from the physical trauma and possible bacterial infection caused by a puncture or laceration.
- To prevent accidents from punctures or lacerations, always keep needles, scalpel blades, and other sharps capped or sheathed until ready for use.
- Place the sharp in a red sharps container immediately after use; do not attempt to recap the needle unless the physical danger from sticks or lacerations cannot be avoided by any other means.

Chemical Hazards

- Every chemical, even common ones such as cleaning supplies, can cause harm.
- Some chemicals can contribute to health problems, whereas others may be flammable and pose a fire threat.
- The most common chemicals used in the veterinary workplace are insecticides, medications, and cleaning agents.
- Veterinary hospitals must follow the guidelines of OSHA's Right to Know Law.
- This law requires that you be informed about all chemicals to which you may be exposed while doing your job.
- The Right to Know Law also requires you to wear all safety equipment that is prescribed by the manufacturer when handling a chemical; it is not optional; you must wear what is prescribed.
- The safety equipment must be provided by the employer at no cost to you.

Hazardous Materials Plan

- A strategic component of the Right to Know Law is the hazardous materials plan.
- This plan describes the details of the practice's Safety Data Sheet (SDS) filing system and the secondary container labeling system.

- There must be an up-to-date list of chemicals that are known to be on the hospital premises.

Container Labels

- When you receive a supply of chemicals from the distributor, every bottle is identified with a label containing directions and appropriate warnings.
- Sometimes it is necessary to dilute a chemical or pour it into smaller bottles for use.
- These smaller bottles are known as secondary containers.
- All secondary containers must have a label that indicates the contents and appropriate safety warnings.

Electrical Hazards

- Only persons trained to perform maintenance duties should repair electrical outlets, switches, fixtures, or breakers.
- Extension cords should be used only for temporary supply applications and should always be of the three-conductor, grounded type.
- Never run extension cords through windows or doors that could close and damage the wires.
- Never run extension cords across aisles or floors, which create a tripping hazard.

Fire and Evacuation

- Materials such as gasoline, paint thinner, and ether should never be stored inside the hospital, except in an approved storage cabinet designed for flammables.
- Some components of specialty dental and large animal acrylic repair kits are also flammable.
  - Very small amounts of these components can usually be safely stored in an area with good ventilation, free from flames or sparks.
- Flammable items, particularly newspapers, boxes, and cleaning chemicals, must always be stored at least 3 feet away from any ignition source, such as a water heater, furnace, or stove.
- Know the location of all fire extinguishers on the premises and how to use them.
- The National Fire Protection Association (NFPA) recommends that you never attempt to fight a fire if any of the following conditions apply:
  - The fire is spreading beyond the immediate area where it started or has already become a large fire.
  - The fire could block your escape route.
  - You are unsure of the proper operation of the extinguisher.
  - You doubt that the extinguisher is designed for the type of fire at hand or is large enough to suppress the fire.
- Make sure that emergency exits are always unlocked and free from obstructions.

Personal Safety

- Workers in emergency or 24-hour practices should use the barriers that are usually available. Use the buzzer to control access through the front door and one-way locks on the remaining doors.

- In any situation in which someone demands money or drugs while threatening your personal safety, do not attempt to withhold whatever they demand.
- Cooperate with the demands, but do not go with the person, even to the parking lot. Attempt to contact the police if this can be done safely without the intruder's knowledge; otherwise, do it immediately after the intruder has left the premises.

RECOMMENDED READINGS

AVMA: *Zoonosis update*, Schaumberg, IL, 2010, American Veterinary Medical Association.

Birchard SJ, Sherding RG: *Saunders manual of small animal practice*, ed 3, St Louis, 2006, Saunders.

Bonagura JD: *Kirk's current veterinary therapy XV: Small animal practice*, St Louis, 2013, Saunders.

Case, LP, Daristotle, L, Hayek, MG, Raasch, MF: *Canine and feline nutrition*, ed 3, St Louis, 2011, Mosby.

Colville JL, Berryhill DL: *Handbook of zoonoses*, St Louis, 2007, Mosby.

Morris ML, Hand, MS, Thatcher, CD et al.: *Small animal clinical nutrition*, ed 5, Topeka, 2010, Mark Morris.

Seibert Jr. PJ: *The complete veterinary practice regulatory compliance manual*, ed 6, Calhoun, 2014, SafetyVet.

Summers A: *Common diseases of companion animals*, ed 3, St Louis, 2014, Mosby.

Tizard IR: *Veterinary immunology: An introduction*, ed 8, St Louis, 2008, Saunders.

Zachary JF, McGavin MD: *Pathologic basis of veterinary disease*, ed 5, St Louis, 2012, Mosby.

Surgical Preparation and Assisting

KEY TERMS

Analgesia	General anesthesia	Ovariohysterectomy	Sedation
Anamnesis	Hypercarbia	Pain	Sterilization indicators
Anesthesia	Laparotomy	Peritonitis	Suture
Aseptic technique	Laryngoscope	Pressure manometer	Tidal volume
Autoclave	Mayo stand	Pulse deficit	Vaporizer
Breathing circuit	Narcosis	Pulse oximeter	Vasoconstriction
Electrocautery	Nociception	Pulse quality	Ventilation
Esophageal stethoscope	Non–rebreathing system	Rebreathing system	
Eviscerate	Nosocomial infection	Reservoir bag	
Flow meter	Orchiectomy	Scavenging system	

LEARNING OBJECTIVES

After reviewing this chapter, the reader will be able to:

1. Describe and explain surgical terminology.
2. Discuss principles of aseptic technique.
3. Give examples of methods used to disinfect or sterilize surgical instruments and supplies.
4. Describe procedures for preparing the surgical site and surgical team.
5. Identify surgical instruments and explain their uses and maintenance.
6. Compare and contrast types of suture needles and suture materials.
7. Define the role of veterinary staff members in anesthesia and perioperative pain management.
8. Describe the equipment used for anesthetizing animals.
9. Prepare and maintain anesthetic machines and the associated equipment.
10. List and describe the steps involved in anesthetizing animals for induction.
11. Explain the procedures used in medicating and monitoring animals before, during, and after anesthesia.
12. Prepare a small animal patient, anesthetic equipment, anesthetic agents, and accessories for general anesthesia.

INTRODUCTION

- The role of the veterinary assistant in surgical procedures is diverse, and the specific duties performed may vary in different locations depending on the laws in each location.
- During the presurgical period, the veterinary assistant may be responsible for preparation of the patient, surgical instruments and equipment, and surgical environment.
- During surgery, the veterinary assistant may aid the veterinary technician with monitoring the anesthetized patient.
- The veterinary assistant is often responsible for obtaining and opening surgical packs, suture materials, and other supplies for the surgeon.
- In the postsurgical period, the veterinary assistant is frequently responsible for postoperative patient care and monitoring, instructing clients on patient care during the recovery period, and removing sutures.

SURGERY SUITE

- The American Animal Hospital Association (AAHA) recommends three distinct and separate areas for a surgical facility—the preparation area, scrub area, and surgery room.
- Although AAHA certification is not a legal requirement for veterinary facilities, a surgical facility should create the best environment for the patient.
- Some state licensing boards have specific requirements regarding surgical facilities that a veterinary hospital must meet to pass inspection and to receive authorization to offer surgery.

Preparation Area

- Ideally, the preparation area should be adjacent to the surgery room.
- The prep room can be used for patient preparation and the storage of surgical supplies.
- The surgeon and veterinary technician can use the preparation area to scrub and gown for surgery if a separate scrub area is not available.
- The prep area is used for clipping the patient.

- Procedures classified as dirty should be done in the prep area.
  - Procedures such as abscessed wound care, débridement of old wounds, and treatment of impacted anal sacs are often defined as dirty.

Scrub Area

- The scrub area may be a small area with the scrub sink, autoclave, and room to gown and glove.
- This is a transitional area in which the veterinarian and staff can prepare to move into the surgery room.

Surgery Room

- Ideally, the surgery room is a separate room that should be used only for surgery.
- The AAHA recommends that the surgery room be easily cleanable and be closed off as needed.
- Closing the door minimizes traffic, maximizes cleanliness, and helps ensure that the surgery room is used only for aseptic procedures.
- The room should be a dedicated room reserved for sterile surgical procedures.
- The surgery room should be large enough that personnel can easily move around the surgery table without contaminating the surgical field or the surgeon.
- If present, cabinets should be off the floor and constructed of nonporous material.
- The cabinets that hold sterile supplies should have doors that can be closed to protect the packs and other supplies from dust, debris, and other contaminants.
- The surgery room should also be free of clutter and items that may collect dust or harbor bacteria.
- If possible, the air pressure should be greater in the surgery room to reduce the influx of bacteria from the rest of the veterinary facility.

PRINCIPLES OF ASEPSIS

- Aseptic technique is the term used to describe all the precautions taken to prevent contamination, and ultimately infection, of a surgical wound.

Contamination and Infection

- Contamination of an object or a wound implies the presence of microorganisms within or on it.
- Contamination of a wound can, but does not necessarily, lead to infection.
- With infection, microorganisms in the body or a wound multiply and cause harmful effects. Fungal, protozoal, viral, and bacterial organisms can all cause contamination of the surgical area and harmful effects to the patient.
- Four main factors determine whether infection occurs:
    1. Number of microorganisms: There must be a sufficient number of microorganisms to overcome the defenses of the animal.
    2. Virulence of the microorganisms: This is their ability to cause disease.
    3. Susceptibility of the animal: Some individuals have a greater natural resistance to infection than others.
    4. Route of exposure to the microorganisms: Some routes of exposure are more likely to result in infection than others.
- Improper application of methods of sanitation, sterilization, and disinfection can lead to microbial resistance and increase the risk of nosocomial (hospital-acquired) infection.

Rules of Aseptic Technique

- During surgery, aseptic technique protects the exposed tissues of the patient from four main sources of potential contamination: the operative personnel, surgical instruments and equipment, the patient itself, and the surgical environment.
- Proper operating room conduct and adherence to a few general rules will help minimize the possibility of contamination.
    - Be aware of which items are sterile and which are nonsterile.
    - Group sterile items together in the operating room.
    - Keep sterile items separate from nonsterile items.
    - Restrict body movements to reduce air currents.
    - Only sterile items should touch patient tissues.
    - When the sterility of an item is in question, always consider it contaminated.

Sterilization and Disinfection

- Sterilization refers to the destruction of all microorganisms (e.g., bacteria, viruses, spores) on a surface or object.
    - It usually refers to objects that come into contact with sterile tissue or enter the vascular system (e.g., instruments, drapes, catheters, needles).
- Disinfection is the destruction of most pathogenic microorganisms on inanimate (nonliving) objects; antisepsis is the destruction of most pathogenic microorganisms on animate (living) objects.
- Antiseptics are used to kill microorganisms during patient skin preparation and surgical scrubbing; however, the skin cannot be sterilized.
- Most disinfectants are microbicidal—that is, they kill microbes. Some disinfectants are bacteriostatic; they inhibit the growth of microbes.
- Common antimicrobial agents are listed in Table 7.1.
- Disinfectants can be classified according to their spectrum of activity as the following:
    - Bactericidal (kills bacteria)
    - Bacteriostatic (inhibits growth of bacteria)
    - Sporicidal (kills spores)
    - Virucidal (kills viruses)
    - Fungicidal (kills fungi)

Mode of Action

- Different physical and chemical methods destroy or inhibit microorganisms in several ways. Some act by damaging microbial cell walls or membranes.

TABLE 7.1 Common Antimicrobial Chemical Agents

Agents	Major Mode of Action	Applications
Soaps	Disrupt cell membranes and increase permeability	Cleansing, mechanical removal of microorganisms
Detergents	Disrupt cell membranes by combining with lipids and proteins; leak N and P compounds out of cells	Cleansing, bactericidal action
Quaternary ammonium compounds	Cause changes in cell permeability; neutralize phospholipids	Disinfection of surfaces
Biguanide compounds (e.g., chlorhexidine)	Alter cell wall permeability, protein precipitation; rapid action, broad spectrum	Routine skin preparation
Povidone-iodophor compounds	Damage cell wall, form reactive ions and protein complexes; rapid action	Routine skin preparation

Continued

TABLE 7.1 Common Antimicrobial Chemical Agents—cont'd

Agents	Major Mode of Action	Applications
Phenol, cresols, Lysol, hexylresorcinol	Bactericidal; denaturation and precipitation of proteins	Disinfection of laboratory equipment, instruments, bench tops, garbage pails, toilets
Bisphenols (e.g., hexachlorophene)	Bacteriostatic	Deodorants in soaps, inhibition of gram-positive bacteria; require repeated use
Cl_2 and sodium hypochlorite (bleach)	Bactericidal, oxidation of -SH and $-NH_2$ groups	Purification of water, kennel sanitation
Iodine	Bactericidal; oxidation of indole nucleus of enzymes or coenzymes	Skin disinfection, especially as tincture
H_2O_2 (hydrogen peroxide)	Bacteriostatic; mildly bactericidal	Antisepsis of cuts, minor wounds
$HgCl_2$ (zinc)	Highly bacteriostatic; precipitation of proteins	Antisepsis of cuts, minor wounds
$AgNO_3$ (silver nitrate)	Chemical cauterizing agent	Stops minor bleeding

Adapted from Sirois M: Principles and practice of veterinary technology, ed 3, St Louis, 2011, Mosby.

- Others act by interfering with microbial cell enzyme activity or metabolism or by destroying microbial cell contents by oxidation, hydrolysis, reduction, coagulation, protein denaturation, or the formation of salt.
- The effectiveness of all microbial control methods depends on the following factors:
  - Time: Most methods have minimum effective exposure times.
  - Temperature: Most methods are more effective as the temperature increases.
  - Concentration and preparation: Chemical methods require appropriate concentrations of agent; disinfectants may be adversely affected by mixing with other chemicals.
  - Organisms: These are the type, number, and stage of growth of target organisms.
  - Surface: The physical and chemical properties of the surface to be treated may interfere with the method's activity; some surfaces are damaged by certain methods.
  - Organic debris or other soils: If present, these will dilute, render ineffective, or interfere with many control methods.
  - Method of application: Items may be sprayed, swabbed, or immersed in disinfectants; cotton and some synthetic materials used to apply or store chemicals may reduce their activity.
- Methods used for the control of microorganisms consist of chemical and physical methods. Physical methods include dry heat, moist heat, radiation, filtration, and ultrasonic vibration.
- Of these methods, only moist heat, in the form of steam under pressure, is routinely used for sterilization in the veterinary clinic.
- Chemical control methods include the application of soaps, detergents, disinfectants, and gases.

Quality Control for Sterilization and Disinfection

- The effectiveness of any method of microbial control must be monitored regularly. Verification of the effectiveness of microbial control should be performed at least monthly.
- Failure to achieve sterility may be caused by improper cleaning (if an item cannot be disassembled and all surfaces cleaned, it cannot be sterilized), mechanical failure of the sterilizing system, improper use of sterilizing equipment, improper wrapping, poor loading technique, and/or failure to understand the underlying concepts of sterilization processes.

Indicators

- Chemical indicators, or sterilization indicators, are generally paper strips or tape impregnated with a material that changes color when a certain temperature or chemical exposure is achieved (Fig. 7.1).
- Most also indicate that a specific duration of exposure has been achieved, which is critical to the sterilization process.
- Chemical indicators can be used with autoclaves and ethylene oxide systems and must be placed deep inside packs before sterilization.
- Indicator tape is often used to secure surgical packs and mark smaller packages of sterilized items.
- The tape incorporates an indicator that changes color when the sterilization temperature or duration of chemical exposure has been reached.
- The color change in the tape does not allow for any evaluation of duration of exposure to sterilization conditions.

Biologic Testing

- Because the purpose of the sterilization procedures is to eliminate the hardiest microorganisms, the presence or absence of bacterial spores can help verify proper sterilization conditions.

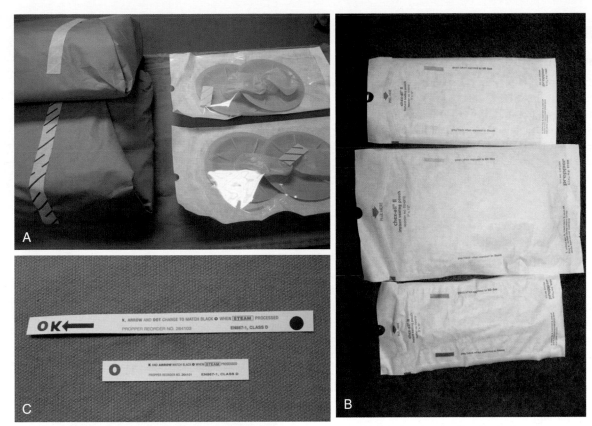

FIGURE 7.1 (A) Surgical packs *(left)* and sterilization pouches *(right)* showing sterilization indicator tape before *(top)* and after *(bottom)* sterilization. The pack was autoclaved and the pouch was gas-sterilized. (B) Sterilization pouches showing paper side indicators before processing *(top)*, after ethylene oxide (EO) gas sterilization *(middle)*, and after autoclave sterilization *(bottom)*. (C) Sterilization indicators typically packed inside surgical instrument packs after *(top)* and before *(bottom)* autoclave sterilization.

- To perform a biologic test of sterility conditions, commercially available bacterial spores are exposed in an autoclave or to ethylene oxide and then cultured.
  - Bacterial spores should be killed by sterilization so that no bacterial colonies should be present after culturing.
- Another test used to verify sterility is the surface sampling technique.
  - The procedure involves swabbing the test surface (i.e., surgical equipment) with a sterile swab.
  - The swab is then transferred to a suitable media plate for growth.
  - This method is recommended for ensuring proper disinfection of surgical suites in veterinary clinics.

Steam Sterilization

- Pressurized steam is the most efficient and common method of sterilization used in veterinary clinics.
- Steam destroys microbes via cellular protein denaturation.
- If steam is contained in a closed compartment under increased pressure, the temperature increases as long as the volume of the compartment remains the same.

- If items are exposed long enough to steam at a specified temperature and pressure, they become sterile.
- The unit used to create this environment of high-temperature, pressurized steam is called an **autoclave**.
- Gravity displacement autoclaves use water that is heated in a chamber; the steam generated gradually displaces the air contained within the chamber.
- A prevacuum autoclave is a much larger and more costly machine that is equipped with a boiler to generate steam and a vacuum system.
  - Air is forced out of the loaded chamber by means of the vacuum pump.
  - Steam at a temperature of 250°F (121°C) or higher is introduced into the chamber; the steam immediately fills the chamber to eliminate the vacuum.
- Autoclaves are safe for most surgical instruments and equipment, drapes and gowns, suture materials, sponges, and some plastics and rubber items.
- Complete sterilization of most items is achieved after 9 to 15 minutes of exposure to a temperature of 250°F (121°C).

SURGICAL INSTRUMENTS

Scalpels and Blades

- Scalpels are the primary cutting instrument used to incise tissue.
- Reusable scalpel handles with detachable blades are most commonly used in veterinary medicine; disposable handles and blades are also available.
- Blades are available in various sizes and shapes, depending on the task for which they are used.

Laser Scalpel

- Laser is an acronym for *l*ight *a*mplification by the *s*timulated *e*mission of *r*adiation.
- The most commonly used surgical laser is a carbon dioxide laser, which produces an invisible beam of light that vaporizes the water normally found in the skin and other soft tissue.
- Lasers have the unique ability both to coagulate and cut tissue.
- Although there are a variety of lasers, the most common types used in veterinary practice are carbon dioxide (CO_2) and diode.
- Because the laser seals nerve endings and small blood vessels as it cuts, it results in less bleeding and less pain for the patient.
- Laser surgery is commonly used in soft tissue surgical procedures, such as spaying, neutering, amputations, oral and dental procedures, dermatology, and avian and exotic procedures.

Electroscalpel

- The electroscalpel functions by passing an electrical current through the unit to the patient's tissues. This causes microcoagulation of tissue proteins as the unit cuts the tissue.

Scissors

- Scissors are available in a variety of shapes, sizes, and weights and are generally classified according to the type of points (blunt-blunt, sharp-sharp, sharp-blunt), blade shape (straight, curved), or cutting edge (plain, serrated; Fig. 7.2).
- Curved scissors offer greater maneuverability and visibility, whereas straight scissors provide the greatest mechanical advantage for cutting tough or thick tissue.
- Metzenbaum or Mayo scissors are most commonly used in surgery.
  - Metzenbaum scissors are more delicate and should be reserved for fine, thin tissue.
  - Mayo scissors are used for cutting heavy tissue, such as fascia.
- Suture scissors used in the operating room are different from suture removal scissors.
  - The latter have a concavity at the top of one blade that prevents the suture from being lifted excessively during removal.

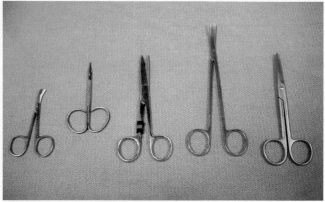

FIGURE 7.2 *Left to right,* Suture removal, tenotomy, sharp-sharp suture, Metzenbaum, and Mayo scissors.

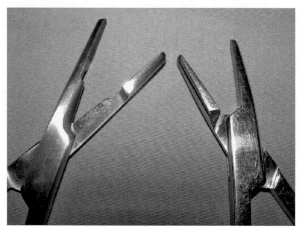

FIGURE 7.3 Needle holders: *Left,* Olsen-Hegar, *right,* Mayo-Hegar. (From Tighe MM, Brown M: *Mosby's comprehensive review for veterinary technicians*, ed 5, St Louis, 2020, Elsevier.)

- Delicate scissors, such as tenotomy scissors or iris scissors, are often used in ophthalmic procedures and other surgeries in which fine, precise cuts are necessary.
- Bandage scissors have a blunt tip that when introduced under the bandage edge, reduce the risk of cutting the underlying skin.

Needle Holders

- Needle holders are used to grasp and manipulate curved needles (Fig. 7.3).
- Mayo-Hegar and Olsen-Hegar needle holders have a ratchet lock just distal to the thumb. Castroviejo needle holders have a spring and latch mechanism for locking.
- Mathieu needle holders have a ratchet lock at the proximal end of the handles of the holder, permitting locking and unlocking simply by a progressive squeezing together of the needle holder handles.

Forceps

Tissue Forceps

- Tissue forceps are used to clamp and hold tissue and blood vessels.

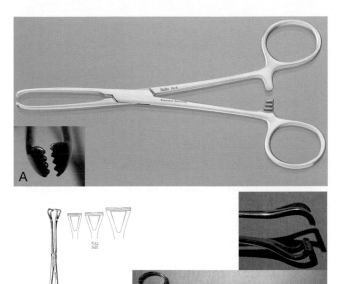

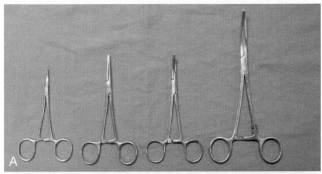

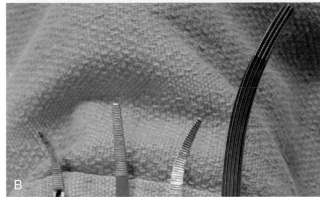

FIGURE 7.4 Tissue forceps: (A) Babcock. (B) Allis. (From Sonsthagen TF: *Veterinary instruments and equipment: A pocket guide*, ed 3, St Louis, 2014, Elsevier.)

FIGURE 7.5 (A) Hemostatic forceps *(left to right):* mosquito, Kelly, Crile, and Rochester-Carmalt. (B) Hemostatic forceps, close-up view *(left to right):* mosquito, Kelly, Crile, and Rochester-Carmalt. (From Sirois M: *Elsevier's veterinary assistant textbook*, ed 2, St Louis, 2017, Mosby.)

- Thumb forceps are tweezer-like, nonlocking tissue forceps used to grasp tissue.
  - They are available in a variety of shapes and sizes; tips (grasping ends) may be pointed, flattened, rounded, smooth, or serrated or have small or large teeth.
- The most commonly used tissue forceps, Brown-Adson, have small serrations on the tips that cause minimal trauma but hold tissue securely.
- Allis tissue forceps and Babcock forceps (Fig. 7.4) are also used for tissue grasping and retraction.

Hemostatic Forceps
- Hemostatic forceps, commonly called hemostats, are crushing instruments used to clamp blood vessels.
  - They are available with straight or curved tips and vary in size from smaller (3-inch) mosquito hemostats with transverse jaw serrations to larger (9-inch) angiotribes.
- Serrations on the jaws of larger hemostatic forceps may be transverse, longitudinal, or diagonal or a combination of these.
- Serrations usually extend from the tips of the jaws to the box locks, but in Kelly forceps, transverse (horizontal) serrations extend over only the distal portion of the jaws.
- Similarly sized Crile forceps have transverse serrations that extend over the entire jaw length (Fig. 7.5).
- Kelly and Crile forceps are used on larger vessels.
- Rochester-Carmalt forceps are larger crushing forceps often used to control large tissue bundles (e.g., during ovariohysterectomy).
  - They have longitudinal grooves with cross grooves at the tip ends to prevent tissue slippage.

Hemostatic Techniques and Materials
- Hemostasis, or the arrest of bleeding, allows visualization of the surgical site and prevents life-threatening hemorrhage.
- Low-pressure hemorrhage from small vessels is controlled by applying pressure to the bleeding points with a gauze sponge.
- Large vessels must be ligated (tied off) by the veterinarian.
- Hemostatic agents used to control hemorrhage during surgery include bone wax and hemostatic materials made of gelatin or cellulose (e.g., Surgicel, Gelfoam).
- The veterinarian may use metal clips or staples for vessel ligation.
- Electrocoagulation can be used to achieve hemostasis in vessels smaller than 2 mm in diameter.
  - The term **electrocautery** is often erroneously used in place of electrocoagulation.
  - With electrocautery, the needle tip or scalpel is heated before it is applied to the tissue; with electrocoagulation, heat is generated in the tissue as a high-frequency current is passed through it. Excessive use of electrocautery or electrocoagulation retards healing.

Retractors
- Retractors are used to retract tissue and improve exposure.
- The ends of handheld retractors may be hooked, curved, spatula-shaped, or toothed. Some handheld retractors may be bent (i.e., malleable) to conform to the structure being retracted or area of the body in which retraction is being performed.

- Senn (rake) retractors are double-ended retractors; one end has three finger-like, curved prongs; the other end is a flat, curved blade.
- Self-retaining retractors maintain tension on tissues and are held open with a box lock (e.g., Gelpi, Weitlaner) or other mechanism (e.g., set screw as with Balfour retractors and Finochietto retractors).

Miscellaneous Instruments

- Instruments are available to suction fluid, clamp drapes or tissues, cut and remove bone pieces (rongeurs), hold bones during fracture repair, scrape surfaces of dense tissue (curettes), remove periosteum (periosteal elevators), cut or shape bone and cartilage (osteotomes and chisels), and bore holes in bone (trephines).

SUTURES AND OTHER MATERIALS USED IN WOUND CLOSURE

Sutures

Suture Characteristics

- The word suture refers to any strand of material used to approximate tissues or ligate blood vessels.
- The ideal suture material is easy to handle; reacts minimally in tissue; inhibits bacterial growth; holds securely when knotted; resists shrinking in tissues; is noncapillary, nonallergenic, noncarcinogenic, and nonferromagnetic; and is absorbed with minimal reaction after the tissue has healed.
  - Such an ideal suture material does not exist; therefore surgeons must choose one that most closely approximates the ideal for a given procedure and/or tissue to be sutured.
- Monofilament sutures are made of a single strand of material.
  - They create less tissue drag than multifilament suture material and do not have interstitial spaces that may harbor bacteria.
  - Care should be used in handling monofilament sutures because nicking or damaging them with forceps or needle holders weakens them and predisposes to breakage.
- Multifilament sutures consist of several strands that are twisted or braided together.
  - Multifilament sutures are generally more pliable and flexible than monofilament sutures.
  - They may be coated to decrease tissue drag and enhance handling characteristics.
- The most commonly used standard for suture size is the USP (U.S. Pharmacopeia) standard, which denotes suture diameters from fine to coarse according to a numeric scale; size 10-0 material has the smallest diameter (finest), and size 7 has the largest diameter (most coarse).
- USP uses different size notations for various suture materials (Table 7.2).
- The smaller the suture diameter, the lower its tensile strength.

TABLE 7.2 Systems Used to Indicate Suture Sizes

Diameter (mm)	Metric Gauge	Synthetic Suture Materials (USP)	Surgical Gut (USP)	Wire Gauge (Brown and Sharpe)
0.02	0.2	10-0		
0.03	0.3	9-0		
0.04	0.4	8-0		
0.05	0.5	7-0	8-0	41
0.07	0.7	6-0	7-0	38–40
0.1	1	5-0	6-0	35
0.15	1.5	4-0	5-0	32–34
0.2	2	3-0	4-0	30
0.3	3	2-0	3-0	28
0.35	3.5	0	2-0	26
0.4	4	1	0	25
0.5	5	2	1	24
0.6	6	3,4	2	22
0.7	7	5	3	20
0.8	8	6	4	19
0.9	0	7		18

Adapted from Sirois M: Principles and practice of veterinary technology, ed 3, St Louis, 2011, Mosby.

- Stainless steel wire is usually sized according to the metric or USP scale or by the Brown and Sharpe wire gauge.

Absorbable Suture Materials

- Absorbable suture materials lose most of their tensile strength within 60 days after placement in tissue and eventually are absorbed from the site and replaced by healthy tissue during the healing process.
- Absorbable sutures are used when sutures must be buried within body cavities.
  Surgical Gut
- Surgical gut is commonly called catgut.
- Surgical gut is made from the submucosa of sheep intestine or the serosa of bovine intestine and is composed of approximately 90% collagen.
- Plain surgical gut is broken down by phagocytosis and elicits a marked inflammatory reaction compared with other materials.
- Tanning, by exposure to chrome or aldehyde, slows absorption.
  - Surgical gut so treated is called chromic surgical gut.
- Surgical gut is rapidly absorbed from infected sites or where it is exposed to digestive enzymes.

Synthetic Absorbable Materials

- Synthetic absorbable materials (e.g., polyglycolic acid, polyglactin 910, polydioxanone, polyglyconate) are generally broken down by hydrolysis.
- There is minimal tissue reaction to synthetic absorbable suture materials.
- The rate of tensile strength loss and rate of absorption are fairly constant in different tissues.

Nonabsorbable Suture Materials

- There are four basic groups of nonabsorbable suture materials: organic sutures, braided synthetic sutures, monofilament synthetic sutures, and metallic sutures.

Organic Nonabsorbable Materials

- Silk is the most common organic nonabsorbable suture material and is used as a braided multifilament suture that is uncoated or coated.
- Silk has excellent handling characteristics and is often used in cardiovascular procedures; however, it does not maintain significant tensile strength after 6 months in tissues and is therefore contraindicated for use with vascular grafts.
  - It also should be avoided in contaminated sites because it increases the likelihood of wound infection.
- Cotton suture has less tissue reaction than silk but it supports bacterial growth and is not generally used for skin closure.

Synthetic Nonabsorbable Materials

- Synthetic nonabsorbable suture materials are available as braided multifilament (e.g., polyester, coated caprolactam) or monofilament (e.g., polypropylene, polyamide, polyolefins, polybutester) threads.
  - They are typically strong and induce minimal tissue reaction.
- Nonabsorbable suture materials consisting of an inner core and outer sheath (e.g., Supramid) should not be buried in tissues because the outer sheath tends to degenerate, allowing bacteria to migrate to the inner core.

Metallic Sutures

- Stainless steel is the most commonly used metallic suture and is available as monofilament wire or twisted multifilament wire.
- The tissue reaction to stainless steel is generally minimal; however, the knot ends evoke an inflammatory reaction.

Suture Needles

- Suture needles are available in a wide variety of shapes and sizes.
- The type of suture needle used depends on the characteristics of the tissue to be sutured (e.g., penetrability, density, elasticity, thickness), wound topography (e.g., deep, narrow), and characteristics of the needle (e.g., type of eye, length, diameter).
- Most surgical needles are made from stainless steel because it is strong and corrosion-free and does not harbor bacteria.

- The three basic components of a suture needle are the attachment end (swaged or eyed), body, and point (Fig. 7.6A).
- With swaged needles, the needle and suture are joined in a continuous unit, minimizing tissue trauma and increasing ease of use.
- Suture material must be threaded onto eyed needles; because a double strand of suture is pulled through the tissue, a larger hole is created than when a swaged needle is used.
- Eyed needles may be closed (round, oblong, or square) or French (with a slit from the inside of the eye to the end of the needle for ease of threading; see Fig. 7.6B).
- Eyed needles are threaded from the inside curvature.
- The needle body comes in a variety of shapes (see Fig. 7.6C); tissue type and depth and size of the wound determine the appropriate needle shape.
- Straight (Keith) needles are generally used in accessible places in which the needle can be manipulated directly with the fingers (e.g., placement of purse-string sutures in the rectum).
- Curved needles are manipulated with needle holders.
- One-fourth (¼) circle needles are primarily used in ophthalmic procedures.
- Three-eighths (⅜) and one-half (½) circle needles are the most commonly used surgical needles in veterinary medicine (e.g., abdominal closure).
- A one-half or five-eighths (⅝) circle needle, despite requiring more wrist manipulation, is easier to use in confined locations.
- The needle point (cutting, taper, reverse-cutting; see Fig. 7.6D) determines the sharpness of a needle and type of tissue in which the needle is used.
- Cutting needles generally have two or three opposing cutting edges and are used in tissues that are difficult to penetrate (e.g., skin).
- With conventional cutting needles, the third cutting edge is on the inside (concave) curvature of the needle.
- Reverse-cutting needles have a third cutting edge located on the outer (convex) curvature of the needle.
- Side-cutting needles (spatula needles) are flat on the top and bottom and are generally used in ophthalmic procedures.
- Tapered needles (round needles) have a sharp tip that pierces and spreads tissues without cutting them.
  - They are generally used in easily penetrated tissues (e.g., intestine, subcutaneous tissues, fascia).
- Tapercut needles have a reverse-cutting edge tip and a taper point body.
  - They are generally used for suturing dense, tough fibrous tissue (e.g., tendon) and for some cardiovascular procedures (e.g., vascular grafts).
- Blunt point needles have a rounded blunt point that can dissect through friable tissue without cutting.
  - They are occasionally used for suturing soft parenchymal organs (e.g., liver, kidney).

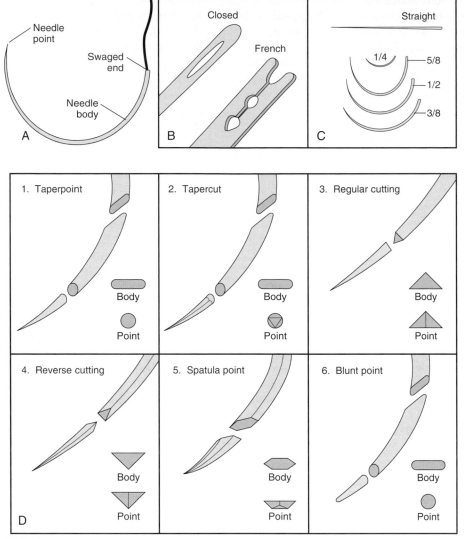

FIGURE 7.6 (A) Basic components of a needle. (B) Types of eyed needles. (C, D) Needle body shapes and sizes. (From Sirois M: *Elsevier's veterinary assistant textbook*, ed 2, St Louis, 2017, Mosby.)

Other Materials

Tissue Adhesives
- Cyanoacrylates (known as Super Glue) are commonly used for tissue adhesion during some procedures (e.g., declawing, tail docking, ear cropping).
- A variety of products are available for use in veterinary patients.
  - These adhesives rapidly polymerize in the presence of moisture and produce a strong flexible bond.
- Adhesion of tissue edges generally takes less than 15 seconds but may be delayed by excessive hemorrhage.

Skin Staples
- Metal staples (skin staples or Michel clips) are used to appose wound edges or attach drapes to the skin.
- Care must be used to ensure that the staple is appropriately bent so that when staples are used for skin closure, they cannot be easily removed by the animal.
- A special staple remover facilitates clip removal after healing.

Surgical Mesh
- Surgical mesh may be used to repair hernias (e.g., perineal hernias) or reinforce traumatized or devitalized tissues (abdominal hernias).
- Occasionally, it is used to replace excised traumatized or neoplastic tissues.
- Surgical mesh is available in nonabsorbable or absorbable forms.

CARE AND MAINTENANCE OF SURGICAL INSTRUMENTS AND SUPPLIES

- Good surgical instruments are a valuable investment and must be used and maintained properly to prevent corrosion, pitting, and/or discoloration.

- Instruments should be rinsed in cool water as soon after the surgical procedure as possible to avoid drying of blood, tissue, saline, or other foreign matter on them.
- Many manufacturers recommend that instruments be rinsed, cleaned, and sterilized in distilled or deionized water because tap water contains minerals that may cause discoloration and staining.
- If tap water is used for rinsing, instruments should be dried thoroughly to avoid staining. Instruments with multiple components should be disassembled before cleaning.
- Delicate instruments should be cleaned and sterilized separately.
- All surgical supplies and equipment that come into contact with the patient or other surgical equipment, such as Mayo instrument stands, must be cleaned and disinfected before use.

Instrument Cleaning

- Ultrasonic and enzymatic methods of cleaning are effective and efficient.
- Before putting soiled instruments in an ultrasonic cleaner, they should be washed in cleaning solution to remove all visible debris.
- Dissimilar metals (e.g., chrome and stainless steel) should not be mixed in the same cycle.
- All instruments should be placed in the ultrasonic cleaner with their ratchets and box locks open.
- Instruments must not be left in the ultrasonic cleaner for longer than the cleaning cycle because this could lead to rust.
  - They should be removed from the cleaner, rinsed, lubricated, and dried at the completion of the cycle.
- If an ultrasonic cleaner is not available, instruments should be manually cleaned as thoroughly as possible, paying particular attention to box locks, serrations, and hinges.
- Nylon brushes and a cool cleaning solution may be used for most instruments.
- Rasps and serrated parts of instruments may require a wire brush.
- A cleaning solution with a neutral pH should be used to avoid staining.
- Enzymatic solutions may be used to remove proteinaceous materials from general surgical instruments and endoscopic equipment.
- Autoclaving is not a substitute for proper instrument cleaning.
- If residual organic debris remains on the instruments, they will not become sterile when autoclaved.

Instrument Lubricating and Autoclaving

- Before they are autoclaved, instruments with box locks and hinges and power equipment should be lubricated with instrument milk or surgical lubricants.

- All instruments should be allowed to thoroughly air-dry before packing them into a surgical pack.
- Before they are packed, instruments are separated and placed in order of their intended use.
- Specific guidelines should be followed when preparing packs for steam and gas sterilization to allow maximal penetration.
- Small items may be wrapped, sterilized, and stored in self-sealing (peel and seal) or heat-sealable paper or plastic peel pouches or in regular cloth, muslin, or drape wrapping material.
- Packed instruments can be placed in a tray or wrapped individually.
- The pack is wrapped using at least two layers of material.
  - A presterilization wrap for steam sterilization consists of two thicknesses of two-layer muslin or nonwoven (paper) barrier materials.
  - The poststerilization wrap (after sterilization and proper cool-down period) consists of a waterproof, heat-sealable plastic dust cover; this wrap is not necessary if the item is used within 24 hours of sterilization.
- Always take care to wrap packs tightly so that the drape material does not contact the inner wall of the autoclave.
- The instrument pack is sealed with autoclave tape and labeled with the date, contents, and initials of the person preparing the pack.
- Autoclave tape provides verification that the outside of the pack was exposed to appropriate sterilization temperatures.
- Individual instruments can also be placed into sterilization pouches.
  - These pouches usually incorporate a chemical sterilization indicator.
  - Double wrapping in pouches can be used for particularly delicate or sharp instruments. Always mark items with the date that the item was autoclaved.
- For steam and gas sterilization, instruments should be organized on a lint-free towel placed on the bottom of a perforated metal instrument tray.
- A chemical sterilization indicator is included in every pack to provide verification that the inside of the pack was exposed to appropriate sterilization temperatures for the correct amount of time.
- Instruments with box locks should be autoclaved opened.
- A 3- to 5-mm space between instruments is recommended for proper steam or gas circulation. Complex instruments should be disassembled when possible, and power equipment should be lubricated before sterilization.
- Items with a lumen should have a small amount of water flushed through them immediately before steam sterilization because water vaporizes and forces air out of the lumen.
  - Conversely, moisture left in tubing placed in a gas sterilizer may decrease the sterilization efficacy.

- Containers (e.g., saline bowl) should be placed with the open end facing up or horizontally; containers with lids should have the lid slightly ajar.
- Multiple basins should be stacked with a towel between each.
- A standard count of radiopaque surgical sponges should be included in each pack.

Wrapping Instrument Packs

- Packs may not be completely sterilized if they are wrapped too tightly or improperly loaded in the autoclave or gas sterilizer container.
- Instrument packs should be positioned vertically (on edge) and longitudinally in an autoclave. Heavy packs should be placed at the periphery, where steam enters the chamber.
- Allow a small amount of air space between each pack to facilitate steam flow (1 to 2 inches between each pack and surrounding walls).
- Load linen packs so that the fabric layers are oriented vertically, on edge.

Sterilization

Gas Sterilization

- Ethylene oxide is the most common form of gas sterilization used in the veterinary hospital.
  - It is a flammable explosive liquid that becomes an effective sterilizing agent when mixed with carbon dioxide or Freon.
- Equipment that cannot withstand the extreme temperature and pressures of steam sterilization (e.g., endoscopes, cameras, plastics, power cables) can be safely sterilized with ethylene oxide.

- Environmental and safety hazards associated with ethylene oxide are numerous and severe.
- It is critical to the safety of the patient and hospital personnel that all materials sterilized with ethylene oxide be aerated according to instructions provided by the manufacturer of the ethylene oxide gas sterilization unit.
- Porous materials or those that will be used as implants in patients should generally be aerated for 24 hours after gas sterilization.
- Items should be clean and dry before ethylene oxide sterilization; moisture and organic material bond with ethylene oxide and leave a toxic residue.
- Items are packed and loaded loosely to allow gas circulation.
- Complex items (e.g., power equipment) are disassembled before processing.
- Items that cannot be sterilized with ethylene oxide include acrylics, some pharmaceutical items, and solutions.

Cold Chemical Sterilization

- Liquid chemicals used for sterilization must be noncorrosive to the items being sterilized.
- These items are usually placed in a special tray kept in the surgery area.
- Glutaraldehyde solution is noncorrosive and provides a safe means of sterilizing delicate, lensed instruments (e.g., endoscopes, cystoscopes, bronchoscopes).
- Most equipment that can be safely immersed in water can be safely immersed in 3% glutaraldehyde.
  - Table 7.3 lists some commonly used cold sterilization agents.

TABLE 7.3 Antimicrobial Activity of Commonly Used Cold Sterilants

Agent	DESTRUCTIVE ACTION AGAINST				
	Bacteria	Tubercle bacilli	Spores	Fungi	Viruses
Alcohol, ethyl (70%–90%)	+	+	0	+	±
Alcohol, isopropyl (70%–90%)	++	+	0	+	±
Alcohol, iodine (2%)	++	+	±	+	+
Formalin (37%)	+	+	+	+	+
Glutaraldehyde (buffered, 2%; Cidex)	++	+	++	+	+
Iodine (2%–5% aqueous)	++	+	±	+	+
Iodophors (1%; povidone-iodine complex)	+	+	±	±	+
Mercury-containing (e.g., Merthiolate)	±	0	0	+	±
Phenolic derivatives (0.5%–3%)	+	+	0	+	±
Quaternary ammonium cation (quat; e.g., benzalkonium chloride, 1:750–1:1000)	++	0	0	+	0

Adapted from Sirois M: Principles and practice of veterinary technology, ed 3, St Louis, 2011, Mosby.
++, Very good; +, good; ±, fair (greater concentration or more time needed); 0, no activity.

TABLE 7.4 Recommended Storage Times for Sterilized Packs*

Wrapper	Shelf Life
Double-wrapped, two-layer muslin	4 wk
Double-wrapped, two-layer muslin, heat-sealed in dust covers after sterilization	6 mo
Double-wrapped, two-layer muslin, tape-sealed in dust covers after sterilization	2 mo
Double-wrapped nonwoven barrier materials (paper)	6 mo
Paper, plastic peel-back pouches, heat-sealed	1 yr
Plastic peel-back pouches, heat-sealed	1 yr

Adapted from Sirois M: *Principles and practice of veterinary technology, ed 3,* St Louis, 2011, Mosby.
*Note that sterilized items from hospitals adopting event-related sterility assurance have an indefinite shelf-life.

- Items for sterilization should be clean and dry; organic matter (e.g., blood, pus, saliva) may prevent penetration of instrument crevices or joints, and residual water causes chemical dilution.
- Immersion times suggested by the manufacturer should be followed (e.g., for sterilization in 3% glutaraldehyde, 10 hours at 68°F [20°C] to 77°F [25°C]; for disinfection, 10 minutes at 68° to 77°F [20° to 25°C]).
- After the appropriate immersion time, instruments should be rinsed thoroughly with sterile water and dried with sterile towels to avoid damaging the patient's tissues.

Folding and Wrapping Gowns and Drapes

- Surgical gowns must be folded so that they can be easily donned without breaking sterile technique.
- Fan folding (accordion folding) allows compact storage and simple unfolding.
- Fold a hand towel and place it on top of the folded gown, leaving one corner turned back to allow it to be easily grasped.
- Wrap the gown and towel in two layers of paper or cloth wrap as described.
- Drapes should be folded so that the fenestration (or the center of an unfenestrated drape) can be properly positioned over the surgical site without contaminating the drape.
- Fan-fold the drape so that the fenestration is on the ventral outermost aspect of the drape. Wrap it in two layers of paper or cloth wrap, as described.

Storing Sterilized Items

- Packs are allowed to cool and dry individually on racks when removed from the autoclave; placing instrument packs on top of each other during cooling may promote condensation of moisture, resulting in contamination via strike-through (wick action).
- After sterile packs are completely dry, they should be stored in waterproof dust covers in closed cabinets, rather than uncovered on open shelves, to protect them

from moisture or exposure to particulate matter, such as dust-borne bacteria.
- Sterile packs are labeled with the date on which the item was sterilized and a control lot number to trace an unsterile item.
- Heat-sealed waterproof dust covers are placed on items not routinely used.
- The shelf life of a sterilized pack varies with the type of outer wrap (Table 7.4).

Basic Surgical Terminology

- Surgical procedures are described using anatomic terms combined with word roots (suffixes; see Chapter 1).
- The most common suffixes used for describing surgical procedures are presented in Box 7.1.

Incisions
Abdominal Incisions

- Entry into the abdomen is usually gained by any of four common abdominal incisions.
- Named according to its location, each incision offers different advantages and a different exposure of the abdomen (Fig. 7.7).
- A ventral midline incision is located on the ventral midline of the animal and offers excellent exposure of the entire abdominal cavity.
- A paramedian incision is located lateral and parallel to the ventral midline of the animal and is usually used when exposure of only one side of the abdomen is needed, such as for removal of a cryptorchid (retained) testis.
- A flank incision is generally performed on a standing animal or one in lateral recumbency.
  - It is oriented perpendicular to the long axis of the body, caudal to the last rib.
  - A flank incision provides good exposure of the organ(s) immediately deep to (beneath) the incision but does not allow exploration of much of the

> **BOX 7.1** Common Suffixes Used to Describe Surgical Procedures
>
> - *-ectomy* = to remove (excise). For example, a splenectomy is a surgical procedure to remove the spleen.
> - *-otomy* = to cut into. For example, a cystotomy (incision into the urinary bladder) is often performed to remove urinary calculi (bladder stones).
> - *-ostomy* = surgical creation of an artificial opening. For example, a perineal urethrostomy is a surgical procedure often performed on male cats for relief of urethral obstruction. It involves excision of the penis (penectomy) and creation of a widened, new urethral opening.
> - *-rrhaphy* = surgical repair by suturing. For example, abdominal herniorrhaphy is the surgical repair of an abdominal hernia by suturing the defect in the abdominal musculature.
> - *-pexy* = surgical fixation. For example, gastropexy (suturing of the stomach to the abdominal wall to fix it in place) is often performed in cases of gastric torsion.
> - *-plasty* = surgical alteration of shape or form. For example, pyloroplasty enlarges the pyloric orifice of the stomach to facilitate gastric emptying.

From Sirois M: Principles and practice of veterinary technology, ed 3, St Louis, 2011, Mosby.

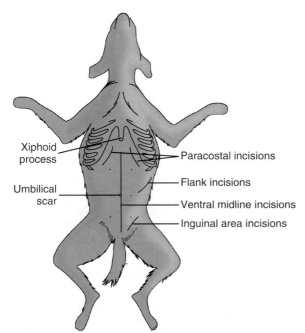

FIGURE 7.7 Surgical incisions for abdominal procedures. (From Sirois M: *Elsevier's veterinary assistant textbook*, ed 2, St Louis, 2017, Mosby.)

Xiphoid process
Umbilical scar
Paracostal incisions
Flank incisions
Ventral midline incisions
Inguinal area incisions

remainder of the abdomen. It is therefore useful for such procedures as nephrectomy, in which the organ in question lies directly beneath the incision.

- A paracostal incision is oriented parallel to the last rib and offers good exposure of the stomach and spleen in monogastric animals.

Thoracic Incisions

- Thoracic surgery may be indicated because of pathology in the chest or traumatic injuries. Two common incisions are used in veterinary medicine.
- A median sternotomy is used for many cardiac procedures or when all lung fields need to be visualized or approached.
  - This incision is along the patient's midline, on the ventral thorax, moving cranially from the xiphoid process or caudally from the first sternebrae, always leaving two to three sternebrae intact.
- A lateral intercostal thoracotomy may be used if only one side of the chest needs to be approached, such as in cases of lung lobe torsion or mass.
  - This is done on the side of the patient's thorax, perpendicular to the spine and between the ribs.

Common Surgical Procedures

Soft Tissue Procedures

- An **ovariohysterectomy**, commonly referred to as a spay, involves removal of the ovaries and uterus.
- A cesarean section is a method of delivering newborn animals in cases of dystocia (difficult labor).
  - It consists of an abdominal incision (flank or ventral midline) and then an incision into the uterus through which the newborn(s) is (are) delivered.
- An **orchiectomy** (castration) is the surgical removal of the testes.
- A lateral ear resection is often performed in animals with chronic external ear infection.
  - It involves removal of the lateral wall of the vertical portion of the external ear canal to allow improved **ventilation** and establish drainage for exudates.
- A **laparotomy** is an incision into the abdominal cavity, often through the flank.
- A celiotomy is another term for laparotomy.
- A cystotomy is an incision into the urinary bladder, frequently for the removal of urinary calculi (bladder stones).
- A gastrotomy is an incision into the stomach.
- Gastropexy involves suturing of the stomach to the abdominal wall to fix it in place. This procedure is frequently done in cases of gastric torsion.
- A splenectomy is the removal of the spleen.
- A thoracotomy is an incision into the thoracic cavity (chest).
- A herniorrhaphy is the surgical repair of a hernia by suturing the abnormal opening(s) closed.
- An enterotomy is an incision into the intestine, often for removal of a foreign body.

- An intestinal anastomosis involves removal of a portion of the intestine (resection) and suturing the cut ends together to restore the continuity of the intestinal tube (anastomosis).
- A perineal urethrostomy involves incision into the urethra and suturing of the splayed urethral edges to the skin to create a larger urethral orifice. This procedure is frequently performed on male cats with recurrent urethral obstruction.
- A urethrotomy is an incision into the urethra, most commonly to retrieve stones that have traveled out of the bladder and become lodged in the urethra.
- A mastectomy involves removal of part or all of one or more mammary glands.

Orthopedic (Bone) Procedures

- An onychectomy is the surgical removal of a claw, commonly called declawing.
- An intervertebral disc fenestration is done to remove prolapsed intervertebral disc material causing pressure on the spinal cord.
- An intramedullary bone pinning involves insertion of a metal rod (bone pin) into the medullary cavity of a long bone to fix fracture fragments in place.
- Joint stabilization via lateral suture technique or tibial tuberosity advancement is performed when the cranial cruciate ligament in the stifle joint has ruptured.
- A femoral head ostectomy involves amputation of the head of the femur. It is usually performed in animals with severe damage to the femoral head or neck or with a damaged acetabulum.

PREOPERATIVE AND POSTOPERATIVE CONSIDERATIONS

Preoperative Evaluation

- Anesthesia and surgery are stressful events that put an animal's life at risk.

- The role of a proper preoperative evaluation is to gather enough pertinent information to minimize that risk.
- That information can be gathered through a patient history, physical examination, and appropriate laboratory tests.
- The veterinary assistant will work closely with the veterinary technician who is performing the evaluation.

Patient Evaluation

- Patient evaluation means to judge a patient's medical history and physical condition carefully to determine health status and predict potential complications.
- This is the most important step because all anesthetic decisions are based on health status.
- Patient evaluation includes consideration of patient characteristics, medical history, physical examination, and laboratory test results.
  - Patient characteristics include species, breed, age, and gender.
  - Patient medical history should include signalment and anamnesis (medical history), including the vaccine status, medical and surgical history, injuries, diseases, past anesthetic complications, changes in the patient's condition since last observed, purpose of the appointment (including specific location), observance of fasting recommendations, and concurrent medication.
- The physical examination includes general body condition scoring and evaluation of the cardiovascular, respiratory, hepatic, renal, and central nervous systems (Table 7.5).
- Preanesthetic laboratory tests may include hematocrit (packed cell volume [PCV]), total plasma protein, liver enzyme (e.g., alanine aminotransferase [ALT]), bile acid, blood urea nitrogen (BUN), blood glucose, and electrolyte levels; blood smear; heartworm status; fecal analysis; acid–base balance; urinalysis; blood gas values; and blood coagulation screens, depending on the condition and age of the animal.

TABLE 7.5 Preanesthetic Physical Examination Checklist

System	Check	Note Signs
General body condition	Temperature, weight, body score, skin turgor, temperament	Obesity, dehydration, cachexia, hypothermia, hyperthermia, pregnancy, recent changes in weight, aggressiveness
Central nervous system	Level of consciousness	Bright, alert, responsive (BAR); quiet, alert, responsive (QAR); obtunded, depressed, lethargic, stuporous, comatose, seizures, syncope
Cardiovascular	Heart rate and rhythm, arterial blood pressure quality and regularity, concurrent pulse and auscultation, capillary refill time (CRT)	Cyanosis or icterus, pale mucous membranes, prolonged CRT, heart murmurs, weak or irregular pulse, arrhythmias
Respiratory	Respiratory rate, depth and effort, character, mucous membrane color	Pallor, cyanosis, increased effort or rate, abnormal lung sounds (e.g., wheezing, crackles), dyspnea, nasal discharge

Continued

TABLE 7.5 Preanesthetic Physical Examination Checklist—cont'd

Hepatic	Color	Jaundice, failure of blood to clot, coma, seizures
Renal	Volume and discharges	Vomiting, polyuria-polydipsia, oliguria-anuria, hematuria
Gastrointestinal	Abnormalities	Diarrhea, vomiting, distention
Musculoskeletal	Stance, activity	Weakness, abnormal gait, recumbency
Exterior surfaces	Integument, coat condition, lymph nodes, mammary glands, body openings	Wounds, parasites, tumors, lesions, exudates, hair loss, roughness, redness, inflammation, enlarged lymph nodes, discharges, odors, vaginal discharge
EENT	Ears, eyes, nose, and throat	Discharges, inflammation, swelling, abnormal pupil size and response, redness, odor, stridor, dental tartar
Abdominal palpation	Abnormalities	Hardness, pain, distention

Adapted from Sirois M: Principles and practice of veterinary technology, ed 3, St Louis, 2011, Mosby.

- Thoracic radiography and electrocardiography also may be useful in evaluating a patient.

Patient Preparation

- Patient preparation requirements vary depending on the anticipated procedure. It is also important to prepare for the possibility of unanticipated situations.
- Standard practice is to withhold food for 8 to 12 hours and water for 2 to 4 hours before anesthetic induction.
- If food is not withheld, pulmonary aspiration leading to pneumonia, permanent disability, or immediate respiratory arrest and death of the patient may occur.
  - Pediatric or smaller patients should be fasted for shorter time periods.
  - Chronically compromised patients should have their condition stabilized, when possible, before anesthesia.
    - For example, dehydrated patients should receive sufficient intravenous (IV) fluids to restore hydration status.
- It is important to obtain a current and accurate weight for the patient.
- Clipping the surgical site and placing an IV catheter before induction minimize anesthesia time.
- Avoid unnecessary handling of the patient and noisy personnel or equipment.
- Oxygenation before and during induction may be beneficial to patients with cardiopulmonary compromise, especially during mask or chamber induction.
- Preanesthetic checklists should be completed before all procedures to ensure that appropriate items are readily available, important health issues have been addressed, and all persons involved have been informed.

PREPARATION OF THE OPERATIVE SITE

- Surgery puts a patient at risk for nosocomial infections (hospital-acquired infections).

- Because most surgical infections develop from bacteria that enter the incision during surgery, proper preparation of the surgical site is crucial to reduce the likelihood of infection.
- Resident skin flora (particularly *Staphylococcus aureus* and *Streptococcus* spp.) are the most common sources of surgical wound contaminants.
- Although it is impossible to sterilize skin without impairing its natural protective function and interfering with wound healing, proper preoperative preparation reduces the likelihood of infection.

Hair Removal and Skin Scrubbing

- Before preparing the patient for surgery, verify the patient's identity, surgical procedure being performed, and surgical site.
- It may be useful to bathe the animal the day before the surgical procedure to remove loose hair, debris, and external parasites.
- Preparing patients for surgery includes clipping hair and scrubbing the skin at the surgical site. These procedures should be performed outside of the surgical suite.
- The extent and location of hair removal are based on the type of surgical procedure to be performed (Fig. 7.8).
- Hair should be liberally clipped around the proposed incision site so that the incision can be extended, if needed, while still remaining within a sterile field.
- A general guideline is to clip 20 cm on each side of the incision.
- The hair can be removed most effectively with an Oster-type clipper and a no. 40 clipper blade.
  - The higher the blade number, the shorter the remaining hair.
- Clippers should be held using a pencil grip, and initial clipping should be done with the grain of the hair growth pattern with the blade parallel to the skin surface.
- Subsequent clipping should be against the pattern of hair growth to obtain a closer clip.

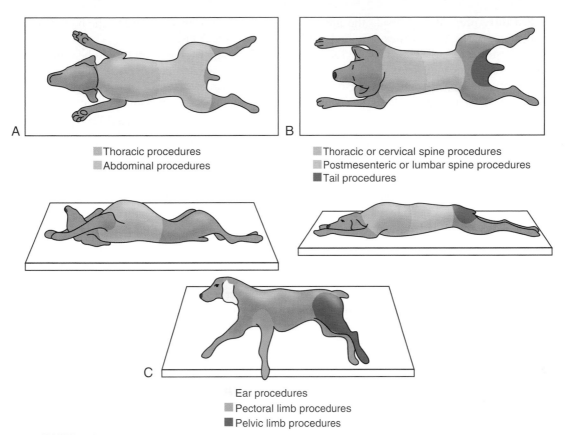

Thoracic procedures
Abdominal procedures

Thoracic or cervical spine procedures
Postmesenteric or lumbar spine procedures
Tail procedures

Ear procedures
Pectoral limb procedures
Pelvic limb procedures

FIGURE 7.8 Hair removal patterns for selected surgical procedures. (A) Dorsal recumbency. (B) Sternal recumbency. (C) Lateral recumbency. (From Sirois M: *Elsevier's veterinary assistant textbook*, ed 2, St Louis, 2017, Mosby.)

- Depilatory creams are less traumatic than other hair removal methods, but they induce a mild dermal lymphocytic reaction.
  - They are most useful in irregular areas in which adequate hair clipping is difficult.
- Razors are occasionally used for hair removal (e.g., around the eye), but they cause microlacerations in skin that may increase irritation and promote infection.
- After hair has been clipped from the site, loose hair is removed with a vacuum.
- To enhance manipulation of limbs during surgery, a hanging leg preparation may be done. This requires that the limb be circumferentially clipped; the limb is hung from an IV pole during preparation to allow the sides of the limb to be scrubbed (Fig. 7.9).
- Before transporting the animal to the surgical site, the incision is given a general cleansing scrub, and ophthalmic antibiotic ointment or lubricant may be placed on the cornea and conjunctiva.
- In male dogs undergoing abdominal procedures, the prepuce may be flushed with an antiseptic solution.
- The skin is scrubbed with germicidal soap to remove debris and reduce bacterial populations in preparation for surgery.

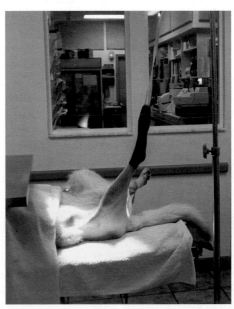

FIGURE 7.9 Manipulation of the limb during orthopedic procedures may be facilitated with a hanging leg preparation. The limb is clipped circumferentially and carefully suspended from an IV pole with tape. The patient is positioned for medial rear limb surgery. (From Sirois M: *Elsevier's veterinary assistant textbook*, ed 2, St Louis, 2017, Mosby.)

- This so-called dirty prep (done outside the operating room) will often consist of chlorhexidine and saline, and the lather step may be left in place for 60 to 120 seconds to ensure adequate contact time.
- Other options for scrubbing solutions include iodophors, alcohols, hexachlorophene, and quaternary ammonium salts.

Positioning

- Before sterile application of the epidermal germicide, the animal is moved to the operating room and positioned so that the operative site is accessible to the surgeon and secured with ropes, sandbags, troughs, or tape.
- The animal is generally placed on a water-circulating heating pad and provided with a warm air-circulating blanket; if electrocautery is being used, a ground plate should be positioned under the patient.
- Anesthetic monitoring equipment is then attached and baseline vital signs evaluated before proceeding with the sterile prep.

Sterile Skin Preparation

- Sterile preparation of the surgical site begins after transporting and positioning the animal on the operating table.
- Sterile patient preparation generally consists of three rounds of alternating antiseptic solution with saline rinse; every pass with gauze moves in a circular motion from the anticipated incision site, radiating outward.
- Frequently, when using povidone-iodine and alcohol, the site is scrubbed alternatively with each solution three times to allow for 5 minutes of contact time.
- Using alcohol between the povidone-iodine scrubs decreases the contact time of povidone-iodine with the skin and may decrease its efficacy.
- When the final povidone-iodine scrub is completed, a 10% povidone-iodine solution should be sprayed or painted on the site.
- If chlorhexidine is the preparation solution, it may be rinsed with saline.
- Because chlorhexidine binds to keratin, contact time is less critical than with povidone-iodine. Two 30-second applications are considered adequate for antimicrobial activity.

PREPARATION OF THE SURGICAL TEAM

Surgical Attire

- All persons entering the operating room suite, regardless of whether a surgery is in progress or not, should be dressed in appropriate surgical attire.
- To minimize microbial contamination from operating room personnel, wear dedicated surgical scrub clothes rather than street clothes in the operating suite.
- With two-piece pant suits, tuck loose-fitting tops into the trousers.

- Tunic tops that fit close to the body may be worn outside the trousers.
- The sleeves of the top should be short enough to allow the hands and arms to be scrubbed. Pants should have an elastic waist or drawstring closure.
- Nonscrubbed personnel should wear long-sleeved jackets over their scrub clothes.
- Jackets should be buttoned or snapped closed during use to minimize the risk of the edges inadvertently contaminating sterile surfaces.
- Scrub clothes should be laundered between wearings and changed if they are visibly soiled or wet to prevent transfer of microorganisms to the environment.
- Wearing scrub clothes outside the surgical environment increases microbial contamination.
- If a scrub suit must be worn outside the surgery room, a laboratory coat or single-use gown should be used to cover it.
- Other surgical attire includes hair coverings, masks, shoe covers, gowns, and gloves.
- Because bacterial shedding from hair increases surgical wound infection rates, complete hair coverage is necessary.
- Even when surgery is not in progress, caps and masks should be worn in the surgical suite.
- Caps should completely cover all scalp and facial hair, and masks should cover the mouth and nostrils.
- Sideburns and/or beards require a hood for complete coverage.
- Skull caps that fail to cover the side hair above the ears and hair at the nape of the neck should not be worn.
- Any comfortable footwear can be worn in the surgery area.
- Shoe covers should be donned when first entering the surgical area and should be worn when leaving it to keep shoes clean.
- New shoe covers are donned when returning to the surgical area.
- Shoe covers are generally made of reusable or disposable materials that are water-repellent and tear-resistant.
- Masks, constructed from lint-free material containing a hydrophilic filter web sandwiched between two outer layers, should be worn whenever entering a sterile area.
  - Their major function is to filter and contain droplets of microorganisms expelled from the mouth and nasopharynx during talking, sneezing, and coughing.
- Masks must be fitted over the mouth and nose and secured in a manner that prevents venting.
- The dorsal aspect of the mask is secured by shaping the reinforcing top edge tightly around the nose.
- Surgical gowns may be reusable and made of woven materials (usually cotton) or disposable.
- Disposable (single-use) gowns are nonwoven and made directly from fibers rather than yarn. Loosely woven cotton is commonly used for reusable gowns.
- Fewer microorganisms contaminate the surgical environment when disposable (single-use) nonwoven materials are used.

Surgical Scrub

- Surgical scrubbing cleans the hands and forearms to reduce the numbers of bacteria that come into contact with the wound from scrubbed personnel during surgery.
- The veterinarian and veterinary technician must perform a hand and arm scrub before entering the surgical suite.
- Objectives of a surgical scrub include mechanical removal of dirt and oil, reduction of the transient bacterial population (bacteria deposited from the environment), and reduction of the skin's resident bacterial population.
- Two accepted methods of performing a surgical scrub are the anatomic timed scrub (5-minute scrub) and the counted brush stroke method (strokes per surface area of skin).

Gowning and Gloving

- Gowns are another barrier between the skin of the surgical team and patient.
  - They should be constructed of a material that prevents passage of microorganisms between sterile and nonsterile areas.
- Gowns should be resistant to fluid, lint accumulation, stretching, and tearing, especially at the forearm, elbow, and abdominal areas, and should be comfortable, economical, and fire-resistant. Reusable or single-use disposable gowns are available.
- Gowning and gloving should occur away from the surgical table and patient to avoid dripping water onto the sterile field and contaminating it.

Anesthetic Equipment and Supplies

- More anesthetic mishaps are attributed to poor planning and preparation than to improper use of drugs.
- Correct selection, preparation, and use of anesthetic equipment are essential for patient safety.
- All equipment should be prepared and checked to be in good working order before the administration of anesthetic compounds; intubation and oxygenation may be required unexpectedly.
- The veterinary assistant will work closely with the veterinary technician who is performing these tasks.

Supplies for Intravenous Fluid Administration

- Placement of an IV catheter is essential for patient safety during anesthesia.
- IV catheters provide immediate access for IV injection and administration of fluids.
- Catheters should be placed before induction of anesthesia, when possible, because most anesthetic agents produce hypotension or vasoconstriction and may complicate catheter placement.
- Appropriately sized catheters, infusion sets, needles, syringes, and other supplies necessary for aseptic catheterization should be arranged for easy access.

Endotracheal Tubes

- Endotracheal intubation ensures a patent airway, facilitates patient ventilation, and provides easy delivery of volatile anesthetics (Fig. 7.10).
- Endotracheal tube (ETT) diameter and length are important. The diameter should be the largest size that will fit into the trachea with ease.
  - If too large, the larynx and trachea may be traumatized.
  - If too small, the patient will have difficulty breathing through the tube.
- A fairly accurate assessment for tube size can be based on the weight of the dog, keeping in mind that body condition, confirmation, brachycephalic breed, obesity, and small size may alter the final size chosen.
- Use a 9- to 9.5-mm tube for a 40-pound (18.2-kg) dog.
- As the weight changes by 5 lb (2.3 kg), change the size of the ETT by 0.5 mm.
- The trachea also can be palpated to feel the approximate size, or an approximation can be made by measuring the nasal septal width with the outer diameter of an ETT.
- Proper length of the ETT is also important.
  - The inserted tip of the tube should not extend beyond (caudal to) the thoracic inlet to prevent bronchial intubation.
  - The adapter end of the tube should not extend more than 1 or 2 inches beyond (rostral to) the mouth to limit mechanical dead space and prevent the rebreathing of exhaled gas.
- The ETT should be clean and free of defects or obstructions.
- If the ETT has an inflatable cuff, it should be checked for leaks.

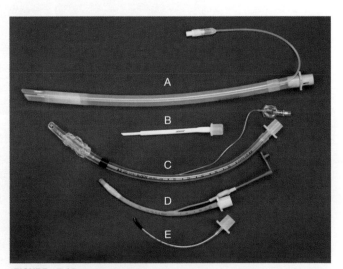

FIGURE 7.10 Endotracheal tube type, material, and size comparison. (A) Cuffed 11-mm silicone rubber tube. (B) 2.5-mm Cole tube. (C) Cuffed 8-mm polyvinyl chloride (PVC) tube. (D) Cuffed 4-mm red rubber tube. (E) Uncuffed 2-mm PVC Murphy tube. (From Sirois M: *Elsevier's veterinary assistant textbook*, ed 2, St Louis, 2017, Mosby.)

Laryngoscope

- The laryngoscope facilitates visualization of the glottis as the ETT passes through into the trachea.
- Laryngoscopes consist of a handle and detachable blade in a variety of sizes and shapes (Fig. 7.11).
- The blade is curved to match the curvature of the tongue and allow even pressure along its length.

Medical Gas Supply

- Medical gases may be delivered from compressed gas cylinders by a central pipeline or direct attachment to the anesthetic machine.
- Medical-grade oxygen and nitrous oxide are the gases commonly used in veterinary medicine, although the benefits of nitrous oxide in veterinary practice are limited.
- The nitrous oxide source must be independent of the oxygen source; nitrous oxide is mixed with oxygen just before passing through the vaporizer.
- The most commonly used sizes of compressed medical gas cylinders are the E cylinder (4.25 × 26 inches) and the H cylinder (9.25 × 51 inches).

- All medical gas cylinders are color coded; oxygen cylinders are green (white in Canada), and nitrous oxide cylinders are blue.
- An alternative to gas cylinders is the oxygen concentrator.
  - The concentrator draws room air in through a filter, extracts nitrogen from the room air, and delivers the filtered air (approximately 95% oxygen) to a reservoir in the machine.
- Pressure regulators attached to the cylinder valve on H cylinders and near the hanger yokes for E cylinders passively reduce oxygen pressure to the normal working pressure of the anesthetic machine to a gauge of 50 pounds per square inch (psi).
- If there is a line pressure gauge, it should be checked before every procedure to verify correct pressure in the intermediate pressure gas lines (40 to 50 psi).
- Pressure reduction is necessary to prevent damage to the anesthetic machine and allow a constant rate of oxygen delivery to the flow meter.
- Cylinder pressure gauges are associated with the pressure regulator and may be used to estimate the relative volume of gas remaining in a cylinder.

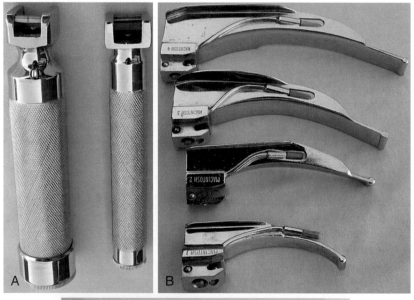

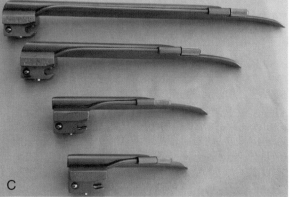

FIGURE 7.11 Laryngoscopes. (A) Laryngoscope handle. (B) MacIntosh laryngeal speculum. (C) Miller laryngeal speculum. (From Sirois M: *Elsevier's veterinary assistant textbook*, ed 2, St Louis, 2017, Mosby.)

- The pressure in a fully charged oxygen cylinder, regardless of size, is almost 2200 psi.

Anesthesia Machines

- Anesthesia machines deliver a mixture of oxygen and inhalation anesthetic to the breathing circuit.
- The components of an anesthesia machine include the oxygen source, pressure regulator, oxygen pressure valve, flow meter, vaporizer, breathing circuit, reservoir bag, circuit manometer, positive-pressure relief valve, carbon dioxide absorbent, and unidirectional dome valves (Fig. 7.12).
- Flow meters deliver a constant gas flow to the vaporizer, common gas outlet, and breathing circuit.
  - Flow meters are common sources of leaks and should be checked at regular intervals for cracks in the flow tube.
  - Excessive tightening easily damages control knobs, leading to expensive repair. Overtightening may prevent the flow meter from closing completely, causing significant leaking in the off position.
- The primary function of a vaporizer is controlled enhancement of anesthetic vaporization. Each vaporizer is designed to be used with a specific inhalant anesthetic

and is color coded—isoflurane is purple, sevoflurane is yellow, and desflurane is blue.
  - Inhalation anesthetic agents are volatile liquids that vaporize at room temperature.
- Precision vaporizers, designed for a specific anesthetic agent, deliver a constant concentration (as a percentage) that is automatically maintained with changing oxygen flow rates and temperature.
- Precision vaporizers are designed to function out of the breathing circuit (vaporizer out of circuit [VOC])—that is, between the flow meter and breathing circuit—so that oxygen from the flow meter flows into the vaporizer before entering the breathing circuit.
- Several hazards are associated with vaporizers:
  - Filling with the incorrect agent can lead to delivery of an excessively high or low concentration of vapor to the patient.
  - Tipping the vaporizer may allow liquid agent to enter the fresh gas line, increasing the anesthetic concentration.
  - Overfilling the chamber decreases the volume of vapor available to mix with fresh gas and may allow liquid anesthetic to reach the common gas outlet line.
  - Leaks are also common at the inlet fitting, outlet fitting, filling port, and drain port.
- Medical gases pass from the anesthetic machine to the patient through tubing known as a breathing circuit.
- Breathing circuits deliver fresh gases (oxygen and anesthetic vapor) to the patient and transport exhaled gases from the patient.
- The breathing circuit is classified as a rebreathing system (circuit), where it is incorporated into the machine and carbon dioxide is eliminated from the circuit by soda lime absorption, or a non–rebreathing system, in which the carbon dioxide is eliminated using high gas flow rates and not a carbon dioxide absorber.

Rebreathing Circuits

- Rebreathing circuits (circle system) are most commonly used in veterinary practice.
- The components of the circle system include a reservoir bag, manometer, positive-pressure relief valve (pop-off valve), carbon dioxide absorbent, unidirectional valves, fresh gas inlet, and removable set of breathing tubes (Fig. 7.13).
- Some circuits also have a negative-pressure relief valve.
- Advantages of the rebreathing circuit include conservation of body heat and fluids; reuse of exhaled oxygen and anesthetic gases; and cost-efficient, lower flow rates.
- Disadvantages of the rebreathing circuit include the danger of hypercarbia (excess carbon dioxide) resulting from malfunction of the carbon dioxide absorbent or unidirectional valves, particularly at flow rates low enough to produce a closed system.

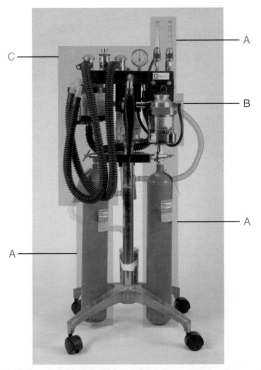

FIGURE 7.12 Small animal anesthesia machine; anesthetic machine systems. (A) Carrier gas supply. Note the two size E compressed gas oxygen cylinders next to the A's at the bottom of this image. (B) Anesthetic vaporizer. (C) Breathing circuit. Note that the scavenging system is not visible in this view. (From Sirois M: *Elsevier's veterinary assistant textbook*, ed 2, St Louis, 2017, Mosby.)

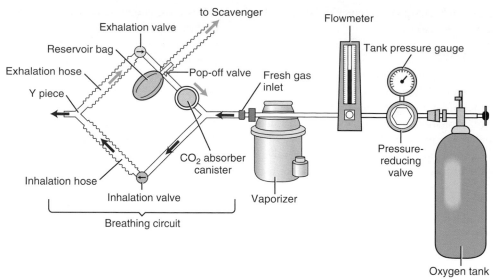

FIGURE 7.13 Diagram of an anesthetic machine with a rebreathing circuit and vaporizer outside the breathing circuit. (From Sirois M: *Elsevier's veterinary assistant textbook*, ed 2, St Louis, 2017, Mosby.)

- The **reservoir bag** (rebreathing bag) provides a gas volume sufficient for the patient to inhale maximally without creating negative pressure in the circuit.
  - It is also used for positive-pressure ventilation or to inflate the lungs when needed.
- Reservoir bag sizes of 0.5 to 5 liters are used for small animals.
- The ideal reservoir bag is five to six times the patient's normal **tidal volume** of 10 mL/kg.
- The circuit manometer is useful to monitor circuit pressure.
- Excessive circuit pressure (>4 cm H_2O) may prevent normal respiration and increase intrathoracic pressure, resulting in decreased venous return and a subsequent drop in cardiac output.
- The positive-pressure relief (pop-off) valve prevents excessive pressure in the rebreathing circuit and allows for the removal of excess waste gases.

- The pop-off valve is equipped with a scavenger interface, permitting connection to a waste gas removal system to prevent waste gas discharge into the room air.
- The carbon dioxide–absorbent canister removes carbon dioxide from the exhaled gases before the gases are returned to the patient.
  - The gases are directed to the canister by the expiratory unidirectional valve of the breathing circuit.
  - The canister contains absorbent granules such as calcium hydroxide, which remove CO_2 from the expired air.
- The absorbent should be changed monthly or after 6 to 8 hours of use, whichever is first. Look for signs to determine whether the granules need to be changed earlier (Table 7.6).
- Precautionary measures to ensure that the absorbent is reasonably fresh include logging of date changed and amount of time used for anesthesia.

TABLE 7.6 Comparison of Fresh and Exhausted CO_2 Granules

Feature	Fresh CO_2 Granules	Exhausted CO_2 Granules
Consistency	$Ca(OH)_2$—chip or crumble with finger pressure	$CaCO_3$—hard and brittle
Color	White	Slightly off white
pH indicator	Pink or white depending on brand	When one-third to half of granules change color to white instead of original pink; violet instead of original white*
Capnographic monitor	[CO_2]—peak inspiration, near 0 mm Hg	[CO_2] → 0 mm Hg (could also result from other causes; e.g., dysfunctional expiratory unidirectional valve)

Adapted from Sirois M: Principles and practice of veterinary technology, ed 3, St Louis, 2011, Mosby.
*May not occur in small patients and returns to original color in a few hours.

- The unidirectional valves maintain one-way flow of gases within the breathing circuit.
- The inhalation or inspiratory unidirectional valve opens so that fresh gas and anesthetic can flow to the patient; the exhalation or expiratory valve passes through the carbon dioxide absorbent before reaching the patient again.
- Corrugated inspiratory and expiratory breathing tubes carry the anesthetic gases to and from the patient.
  - Each tube is connected to a unidirectional valve at one end and the Y piece at the other end. Standard breathing tubes are 22 mm in diameter and 1 m long for small animal patients weighing 7 to 135 kg.
  - Shorter 15-mm-diameter tubes are preferred for patients weighing less than 7 kg.
- The classic setup uses separate inhalation and exhalation tubes connected via a Y piece to the ETT adapter.
- The air intake valve admits room air to the circuit in the event that negative pressure (a partial vacuum) is detected in the breathing circuit, a situation indicated by a collapsed reservoir bag.
- An air intake valve can be present on some machines either separately or integrated into the inspiratory unidirectional valve or pop-off valve.

Nonrebreathing Circuits
- Nonrebreathing circuits do not have a carbon dioxide absorber; exhaled gases are immediately vented from the system through another hose, usually into a reservoir bag, where the gases are released into the scavenging system through an overflow valve.
- Nonrebreathing systems do not resist air; they are recommended for patients less than 7 kg in body weight so that work required to breathe is minimized.
- As with the rebreathing system, the oxygen or nitrous oxide enters the circuit from the tank, through the flow meter, and into the vaporizer, but instead of the fresh gas passing into the circle, as with a rebreathing system, the fresh gas goes directly to the patient.
  - The carbon dioxide absorber canister, pressure manometer, and unidirectional valves are not present in a nonbreathing circuit.
- Nonrebreathing circuits used in veterinary medicine include the Mapleson A (Magill and Lack circuits), modified Mapleson D (Bain coaxial circuit), Mapleson E (Ayre's T-piece and Bain circuits), and Mapleson F circuits (Jackson-Rees' modification of Ayre's T-piece circuit and Norman mask elbow), and the Humphrey ADE circuit, which can switch among Mapleson A, D, and E circuits (Fig. 7.14).

ANESTHESIA

Preanesthetic Medication
- Preanesthetic medication is usually beneficial to the patient and should be considered for all patients.

- Selection of preanesthetics is based on the patient's health status, not on the surgical procedure.
- Various drugs are used for premedication, including calming agents, analgesics, and anticholinergics.

Induction
- A primary goal of proper anesthetic technique is to provide maximum safety for the patient and personnel.
- Recognize that induction is short-term general anesthesia and induction agents are frequently used alone to perform short surgical or diagnostic procedures.
- When gas anesthesia is to be used, anesthetic induction is the transition from the conscious preanesthetic state to the level of anesthesia at which the patient may be intubated.
- It is important to minimize or avoid personnel exposure to anesthetic waste gases (Box 7.2). Anesthetic techniques have evolved to avoid specific problems that were previously encountered.
- Several methods are used for induction before inhalation anesthesia; each has its advantages and disadvantages.
- IV administration of the induction agent is preferred in most cases.
- Anesthetic induction may proceed after a vein is catheterized, the equipment is readied, and the surgeon is available.
- Administration of the induction or maintenance agent should provide a smooth and safe transition to unconsciousness.
- When jaw muscle tone and orolaryngeal reflexes are lost, intubate the patient.

Endotracheal Intubation in Dogs and Cats
- Dogs and cats are placed in a sternal position, with the head and neck extended in a straight line to aid visualization of the larynx.
- The veterinary assistant will position the head by grasping the maxilla behind the canine teeth while the anesthetist places the ETT.
- Lubrication of the cuff with sterile, water-soluble lubricant facilitates intubation and protects the tracheal mucosa from drying where the inflated cuff contacts the mucosa.
- Pulling the tongue forward also helps improve visualization of the glottis.
- Once the tube is placed, the veterinary technician will attach the breathing circuit to the ETT adapter before inflating the cuff.

Maintenance of Anesthesia
- Once the patient is fully anesthetized by the inhalation anesthetic, the induction period is over and the stage of maintenance anesthesia begins.
- The amount of anesthetic needed to maintain an appropriate level of anesthesia is not a constant.

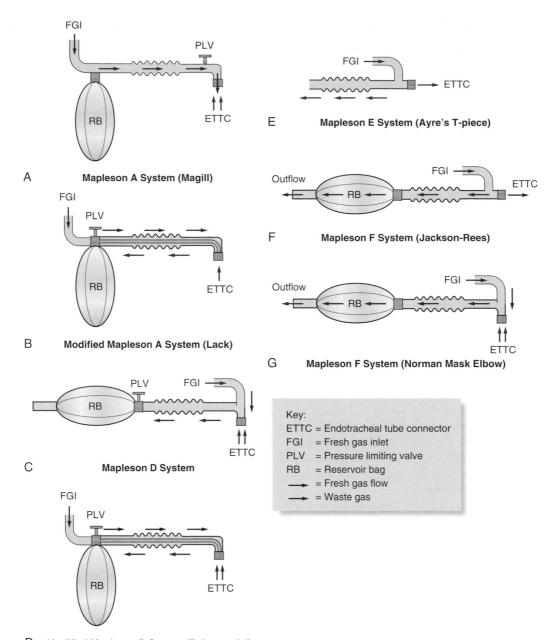

FIGURE 7.14 Nonrebreathing circuits. (From Sirois M: *Elsevier's veterinary assistant textbook*, ed 2, St Louis, 2017, Mosby.)

BOX 7.2 Techniques for Minimizing Exposure to Waste Anesthetic Gases

1. Check for and correct leaks in anesthesia machine and breathing circuit.
2. Use a cuffed endotracheal tube of the proper size; inflate the cuff if needed.
3. Do not disconnect the patient from the breathing circuit immediately after anesthesia; if possible, wait several minutes for gases to dissipate.
4. Connect pop-off valve to a scavenger system, preferably one that discharges outdoors.
5. Connect a nonrebreathing system to a scavenger system.
6. Avoid use of chamber or mask induction techniques.
7. Avoid spilling liquid anesthetic while filling the vaporizer; recap bottle and vaporizer immediately.
8. Maintain adequate ventilation of the area.

Adapted from Sirois M: *Principles and practice of veterinary technology*, ed 3, St Louis, 2011, Mosby.

BOX 7.3 Monitoring of Anesthetic Equipment

1. All anesthetic equipment should be clean, calibrated, maintained in good working order, and functionally checked before and continuously throughout the procedure. Observe the oxygen source, anesthetic machine, and breathing circuit for leaks, and check that carbon dioxide absorbent is not exhausted.
2. During anesthesia, frequently check connections to the patient and anesthetic circuit. Power sources to monitoring equipment and heat sources should be verified throughout the procedure.
3. Verify monitoring device readings with quick, simple observations, such as mucous membrane color, capillary refill time, pulse rate, and pulse quality. If the blood pressure reads zero but the mucous membranes are pink and well perfused, common sense dictates that the blood pressure reading is probably incorrect.

Adapted from Sirois M: Principles and practice of veterinary technology, ed 3, St Louis, 2011, Mosby.

- Anesthetic depth is a product of the amount of drug reaching the brain, degree of painful stimulus applied, and patient's health status.
- Once anesthesia with the inhalant agent is accomplished, the vaporizer setting and oxygen flow are reduced to maintenance levels.
- The anesthetist's attention now focuses on monitoring and support of vital organ function.
- All monitoring instruments are connected and all pertinent information recorded on the patient's anesthetic record.
- Monitoring should be continuous, and data should be recorded every 5 to 10 minutes or when significant changes occur.
- Comprehensive monitoring of the anesthetized patient involves observing anesthetic equipment and evaluating the central nervous system (CNS), pulmonary function, and cardiovascular function.
- Early detection of equipment failure and/or depression of vital organ function allow for the execution of corrective measures, which are more effective than treating complications (Box 7.3).
- Corrective actions to maintain or restore tissue perfusion are determined by integrating information from all body systems.
- The most essential monitor is a well-prepared, highly skilled individual performing continuous monitoring.

Monitoring Physiologic Conditions

- The patient's physiologic conditions are monitored to ensure that excessive derangement of vital functions is not developing.

- A variety of equipment is available for this purpose (Table 7.7).
- The patient's heart rate, heart sounds, pulse quality and rate, mucous membrane color, and capillary refill time are also regularly monitored and recorded.
- Auscultation of the heart while simultaneously palpating the peripheral pulse is an excellent method of recognizing pulse deficits that may result from cardiac arrhythmias.

SURGICAL ASSISTING

- The veterinary technician serves as the sterile surgical assistant and must don a sterile gown and gloves when entering the surgical suite.
- The veterinary assistant serves as the circulating assistant (nonsterile) and should be available to place needed supplies and equipment on the Mayo stand.
- All personnel should have their cap and mask on before placing sterile items on the Mayo stand.
- Materials should be opened facing away from the body and allowed to fall on the stand so that the assistant's arms are not directly over the top of the Mayo stand.
- The surgical assistant should arrange the instruments and supplies on the Mayo stand before the start of surgery.
- The assistant may also be responsible for operating the surgical suction and passing and holding instruments for the surgeon.
- The assistant must be familiar with the procedure to be performed and be able to anticipate the instruments and supplies that the surgeon may need.
- The veterinary assistant may also be responsible for ensuring that the surgical lighting is focused on the surgical site.
- When a body cavity is opened, sponges should be counted at the beginning of the procedure (before the first incision) and before closure to ensure that none have been inadvertently left in the body cavity.
- Contaminated instruments or soiled sponges should not be placed back on the instrument table.

Draping and Organizing the Instrument Table
Organizing the Instrument Table

- Instrument tables should be height-adjustable to allow them to be positioned within reach of surgical personnel.
- The instrument packs should not be opened until the animal has been positioned on the surgical table and draped.
- Large, water-impermeable table drapes should be used to cover the entire instrument table. To open these drapes, the drape and outer wrap are positioned on the instrument table, the exposed undersurface of the drape is gently grasped, and the ends and then the sides are unfolded.
- Once the drape has been opened, nonsterile personnel should not reach over it.

TABLE 7.7 Monitoring Equipment Used in Veterinary Medicine

Monitoring Device	Overview	Concerns
Stethoscope	Always accessible; evaluates heart rate (HR), rhythm, and sounds	More difficult to hear beat in anesthetized patient
Esophageal stethoscope	Amplifies heartbeat, audible from a distance, can alert to possible arrhythmia, inexpensive	Does not give quantitative information; if sounds are muffled, difficult to hear; complicated if mouth or throat surgery
Electrocardiograph	Monitors HR and rhythm	Heart can stop beating even though electrical activity continues
Pulse oximeter	Detects changes in oxygen saturation of hemoglobin by calculating the difference between levels of oxygenated and deoxygenated blood; also determines HR; during oxygenation saturation, level should be >95%; probe transmissive—place over nonpigmented skin that allows light transmission (e.g., tongue, lip) or reflective (in hollow organ; rectum or esophagus)	To help minimize signal loss, light source must be oriented toward the tissue; decreased signal strength in hypotension, hypothermia, and altered vascular resistance; inaccurate if carboxyhemoglobin or methemoglobin is present
Apnea monitor	Sensor placed between ETT connector and breathing circuit; audible beep is heard when the patient breathes, and the difference in temperature between warm expired and cold inspired air is monitored; will hear an alarm if no breath for a preset time period	Increased mechanical dead space can be a problem in smaller animals if not using a special ETT connector; does not warn of inadequate respiratory depth; alarm may sound with decreased tidal volume (V_T) or hypothermic patient
Ultrasonic Doppler	Monitors HR and rhythm by detecting flow of blood through small arteries; converts into an audible beep; when combined with cuff and sphygmomanometer, can indirectly determine systolic BP; fairly accurate in dogs	Must clip hair, cover skin with ultrasonic gel, be parallel to and directly over artery, and use firm contact; if using cuff, must be 30%–50% of circumference of the extremity; manually performed so is labor-intensive; probe is expensive and easily damaged; underestimates systolic BP in cats by 15 mm Hg; prone to artifacts and technical problems such as movement, shivering, contact pressure
Oscillometric BP monitor	Monitors HR and indirect BP; cuff with an internal pressure-sensing bladder is placed around tail or leg, then connected to computerized base that automatically inflates and deflates the cuff and interprets the signals sent by machine; more expensive but measures BP automatically and, in addition to systolic pressure, notes diastolic and MAP	Expensive and not as accurate in animals <7 kg; also prone to artifacts and technical problems as well as hypotension, tachycardia, and arrhythmias; best to keep the cuff at the same horizontal plane as the heart; inaccurate at low BPs
Capnometer	Determines respiratory rate and end-tidal CO_2 by estimating partial CO_2 in bloodstream at the end of expiration, when CO_2 levels of the expired gas are approximately equal to alveolar and arterial CO_2 ($Paco_2$); the fitting is placed between ETT and breathing circuit; monitor measures CO_2 in inspired and expired air; one of the best indicators of adequate respiration; levels for anesthetized patients should be 40–45 mm Hg	Abnormal readings if lung, cardiovascular, or tissue disease; hypoventilation; abnormal breathing problems; or malfunctioning equipment; interpretation of capnogram is complex; levels higher than normal indicate hypoventilation; lower levels indication of hyperventilation
Central venous pressure	Monitors hydration and efficacy of fluid therapy by inserting catheter into anterior vena cava; catheter is connected to water manometer for measurement of mean right arterial pressure	Invasive; best used in conjunction with other parameters and to monitor trends; zero mark of manometer must be at level of distal catheter tip

Adapted from Sirois M: Principles and practice of veterinary technology, ed 3, St Louis, 2011, Mosby.
Note: If alarm signals occur when using monitoring equipment, it is important to confirm by physically examining the patient.
MAP, Mean arterial pressure.

- Mayo stands are often used in procedures that require additional instruments (e.g., bone plating); specially designed Mayo stand covers are available to cover these tables.
- The instrument layout is generally determined by the surgeon's preference, but grouping similar instruments (e.g., scissors, retractors) facilitates their use.

Draping

- Once the animal has been positioned and the skin prepared, the animal is ready to be draped. The drapes maintain a sterile field around the operative site.
- If electrocautery is being used, sufficient time should elapse between skin preparation and application of the drapes to permit complete evaporation of flammable substances (e.g., alcohol) from the skin.
- If an abdominal incision extends to the pubis in males, the prepuce should be clamped to one side with a sterile towel clamp.
- Draping is performed by a gowned and gloved surgical team member (veterinarian and/or veterinary technician) and begins with placement of field drapes (quarter drapes) to isolate the unprepared portion of the animal.
  - These towels should be placed one at a time at the periphery of the prepared area.
  - Field (quarter) drapes may be lint-free towels or disposable nonabsorbent towels.
- Drapes should not be flipped, fanned, or shaken because rapid movement of drapes creates air currents onto which dust, lint, and droplet nuclei can migrate.
- Drapes, supplies, and equipment extending over or dropping below the table level should be considered nonsterile because they are not within the surgeon's visual field and their sterility cannot be verified.
- Towels are secured at the corners with Backhaus towel clamps.
- When the animal and incision site are protected by field drapes, final draping can be performed.
  - A large drape is placed over the animal by the veterinarian or veterinary technician and the entire surgical table to provide a continuous sterile field.
- Cloth drapes should have an appropriately sized and positioned opening that can be placed over the incision site while the drape covers the remaining surfaces.

Unwrapping or Opening Sterile Items

Unwrapping Sterile Linen or Paper Packs

- If you are right-handed, hold the pack in your left hand (and vice versa).
- Using the right hand, unfold one corner of the outside wrap at a time, being careful to secure each corner in the palm of the left hand to keep it from recoiling and contaminating the contents; hold the final corner with your right hand.
- When the pack is fully exposed and all corners of the wrap secured, gently pass the pack to sterile personnel or set the pack on the table cover, being careful not to allow your hand and arm to reach across or over the sterile field.

Unwrapping Sterile Items in Paper or Plastic or Plastic Peel-Back Pouches

- Identify the edges of the peel-back wrapper and carefully separate them.
- Peel the edges of the wrapper back slowly and symmetrically to ensure that the sterile item does not contact the torn edge of the wrapper, which is nonsterile.
- If the item is small, place it on the sterile area as described, being careful not to lean across the sterile table.
- If the item is long or cumbersome, have a sterile team member grasp it and gently pull it from the peel-back wrapper, taking care not to brush the item against the peeled edge of the wrapper.

RECOVERY

- Recovery means to restore to a normal state; it begins when the administration of anesthetic is discontinued.
- Pain relief and maintenance of a patent airway are important during recovery.
- The critical period has passed when the body temperature is normal, sternal recumbency is achieved, and oropharyngeal reflexes are restored.
- Observation should continue until the patient can stand and is free of all drug effects.
- When recovering, the patient should be maintained on 100% oxygen to ensure oxygenation and allow exhaled anesthetic gases to enter the scavenger system rather than the room air.
- As the patient begins to awaken, the ETT cuff should be deflated and the tie undone.
- When the patient exhibits swallowing reflexes, the ETT should be gently removed.
- Recovery is considered adequate, but not complete, when the body temperature is normal, the patient's vital signs are stable, and sternal recumbency is maintained.
- Observation should continue until the patient can stand and walk without assistance.

Postoperative Evaluation

- The postoperative period should be considered critical for all patients.
- Because of the possibility of unforeseen complications, it is essential that patients be continually monitored after any type of surgery.
- After surgery, every patient should have its rectal temperature measured hourly until it reaches 100°F (37.8°C) and then every 4 to 12 hours based on orders prepared by the doctor.
- A 1° or 2°F increase in rectal temperature for the first few postoperative days is a normal physiologic response to the trauma of major surgery.

- A higher or more prolonged temperature increase may indicate infection.
- Daily monitoring of a surgical patient's body weight provides a measure of the animal's nutritional status and general body condition.
- One of the most frequently neglected aspects of postoperative patient care is provision of adequate nutrition.
- The healing process after surgery increases an animal's nutritional needs, particularly for protein.
- An animal's behavior during the immediate postoperative period can yield important information about the amount of pain it is enduring and possible complications that might be developing.
- If a patient is depressed, the reasons for that state must be determined and appropriate treatment quickly instituted.
- Surgical patients must receive adequate nutrition and fluid intake.
- Animals should begin eating and drinking as soon as possible after surgery. Opioid medications used for pain control may reduce appetite, so encouragement or temptation to eat is sometimes needed by postoperative patients.
- Elimination patterns provide important information about kidney and gastrointestinal (GI) tract function in patients recovering from surgery.
- GI motility and defecation may be reduced if opioids are used for pain management, but this should resolve within 1 or 2 days of discontinuing the medications.

Appearance of the Surgical Wound

- The surgical incision should be examined at least daily by visual inspection as well as gentle palpation during the immediate postoperative period.
- Abnormalities such as excessive or prolonged bleeding, fluid accumulation, dramatic inflammation, and impending dehiscence (opening) of the surgical wound can be detected and corrected early if the incision is carefully evaluated.

Pain Management

- **Pain** is defined as an unpleasant sensory or emotional experience associated with actual or potential tissue damage.
- Physiologic pain results from the stimulation of nerve endings called nociceptors, which are found throughout the tissues.
- Pain may be classified as peripheral, neuropathic, clinical, or idiopathic.
- Nociception (detection of painful stimuli) is different from pain.
- General anesthesia controls the perception of intraoperative pain.
- Unconsciousness or unresponsiveness is not lack of pain; nociception still occurs.
- Pain recognition is difficult because responses to pain vary among species and individuals. Some individuals tolerate considerable discomfort without any reaction;

BOX 7.4 Signs of Pain

1. Changes in behavior and temperament (e.g., shunning or seeking attention, postural changes, inappetence, changes in voiding behavior, reluctance to move, unusual gait)
2. Protection of the affected area (avoids touching; threatens if approached)
3. Vocalization (especially on movement or palpation of affected area)
4. Licking or biting affected area
5. Scratching or shaking affected area
6. Restlessness, pacing
7. Sweating
8. Tachycardia, hyperpnea, peripheral vasoconstriction, muscle tension, hypertension

From Sirois M: Principles and practice of veterinary technology, ed 3, St Louis, 2011, Mosby.

---

other individuals vocalize loudly when given a minor injection (Box 7.4).
- Obvious inflammation (e.g., redness, swelling, heat) is generally accompanied by pain. Animals recovering from anesthesia are not able to exhibit a normal range of behavioral signs and may be experiencing pain long before it becomes apparent to the observer.
- Pain is more easily managed if analgesics are given preemptively, before a patient experiences pain.

Pain Relief Modalities

- Pain relief modalities take advantage of one or more means of preventing or interfering with the development or perception of pain.
- Most of the drugs used for analgesia (pain relief) cause various other dose-dependent effects. The opioid analgesic agents produce a dose-dependent sedation (called narcosis) that may be profound.
- The nonsteroidal antiinflammatory drugs (NSAIDs), especially the older ones, tend to cause GI irritation, ulceration, and bleeding.
- Analgesic agents are needed to suppress the physiologic pain mechanisms that remain active during anesthesia.
- Using several analgesic drugs, each with a different mechanism of action, is called multimodal therapy. This results in lower dosages, which increases safety.

Postoperative Complications

Hemorrhage

- If not quickly corrected, postoperative hemorrhage can lead to serious consequences for an animal, even death from shock.
- External hemorrhage is usually relatively easy to evaluate and control because it is easily visible.
- Internal hemorrhage is not readily apparent and therefore often more serious. An animal can bleed to death

through hemorrhage into the abdominal or thoracic cavity.

- The status of an animal's cardiovascular system should be frequently monitored during the immediate postoperative period for signs that might indicate hemorrhage.

Seroma and Hematoma

- Seromas (accumulations of serum) and hematomas (accumulations of blood) beneath the surgical incision are usually caused by dead space left in the incision that the body naturally fills with fluid.
- Small seromas and hematomas are usually of cosmetic importance only, unless the skin sutures tear out.
- Larger seromas or hematomas may be treated with warm compresses, drainage of the fluid via needle and syringe, and possibly application of a pressure bandage.

Infection

- A persistently or drastically elevated rectal temperature, depressed attitude, poor appetite, or swollen, inflamed incision are all signs of possible postoperative infection.
- Postoperative infections can be superficial, subcutaneous, within a body cavity, or spread throughout the body.
- Superficial infection often results in a draining wound that does not heal well.
- Subcutaneous infections frequently progress to abscess formation. Infection in the abdominal cavity (peritonitis) or thoracic cavity (pleuritis) often results from a penetrating injury or damage to organs in that body cavity.
- Septicemia is a generalized infection that spreads via the bloodstream.

Wound Dehiscence

- Wound dehiscence (disruption of the surgical wound) is one of the most common and serious postoperative complications that can occur. Possible causes of wound dehiscence include the following:
  - Suture failure (loosening, untying, breakage)
  - Infection
  - Tissue weakness (e.g., old or debilitated animals, hyperadrenocorticism, prolonged corticosteroid use)
  - Mechanical stress (e.g., stormy anesthetic recovery, chronic vomiting, chronic cough, excessive activity)
  - Poor nutrition
- Early signs of surgical wound dehiscence are frequently seen within the first 3 or 4 days after surgery.
  - They may include a serosanguineous discharge from the incision, firm or fluctuant swelling deep to (under) the suture line, and palpation of a hernial ring or loop of bowel beneath the skin.
- If only the muscle layer of an abdominal incision breaks down and the skin sutures remain intact, a doughy swelling can be palpated under the skin.

- A bandage should be applied for support, and the suture line should be repaired as soon as possible.
- If both the muscle layer and skin sutures of an abdominal incision break down, the animal can eviscerate (abdominal organs protrude through suture line).
- If evisceration occurs, the involved organs can become bruised and grossly contaminated, and may even be mutilated by the animal itself.
  - This is an acute emergency that must be attended to immediately.
- Carefully gather the exteriorized viscera in a towel moistened with physiologic saline and hold them in place near the incision while others prepare the animal and operating room for the repair.

SUTURE REMOVAL

- Skin incisions are often closed with nonabsorbable suture material.
- These sutures are removed once healing is sufficient to prevent wound dehiscence, usually after 10 to 14 days.
- Skin suture removal is begun by grasping one or both of the suture ends, which were deliberately left long for that purpose, and pulling the knot away from the skin.
- Using suture removal scissors, cut one of the two strands of suture beneath the knot at the skin surface and pull the suture out.
- Skin staples are removed with specially designed staple removers.

RECOMMENDED READINGS

Anonymous: Commentary and recommendations on control of waste anesthetic gases in the workplace, *J Am Vet Med Assoc* 209: 75–77, 1996.

Bassert JM, Thomas J: *McCurnin's clinical textbook for veterinary technicians,* ed 8, St Louis, 2014, Saunders.

Clarke K, Trim C, Hall L: *Veterinary anaesthesia,* ed 11, St Louis, 2014, Saunders.

Fossum TW: *Small animal surgery textbook,* ed 4, St Louis, 2013, Mosby.

Gaynor J, Muir W: *Handbook of veterinary pain management,* ed 3, St Louis, 2014, Elsevier.

Muir WW, Hubbell JAE: *Equine anesthesia: Monitoring and emergency therapy,* ed 2, St Louis, 2008, Mosby.

Muir WW, Hubbell JAE, Skard R, et al.: *Handbook of veterinary anesthesia,* ed 5, St Louis, 2012, Mosby.

Riebold TW: *Large animal anesthesia: Principles and techniques,* ed 2, Ames, 1995, Iowa State University Press.

Sonsthagen TF: *Veterinary instruments and equipment,* ed 3, St Louis, 2013, Mosby.

Tear M: *Small animal surgical nursing: Skills and concepts,* ed 2, St Louis, 2011, Mosby.

Thomas JA, Lerche P: *Anesthesia and analgesia for veterinary technicians,* ed 4, St Louis, 2011, Mosby.

CHAPTER 8 Laboratory Procedures

CHAPTER OUTLINE

KEY TERMS

Acariasis
Arthropod
Azotemia
Bacilli
Centesis
Cestode
Cocci
Control serum
Definitive host

Dermatophyte
Differential white blood
   cell count
Ectoparasite
Electrolyte
ELISA
Endoparasite
Granulocyte
Hemolysis

Icterus
Intermediate host
Lipemia
Microfilaria
Mycology
Myiasis
Oocyst
Packed cell volume
Pediculosis

Polychromasia
Precision
Preprandial samples
Refractometer
Specific gravity
Thrombocyte
Trematode
Urolithiasis
Warble

LEARNING OBJECTIVES

After reviewing this chapter, the reader will be able to:

1. Describe methods used to collect samples for laboratory examination.
2. Describe the preparation of diagnostic samples for laboratory examination.
3. List and describe common procedures used for hematologic examinations.
4. List and describe methods for evaluation of hemostasis in dogs and cats.
5. List and describe equipment needed for clinical chemistry and serology testing.
6. List and describe the types of tests used in clinical chemistry testing.
7. List the biochemical assays commonly performed to asses liver, kidney, and pancreatic function.
8. List the types of immunologic tests and describe the principles used in those tests.
9. Discuss methods used to verify the accuracy of laboratory test results.
10. List and describe methods used to collect samples of body tissues and fluids for laboratory examination.
11. List and describe microbiologic tests commonly performed to identify bacterial and fungal pathogens.
12. List tests commonly performed for analyzing urine specimens.
13. List common internal parasites of dogs and cats.
14. List common external parasites of dogs and cats.
15. Describe procedures used to diagnose parasites.

INTRODUCTION

- Veterinarians depend on laboratory results to help establish diagnoses, track the course of diseases, and offer prognoses to clients.
- Veterinary assistants are often involved in aiding the veterinary technician with the collection and preparation of samples.
- The veterinary assistant must have a thorough knowledge of procedures and equipment used, as well as general knowledge about the tests performed.
- The veterinary practice laboratory can be a significant source of income for the practice. Rapid availability of test results improves patient care and client service.

LABORATORY DESIGN

- The veterinary clinical laboratory should be located in an area that is separate from other hospital operations.
- The area must be well lit and large enough to accommodate laboratory equipment, as well as provide a comfortable work area.
- Countertop space must be sufficient so that sensitive equipment such as chemistry analyzers and cell counters can be physically separated from centrifuges and water baths.
- Room temperature controls should provide a consistent environment, which in turn provides for optimal quality control.
- A draft-free area is preferable to one with open windows or with air conditioning or heating ducts blowing air onto the area.
  - Drafts can carry dust, which may contaminate specimens and interfere with test results.
- The laboratory area needs a sink and a source of running water to provide a place to rinse, drain, and/or stain specimens and reagents and to discard fluids.

- Handling and disposing of hazardous laboratory materials entail legal and ethical responsibilities that have increased substantially in recent decades.
- Adequate storage space must be available for reagents and supplies to avoid clutter on the laboratory counter space.
- Drawers and cabinets should be available so that needed supplies and equipment are conveniently located near the site at which they will be used.
- Some reagents and specimens must be kept refrigerated or frozen.
  - A compact countertop refrigerator is sufficient for most practice laboratories.
  - For long-term storage of fluid samples (e.g., serum, plasma), a chest freezer or freezer that is not self-defrosting should be used.
    - Frost-free freezers remove fluid from frozen samples, making them more concentrated if they are left in the freezer too long.
- Sufficient electrical outlets and circuit breakers must be available; circuits must not be overloaded with ungrounded three-prong adapters or extension cords.
  - An uninterruptible power supply may be necessary if sensitive equipment will be used or if the practice is located in an area subject to frequent power outages.
- The diagnostic laboratory should have Internet access in the laboratory or at another location in the veterinary clinic.
  - Many reference laboratories use email or fax to report the critical results of submitted diagnostic tests.
  - Photographic images such as scanned microscopic images of blood smears and urine sediments may be sent as email attachments to an outside reference laboratory for diagnostic assistance.
  - The Internet also may be a valuable resource for veterinary medical information.

- Two basic determinants are used to assess website quality.
- First, high-quality Internet sites are unbiased—the group providing the information should not have a vested interest (e.g., selling a product) in slanting the information a certain way.
- Second, sources should be staffed by recognized experts in the field, such as those from a government agency, college, or university diagnostic laboratory, or the American Veterinary Medical Association.
- Other signs of the quality of a website include the following:
  - Funding and sponsorship are clearly shown.
  - Timeliness (date of posting, revising, and updating) is clear and easy to locate.
  - Information about the source (e.g., the organization's mission statement) is clear and easy to find.
  - Authors or contributors to references on the site are clearly identified.
  - References and sources for information are listed.
  - Experts have reviewed the site's content for accuracy and completeness.

Safety Concerns and Supplies

- A comprehensive laboratory safety program is essential for ensuring the safety of employees in the clinical laboratory area.
- The Occupational Safety and Health Administration (OSHA) mandates specific laboratory practices that must be incorporated into the laboratory safety policy.
- The safety policy should include procedures and precautions for the use and maintenance of equipment.
- Safety equipment and supplies, such as eyewash stations, fire extinguishers, spill clean-up kits, hazardous and biohazard waste disposal containers, and protective gloves, must be available.
- All employees working in the clinical laboratory must be aware of the location of these items and thoroughly trained in their use.
- Laboratory safety policies must be in writing and placed in an accessible location in the clinical laboratory area.
- Signs should be posted to notify employees that eating, drinking, applying cosmetics, and adjusting contact lenses in the laboratory are prohibited.

LABORATORY MEASUREMENTS AND MATHEMATICS

- Veterinary staff members must have knowledge and skill to perform a variety of calculations in the clinical laboratory.
- Reagent solutions might need to be prepared or diluted, samples must be measured and sometimes diluted, and results must be calculated.
- Concentrations of dilutions are usually expressed as ratios of the original volume to the new volume.

- A ratio is the amount of one number relative to another or the number of parts relative to a whole.
- Ratios may be written in a number of ways—for example, $\frac{1}{2} = 1:2 = 0.5$.
  - These terms express the ratio that is one in two, or one to two, or one half; all three ratios are equal.
- The terms of a ratio are abstract numbers (no units) or of the same unit.
- The only ratio usually expressed as a decimal in veterinary technology is specific gravity.
  - Specific gravity is a ratio expressed in decimal form that represents the weight of a substance relative to the weight of the same volume of water.
- To prepare a 1:10 dilution of a patient sample, combine 10 microliters (μL) of sample with 90 μL of distilled water.
  - This represents a dilution that is 10:100, which reduces mathematically to 1:10.
  - Results from any tests on this 1:10 dilution must then be multiplied by 10 to yield the correct result for the undiluted sample.
- Serial dilutions are sometimes needed when performing certain immunologic tests or when preparing manual calibration curves for some equipment.
  - The dilutions are prepared as described, and the concentration of substance in each dilution is calculated.
  - For example, if a standard solution of bilirubin contains 20 mg/dL and is diluted 1:5, 1:10, and 1:20, the concentration of each dilution would then be 4 mg/dL, 2 mg/dL, and 1 mg/dL, respectively.

EQUIPMENT AND INSTRUMENTATION

- The size of the veterinary practice and the tests routinely performed in the laboratory determine the equipment and instrumentation needed.
- Minimal equipment includes a microscope, refractometer, microhematocrit centrifuge, and clinical centrifuge.
- Additional instrumentation needed, including blood chemistry analyzers, cell counters, and incubators, depends on the type and size of the practice, geographic location of the practice, and special interests of practice personnel.

Microscope

- A high-quality binocular, compound, light microscope is essential, even in the smallest laboratory (Fig. 8.1).
- It may be used to evaluate blood, urine, semen, exudates, and transudates; other body fluids; and feces to detect internal and external parasites and initially characterize bacteria and other miscellaneous specimens.
- A compound light microscope is so named because it generates an image by using a combination of lenses.
- The mechanical stage holds a glass slide to be evaluated and allows it to be manipulated up and down and side to side.

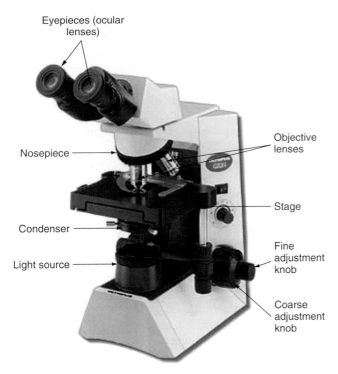

Eyepieces (ocular lenses)

Nosepiece

Condenser

Light source

Objective lenses

Stage

Fine adjustment knob

Coarse adjustment knob

FIGURE 8.1 Binocular microscope for use in the veterinary clinical laboratory. (From Sirois M: *Principles and practice of veterinary technology*, ed 3, St Louis, 2011, Mosby.)

- Coarse- and fine-focus knobs are used to focus the image of the object being viewed.
- The compound light microscope consists of two separate lens systems: the ocular system and the objective system.
- The ocular lenses are located in the eyepieces and most often have a magnification of 10×.
- A monocular microscope has one eyepiece, whereas a binocular microscope, the most commonly used type, has two eyepieces.
  - A binocular head is needed for almost all routine laboratory evaluations.
- Most compound light microscopes have three or four objective lenses, each with a different magnification power.
  - The most common objective lenses are 4× (scanning), 10× (low power), 40× (high dry), and 100× (oil immersion).
  - The scanning lens is not found on all microscopes.
  - An optional fifth lens, a 50× (low oil immersion), is found on some microscopes.
- Total magnification of the object being viewed is calculated by multiplying the ocular magnification power by the objective magnification power.
  - For example, an object viewed under the 40× objective through a 10× ocular lens is 400 times larger in diameter than the unmagnified object.
- The microscope head supports the ocular lenses and may be straight or inclined.

- A microscope with an inclined head has ocular lenses that point back toward the user. This minimizes the need to bend over the microscope to look through the lenses.
- The nosepiece holds the objective lenses and should always rotate easily and provide ready access to the objective lenses for cleaning.
- When viewed through a compound light microscope, an object appears upside down and reversed.
  - The actual right side of an image is seen as its left side, and the actual left side is seen as its right side.
- Movement of the slide by the mechanical stage also is reversed; when the stage is moved to the left, the object appears to move to the right.
- The substage condenser consists of two lenses that focus light from the light source onto the object being viewed.
  - Light is focused by raising or lowering the condenser.
- The aperture diaphragm is usually an iris type, consisting of a number of leaves that are opened or closed to control the amount of light illuminating the object.
- The most common light sources found on compound light microscopes are low-voltage tungsten lamps or higher-quality quartz halogen lamps.
- The light source has a rheostat to adjust intensity.
- Regardless of the features of the individual microscope, care must be taken to follow the manufacturer's recommendations for use and routine maintenance.
- Only high-quality lens tissue should be used to clean the lenses.
- If cleaning solvent is needed, methanol can be used, or a specially formulated lens cleaning solution can be purchased.
- Excess oil may require the use of xylene for cleaning.
- The microscope should be wiped clean after each use and kept covered when not in use.
- A dirty field of study may be caused by debris on the eyepiece.
  - The eyepieces should be rotated one at a time while looking through them; if the debris also rotates, it is located on the eyepiece.
- Cleaning and adjustment by a microscope professional should be performed at least annually.
- Changing a light bulb requires turning off the power and unplugging the microscope.
  - When the defective bulb has cooled, it should be removed and replaced with a new bulb according to the manufacturer's instructions.
  - Replacement bulbs should be identical to those that they are replacing.
  - Avoid touching the replacement bulb directly because oils from the skin can shorten the life of the bulbs.
- Locate the microscope in an area in which it is protected from excessive heat and humidity and where it cannot be moved frequently, jarred by vibrations from centrifuges or slamming doors, or splashed with liquids.

Centrifuge

- The centrifuge is used to separate substances of different densities that are in a solution.
- When solid and liquid components are present in the sample, the liquid portion is referred to as the supernatant and the solid component is referred to as the sediment.
  - The supernatant, such as plasma or serum from a blood sample, can be removed from the sediment and stored, shipped, or analyzed.
- A microhematocrit centrifuge is designed to hold capillary tubes, whereas a clinical centrifuge accommodates test tubes of varying sizes.
- Clinical centrifuges used in veterinary laboratories are one of two types, depending on the style of the centrifuge head.
- A horizontal centrifuge head, also known as the swinging arm type, has specimen cups that hang vertically when the centrifuge is at rest.
  - During centrifugation, the cups swing out to the horizontal position.
  - As the specimen is centrifuged, centrifugal force drives the particles through the liquid to the bottom of the tube.
  - When the centrifuge stops, the specimen cups fall back to the vertical position.
- The second type of centrifuge head available is the angled centrifuge head.
  - The specimen tubes are inserted through drilled holes that hold the tubes at a fixed angle, usually approximately 52 degrees.
  - This type of centrifuge rotates at higher speeds than the horizontal head centrifuge, without excessive heat buildup.
  - The angled centrifuge head is usually configured to accommodate just one tube size.
  - Smaller-sized tubes require the use of an adaptor unless a small-capacity centrifuge is available.
  - Microhematocrit centrifuges are a type of angled centrifuge; the microhematocrit centrifuge is configured to accommodate capillary tubes.
- In addition to a standard on–off switch, most centrifuges have a timer that automatically turns the centrifuge off after a preset time.
- A tachometer or dial to set the speed of the centrifuge is also usually present.
- Some centrifuges do not have a tachometer and always run at maximal speed.
- Most centrifuges have speed dials calibrated in revolutions per minute (rpm) times 1000; thus a dial setting of 5 represents 5000 rpm.
- The centrifuge brake should only be used in cases of equipment malfunction when the centrifuge must be stopped quickly.
- The centrifuge should never be operated with the lid unlatched.

- Always load the centrifuge with the open ends of tubes toward the center of the centrifuge head.
- Tubes must be counterbalanced with tubes of equal size and weight; water-filled tubes may be used to balance the centrifuge.
- The operator's manual should list maintenance schedules of the different components of the centrifuge.
- Some centrifuges require periodic lubrication of the bearings.
- Most need the brushes to be checked or replaced regularly.
- Specimens must be centrifuged for a specific time at a specific speed for maximum accuracy.
- A centrifuge that is run too fast or for too long may rupture cells and destroy the morphologic features of cells in the sediment.
- A centrifuge that is run too slowly or for less than the proper time may not completely separate the specimen or concentrate the sediment.
- Information regarding speed and time of centrifugation should be developed for all laboratory procedures and followed for maximum accuracy.

Refractometer

- A refractometer, or total solids meter, is used to measure the refractive index of a solution.
- Refraction is the bending of light rays as they pass from one medium (e.g., air) into another medium (e.g., urine) with a different optical density.
- The degree of refraction is a function of the concentration of solid material in the medium.
- Refractometers are calibrated to a zero reading (zero refractive index) with distilled water at a temperature between 60° and 100°F (15.6° and 37.8°C).
- The most common uses of the refractometer are determination of the specific gravity of urine or other fluids and the protein concentration of plasma or other fluids.
- The refractometer has a built-in prism and calibration scale.
- Although refractometers can measure the refractive index of any solution, the scale readings in the instrument have been calibrated in terms of specific gravity and protein concentrations (in g/dL).
- The specific gravity or protein concentration of a solution is directly proportional to its concentration of dissolved substances.
- Because no solution can be more dilute or have a lower concentration of dissolved substances than distilled water, the scale calibration and readings (specific gravity or protein concentration) are always greater than zero.
- The refractometer is read on the scale at the distinct light–dark interface (Fig. 8.2).
- Most refractometer models are temperature-compensated between 60° F and 100°F (15.6° and 37.8°C).
  - As long as the temperature remains between these two extremes, even as the refractometer is held in a person's hands, the temperature fluctuation will not affect the accuracy of the reading.

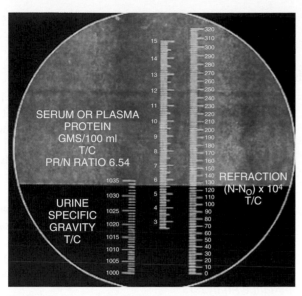

FIGURE 8.2 Reading scale in the refractometer. (From Bassert JM, McCurnin DM: *McCurnin's clinical textbook for veterinary technicians,* ed 7, St Louis, 2010, Saunders.)

- The refractometer should be cleaned after each use.
  - The prism cover glass and cover plate are wiped dry.
  - Lens tissue should be used to protect the optical surfaces from scratches.
- The refractometer should be calibrated regularly—weekly or daily—depending on use.
  - Distilled water at room temperature placed on the refractometer should have a zero refractive index and will read 1.000 on the specific gravity scale.
  - If the light–dark boundary deviates from the zero mark by more than half a division, the refractometer should be adjusted by turning the adjusting screw as directed by the manufacturer.
  - The refractometer should not be used if it has not been calibrated to zero with distilled water.

Chemistry Analyzers

- Various chemistry analyzers are available for use in the veterinary practice laboratory.
- Most chemistry analyzers used in the veterinary practice use the principles of photometry to quantify constituents found in the blood.
- Spectrophotometers are designed to measure the amount of light transmitted through a solution.
- All spectrophotometers contain a light source, prism, wavelength selector, photodetector, and readout device (Fig. 8.3).
  - The light source is typically a tungsten or halogen lamp.
  - The prism functions to fragment the light into its component wavelength segments.
  - The photodetector receives whatever light is not absorbed by the sample.
  - The photodetector signal is then transmitted to the readout device.
  - Depending on the model of the instrument, the readout units may be in percentage transmittance, percentage absorbance, optical density, or concentration units.
- A type of photometer that uses a filter to select the wavelength is referred to as a colorimeter.
- Another type is the reflectometer, which detects light reflected off a test substance rather than transmitted light.
- Some analyzers use principles of electrochemistry to determine analyte concentrations.
- A few analyzers combine electrochemical and photometric methods within self-contained cartridges.
- Electrochemical methods are primarily used for the evaluation of electrolytes and other ionic components.
  - Analyzers are designed with specific electrodes that are configured to allow interaction with just one ion.
  - The most common of these systems is known as a potentiometer.

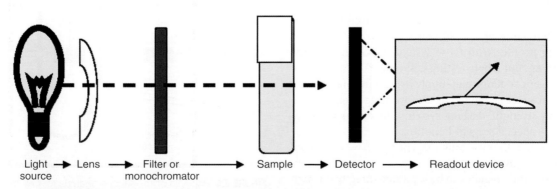

Light source → Lens → Filter or monochromator → Sample → Detector → Readout device

FIGURE 8.3 Principles of spectrophotometry. (From Hendrix CM, Sirois M: *Laboratory procedures for veterinary technicians,* ed 5, St Louis, 2007, Mosby.)

- These systems are designed so that ions diffuse across an area separated by a membrane; the difference in voltage, or electric potential, between the two sides of the membrane can be measured.
- This electrical variation corresponds to the number of active ions present in the sample.

Features and Benefits of Common Types of Chemistry Analyzers

- Most automated analyzers use liquid reagents, dry reagents, or slides that contain dry reagents.
- Dry slide reagents pose little or no handling or storage concerns but tend to be more expensive.
- Analyzers that use dry systems include those with reagent-impregnated slides, pads, or cartridges.
  - Most of these use reflectance assays.
  - They do not require reagent handling, and the performance of single tests is relatively simple.
  - Some dry systems use reagent strips similar to those used for urine chemical testing.
- Liquid systems include those that use a lyophilized (freeze-dried) reagent or an already prepared liquid reagent.
  - These analyzers are the most versatile in that they can perform profiling or single testing with relative ease.
- Liquid reagents may be purchased in bulk or in unitized disposable cuvettes.
- Dry (lyophilized) reagents are available in unitized form.
- The purchase of unitized reagents eliminates the hazards associated with handling these reagents.
- Unitized systems have the advantage of not requiring reagent handling but tend to be the most expensive of all the liquid reagent systems.
- The most common type of lyophilized reagent system for veterinary clinical practice uses rotor technology.
  - The rotors consist of individual cuvettes to which diluted samples are added.
  - Cuvettes are optical-quality reservoirs used in the photometer and may be plastic or glass.
  - Rotor-based systems tend to be accurate and are usually cost-effective for profiles but are not capable of running single tests.
- Bulk liquid reagents are the least expensive but require additional handling and storage space.
- Running profiles with these systems is somewhat time consuming, but single testing is simple.
- Bulk reagent systems may supply reagent in concentrated form that must be diluted or is of working strength.
- Working-strength reagent systems do not usually require any special reagent handling.
- Some systems that use bulk reagent may have a flow cell instead of a cuvette.
  - Sample and reagent can be aspirated directly through the analyzer without the need for transfer of the reactants into cuvettes.

- Dedicated-use analyzers are available for certain tests.
  - These analyzers sample for only one substance, such as blood glucose.

Hematology Analyzers

- Instrumentation designed for veterinary hospital use is available to facilitate the generation of hematologic data for the complete blood count (CBC).
- Instrumentation for the veterinary hospital falls into three general categories: impedance analyzers, laser-based analyzers, and the quantitative buffy coat analysis system.
  - Some manufacturers now provide analyzers that combine several methods for performing a CBC.
  - Some hematology analyzers also have photometric capabilities to determine the hemoglobin level.

Impedance Analyzers

- There are a variety of dedicated veterinary multispecies hematology systems that count cells and determine the hematocrit, hemoglobin concentration, and mean corpuscular hemoglobin concentration (MCHC).
  - Some also provide a partial white blood cell (WBC) differential count.
- Electronic cell counters that use the impedance method are based on the passage of electric current across two electrodes separated by a glass tube with a small opening or aperture (Fig. 8.4).
- Electrolyte fluid on either side of the aperture conducts the current.
- Counting occurs by moving cells through the aperture using a vacuum or positive pressure.
- Because cells are relatively poor conductors of electricity compared with the electrolyte fluid, they impede the flow of current while passing through the aperture.
- These transient changes in current may be counted to determine the blood cell concentration. In addition, the

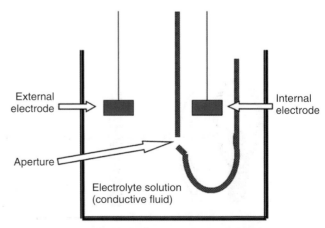

FIGURE 8.4 Principle of impedance analysis for cell counts. (From Hendrix CM, Sirois M: *Laboratory procedures for veterinary technicians*, ed 5, St Louis, 2007, Mosby.)

volume or size of the cell is proportional to the change in current, allowing the system to catalog cell sizes.

- Size information may be displayed in a distribution histogram of the cell population.
- Leukocytes, erythrocytes, and platelets may be enumerated with these systems.
- These instruments are calibrated to count cells in specified size ranges, defined by threshold settings, which prevents erroneous interpretation of small debris and electronic noise as cells, and to separate cell populations properly in the same dilution, such as platelets and erythrocytes.
- Because cell populations vary in size among species, some of the threshold settings are species specific.
- These settings should be established by the manufacturer and are usually set automatically by system software when the user selects the species for analysis in a software menu.
- Erythrocyte analysis on automated systems provides diagnostic information about cell volume and an alternative method for determining the hematocrit (Hct).
- The mean corpuscular volume (MCV) may be directly measured from analysis of the erythrocyte volume distribution.
- The hematocrit is then calculated by multiplying the MCV by the erythrocyte concentration.

Quantitative Buffy Coat System

- The quantitative buffy coat system uses differential centrifugation and estimation of cellular elements by measurements on an expanded buffy coat layer in a specialized microhematocrit tube.
- It provides a hematocrit value and estimates of leukocyte concentration and platelet concentration.
- It extrapolates tube volumes to an estimate of concentration based on fixed cell volumes.
- Partial differential count information is provided in the form of total **granulocyte** and lymphocyte and monocyte categories.
- These systems are best used as screening tools because they provide an estimation of cell numbers rather than an actual cell count.

Laser-Based Analyzers

- These types of analyzers use laser beams to determine the size and density of solid components.
- Cells scatter light differently, depending on the presence or absence of granules and nuclei.
- The degree and direction of light scatter allow the enumeration of monocytes, lymphocytes, granulocytes, and erythrocytes.
- When certain dyes are added to the sample, variations in laser light scatter can also allow the enumeration of mature and immature erythrocytes.

Incubators

- A variety of microbiology tests require the use of an incubator.

- Incubators for the in-house veterinary practice laboratory are available in a variety of sizes and configurations.
- The incubator must be capable of sustaining a constant temperature of 98.6°F (37°C).
- Heat should be provided by a thermostatically controlled element.
- A small dish of water should also be placed inside to maintain proper humidity if built-in humidity controls are not present.
- Larger laboratories may have incubators that automatically monitor temperature and humidity, as well as carbon dioxide and oxygen levels.

Pipettes

- The primary types of pipettes used in the practice laboratory are transfer pipettes and graduated pipettes.
- Transfer pipettes are used when critical volume measurements are not needed.
  - These pipettes may be plastic or glass, and some can deliver volumes by drops.
- Graduated pipettes may contain a single volume designation or have multiple gradations.
- Pipettes with single gradations are referred to as volumetric pipettes and are the most accurate of the measuring pipettes.
- Larger volumetric pipettes are usually designated as TD pipettes, which means that the pipette is designed *to* *d*eliver the specific volume.
  - A small amount of liquid should remain in the tip of the pipette after the volume has been delivered.
- Volumetric pipettes designed to deliver microliter volumes are designated TC, meaning that the pipette is designed *to* *c*ontain the specified volume.
  - These pipettes must only be used to add specified volumes to other liquids and must be rinsed with the other liquid to deliver the specified volume accurately.
- Pipettes that contain multiple gradations are marked as either TD or TD with blow out, depending on whether the fluid remaining in the tip of the pipette should remain or be blown out.
  - TD with blow-out pipettes usually contain a double-etched or frosted band at the top.
- The pipette chosen for a specific application should always be the one that is the most accurate and that measures volumes closest to the volume needed.
  - For example, a 1-mL pipette, rather than a 5-mL pipette, should be chosen if the volume needed is 0.8 mL.
- Pipettes are also designed for measuring liquids at a specified temperature, normally room temperature.
  - Liquids that are significantly colder or warmer will not measure accurately.

Quality Assurance

- Quality assurance refers to the procedures established to ensure that clinical testing is performed in compliance with accepted standards and that the process and results are properly documented.

- Without a comprehensive quality assurance program, the accuracy and precision of laboratory test results cannot be verified.
- A comprehensive quality includes qualifications of laboratory personnel, standard operating procedures for care and use of all supplies and equipment, sample collection and handling procedures, methods and frequency of performance of quality control assays, and record-keeping procedures.

Accuracy, Precision, and Reliability

- Accuracy reflects how closely results agree with the true quantitative value of the constituent.
- Precision is the magnitude of random errors and the reproducibility of measurements.
- Reliability is the ability of a method to be accurate and precise.
- Factors that affect accuracy and precision are test selection, test conditions, sample quality, operator skill, electrical surges, and equipment maintenance.

Analysis of Control Materials

- Control serum is used for assessment of the instrument and operator.
- Producing valid results with control materials provides assurance that the procedure was performed correctly and that all components (e.g., reagents, equipment) are functioning correctly.
- Controls are handled in exactly the same way as patient test samples and should be regularly assayed with each test batch—daily or weekly—at the same time that patient serum samples are assayed.
- After the assay is completed, the control value should fall within the manufacturer's reported range.
  - If it does not, the assays of the patient and control samples must be repeated.
- The results of the analysis of control serum are recorded on a chart or log for each assay.
- Data may be analyzed in two ways: by detecting shifts or trends and by determining whether results for control samples are within the range established by the manufacturer.
- When control values are successively distributed on one or the other side of the mean, the mean has shifted and a systematic error is involved.

Applied Quality Control

- Instrument maintenance is required to prolong the life of the instrument and prevent expensive downtime.
- A notebook listing a schedule with the types of maintenance required for each instrument facilitates instrument maintenance.
  - A page is dedicated to each instrument and includes the following:
    - Instrument name
    - Serial number
    - Model number
    - Purchase date
    - Points to be checked
    - Frequency of checks
    - Record of test readings
    - Changes made to restore accuracy and precision of readings
    - Cost and time associated with necessary repairs and restoration
    - Name or initials of the person performing the maintenance
- Results obtained with the control serum are recorded and kept in a permanent record.
  - The results are graphed so that changes or trends can be detected visually.

LABORATORY RECORDS

- Laboratory records are divided into internal and external record systems.
- Internal records involve tracking assay results and methods.
- The records consist of a standard operating procedure (SOP) and quality control data and graphs.
- The SOP contains the instructions for all analyses run in the laboratory.
- For commercial test kits, insert the instruction sheets accompanying the kit in a three-ring binder, along with pages for any other procedures performed in the laboratory.
- Each procedure not performed with a commercial kit is described on a separate page, including the name of the test, synonyms (if any) for the test, the rationale for use of the procedure, reagent list, and stepwise instructions for a single analysis. Individual pages can be inserted into plastic overlays for protection.
- External records consist of request forms that accompany a sample to the laboratory, report forms for assay results, laboratory log books with individual test results, and a book containing pertinent information on samples sent to reference laboratories.
- The report form should include complete patient identification and presenting signs, test results (including appropriate units), and notation of any extraordinary observations or explanatory comments, if applicable.

HEMATOLOGY SAMPLE COLLECTION

- Careful attention to collection procedures will minimize problems with test accuracy.
- Unless the purpose of the test is to monitor therapy, the blood sample is always collected before any treatment is given.
- Preprandial samples, or samples from an animal that has not eaten for some time, are ideal.
- Postprandial samples, or samples collected after the animal has eaten, may produce many erroneous results.

- Increased amounts of lipid (**lipemia**) may also be present in postprandial blood samples.
- Lipemia also increases the likelihood of hemolysis in the sample and further complicates analyses.
- Improper handling of blood may render a blood sample unusable for analysis or result in inaccurate results.
- Venous blood is preferred for use in hematologic testing and is easily accessible in most species.
- The cephalic vein is the preferred site in dogs and cats when relatively small volumes of blood are needed.
- The saphenous vein (lateral in the dog, medial in the cat) is a reasonable substitute, especially in fractious cats.
- Jugular venipuncture is an efficient way to collect a large volume of blood.
- The veterinary assistant should clip the collection site to remove hair.
- Clean the site with alcohol or another suitable antiseptic and allow it to dry before proceeding with the venipuncture.
- Use only the amount of restraint necessary to immobilize the animal.
- Excitement and stress can cause splenic contraction, which can alter the results of tests performed on red blood cells (RBCs); results of several WBC tests are also affected.

Collection Equipment

- Blood may be collected in a syringe or specialized vacuum device, such as the Vacutainer system.
- When the needle–syringe method is used, the needle chosen should always be the largest one that the animal can comfortably accommodate.
    - For most small animals, 20- to 25-gauge needles work well.
    - The syringe chosen should be one that is closest to the required sample volume.
    - Use of a larger syringe could collapse the patient's vein.
    - Using a large syringe with a small-bore needle can result in **hemolysis** (rupture of RBCs) when the syringe plunger is pulled back with great speed and force.
- Remove the needle before expelling the blood into the collection tube.
    - Erythrocytes (RBCs) may hemolyze (rupture) if forced back through the needle.
- Vacutainers are useful for multiple samples and when blood can be collected from a larger vessel, such as the cephalic or jugular vein.
    - The Vacutainer system consists of a special needle, a needle holder, and vacuum-filled tubes that may be empty (clot tubes) or may contain a premeasured amount of anticoagulant.
    - A fixed amount of blood is drawn into the tube, based on tube size and amount of vacuum in the tube.

- Collapse of veins, especially in smaller animals, may occur because of excessive negative pressure exerted by the vacuum; using small vacuum tubes may remedy this problem.
- Always fill blood collection tubes properly to ensure the correct ratio of blood to anticoagulant.
- Unless otherwise directed, fill the tube approximately two-thirds to three-quarters full. This ensures a proper blood-to-anticoagulant ratio.
- Mix the blood adequately by inverting the tube gently for 10 to 20 seconds after transferring the blood.
- Label the tube with the date and time of collection, owner's name, patient's name, and patient's clinic identification number.

Sample Type
Whole Blood
- Whole blood is composed of cellular elements (erythrocytes, leukocytes, and platelets) and a fluid called plasma.
- To collect a whole-blood sample, place the appropriate amount of blood into a container with the proper anticoagulant and gently mix the sample by inverting the tube multiple times.
- Whole blood may be refrigerated if analysis is to be delayed, but it should never be frozen unless the plasma has been separated from the cellular elements.
- If the blood has been refrigerated, warm the sample to room temperature and mix gently before analysis.

Plasma
- To obtain a plasma sample, collect the appropriate amount of blood in a container with the proper anticoagulant and mix well by gentle inversion.
- Centrifuge the closed container for 10 minutes at 2000 to 3000 rpm to separate the fluid from the cells.
- After the sample is centrifuged, remove the plasma from the cells, being careful not to contaminate the plasma with any pelleted cells, and transfer the plasma into another appropriately labeled container.
- Separate plasma from the cellular elements as soon as possible after collection to minimize any artifactual changes.
- Plasma can be refrigerated or frozen until analysis is performed, depending on the specific requirements of the desired test(s).

Anticoagulants
- Anticoagulants are used when whole blood or plasma samples are required.
- The choice of a particular anticoagulant should be based on the tests needed.
- The most commonly used anticoagulant is ethylenediaminetetraacetic acid (EDTA); heparin may also be used in some cases.
- Tubes that contain EDTA have a lavender or purple rubber stopper.

- EDTA functions as an anticoagulant by binding calcium, which is necessary for clotting to occur.
  - It is preferred for routine hematologic studies because it preserves cell morphology better than other anticoagulants.
- Even if collected in an EDTA tube, blood should be analyzed as quickly as possible, preferably within 2 hours after collection.
- Blood preserved in EDTA remains fresh for several hours or even overnight if stored in a refrigerator at 39.2°F (4°C).
  - However, morphologic changes in the cells, such as cytoplasmic vacuolation, irregular cell membranes, and crenation (shrinkage of RBCs), may occur in stored samples, especially when the ratio of blood to anticoagulant is incorrect.
- Heparin is not a permanent anticoagulant; it inhibits coagulation for only 8 to 12 hours.
- Tubes containing heparin (green-topped tubes) may be used if tests run on whole blood are done promptly.
- Heparin may cause cells to clump and stain poorly.
- Heparin tubes may be a good choice for storing small blood samples from birds because you can use the whole blood for hematologic tests and then collect plasma after spinning the sample.
- Some hematology analyzers require heparinized samples.
- Sodium citrate (blue-topped tubes) anticoagulant is used for coagulation tests.
  - However, it is generally not suitable for routine hematologic studies because it can cause distortion in cell morphology.

Complete Blood Count

- CBCs are indicated for the diagnostic evaluation of disease states, well-animal screening (e.g., geriatric animals), and as a screening tool before surgery.

- A CBC includes total erythrocyte and leukocyte counts, packed cell volume, hemoglobin concentration, differential WBC count, and RBC indices.
- Additional tests that should be included at the time of the CBC are the following:
  - Measurement of total solids
  - Evaluation of serum color and clarity
  - Buffy coat evaluation
  - Platelet estimate
  - Platelet assessment
- Most components of the CBC are performed with automated analyzers.

Packed Cell Volume

- The packed cell volume (PCV), also known as the microhematocrit (mHct), is an expression of the percentage of whole blood occupied by RBCs.
- The PCV assay is usually performed with the microhematocrit technique.
  - A blood-filled capillary tube is centrifuged for 2 to 5 minutes, depending on the type of centrifuge.
  - The blood separates into a plasma layer, a white buffy coat composed of WBCs and platelets, and a layer of packed red cells (Fig. 8.5).
- A low PCV may indicate anemia.
  - There are many causes of anemia, including blood loss, neoplasia, parasitism, and chronic infection.
- PCV values may be erroneously low if the microhematocrit tube contains excessive plasma because of inadequate mixing of the sample.
- Sample dilution because of a low blood-to-anticoagulant ratio may also cause a spurious decrease in the PCV.
- An increased PCV also has several possible causes, including dehydration and splenic contraction in an excited animal.
  - PCV values may be erroneously high because of clots in the sample, failure to mix the EDTA and blood adequately, and insufficient centrifugation time.

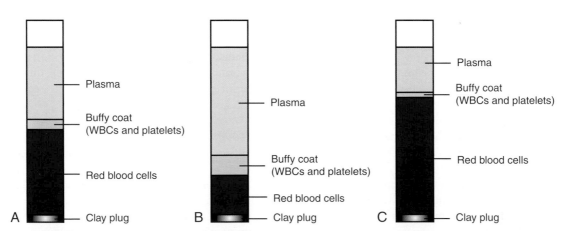

FIGURE 8.5 A, Normal blood. Normal percentage of red blood cells (RBCs) and normal-thickness buffy coat. B, Anemia and leukocytosis. Low percentage of RBCs (anemia) and thicker buffy coat (leukocytosis). C, Polycythemia and leukocytopenia. High percentage of RBCs (polycythemia) and thinner buffy coat (leukocytopenia). (From Colville T, Bassert JM: *Clinical anatomy and physiology for veterinary technicians*, ed 2, St Louis, 2008, Mosby.)

- After determining the PCV, evaluate the plasma for turbidity and color (Box 8.1).
- An icteric, or yellow, plasma layer may occur with liver disease or hemolytic anemia.
- A hemolytic, or red, sample can occur from improper sample collection and handling or with hemolytic anemia (Fig. 8.6).
- Sometimes the buffy coat is red tinged, especially in very sick animals or if there is an increased number of immature RBCs in the circulation.
- Lipemic plasma appears cloudy (turbid) and white, indicating excessive lipids in the blood. This can occur if blood was collected from an animal that was not fasted, or it may be pathologic.
- Icterus, hemolysis, and lipemia may be quantified as slight, moderate, or marked.
- The width of the buffy coat should be assessed.

BOX 8.1 Visual Assessment of Plasma Turbidity and Color

- Normal: Clear and colorless to light straw-yellow
- Icterus: Clear and yellow
- Hemolysis: Clear and red
- Lipemia: Turbid and white

From Sirois M: Principles and practice of veterinary technology, ed 3, St Louis, 2011, Mosby.

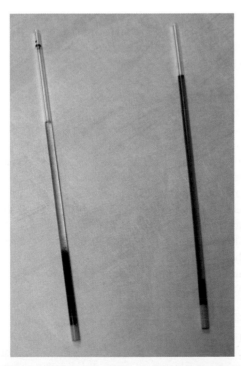

FIGURE 8.6 Icteric *(left)* and hemolyzed *(right)* plasma in a PCV tube. (From Sirois M: *Principles and practice of veterinary technology*, ed 3, St Louis, 2011, Mosby.)

Total Plasma Protein Determination

- The serum or plasma total protein level can be rapidly and reliably measured using a handheld refractometer.
- Accurate plasma protein determination is difficult in lipemic samples because the turbidity produces an indistinct line of demarcation on the scale.
- Hemoglobinemia caused by hemolysis can falsely increase plasma protein levels because of the presence of the heme portion of hemoglobin.
- The yellow color of an icteric sample does not interfere with refractometry.

Erythrocyte Indices

- Erythrocyte indices are calculated values that use the RBC count, hemoglobin measurement, and PCV.
- Erythrocyte indices include the mean corpuscular volume (MCV), mean corpuscular hemoglobin (MCH), and mean corpuscular hemoglobin concentration (MCHC).
- These measurements provide data on the overall size of the RBCs as well as the relative amount of hemoglobin within the individual RBCs.

Differential Blood Film

- Although most veterinary hematology analyzers provide at least a partial differential WBC count, a blood film must still be prepared and evaluated.
- A large number of abnormalities are not routinely reported by automated analyzers.
- These include Heinz bodies, cellular inclusions (e.g., parasites, viral materials), toxic granulation, platelet clumps, polychromasia, target cells, and hypersegmentation.

Evaluating the Blood Film

- The CBC must include a differential blood film that enumerates various types of WBCs present and also describes the morphology of red and white blood cells and platelets.
- A platelet estimate is also performed on the differential blood film.
- In addition to reporting the morphologic changes, a rating system is used to characterize the relative numbers of abnormal cells seen on the differential blood film.
- The preferred sample for preparation of the differential blood cell film is the blood drop on the tip of the needle immediately after the blood is collected.
- This prevents the development of artifacts related to the presence of anticoagulant.
- The two methods of preparing blood smears are the wedge (glass slide) method and the coverslip method.
- Always use precleaned, glass microscope slides and coverslips, and always hold slides by their edges to avoid smudging with grease or fingerprints.
- The wedge method is the most common type of smear used for routine hematology.
- The coverslip method is often preferred for avian blood smears because it renders a thinner film, which facilitates cell identification. It is also less traumatic on fragile avian blood cells.

Performing the Differential

- The evaluation of the differential blood film is the responsibility of the veterinary technician, although the veterinary assistant may aid in preparing the materials for the evaluation.
- The technician will examine the blood smear in a systematic manner.
- The smear is scanned at low power ($100\times$ magnification) to assess overall cell numbers and distribution.
- Platelet clumps (aggregates) and blood parasites (e.g., microfilariae) are sometimes found at the feathered edge and must be noted on the hematology report.
- A monolayer (single layer of blood cells) is located adjacent to the feathered edge.
- Using the oil immersion objective ($1000\times$ magnification), it is here that the differential WBC count takes place.
- The procedure requires that 100 WBCs be counted, identified, and recorded.
  - This is called the relative WBC count.
- Once the relative percentages of each cell type have been determined, the absolute value of each cell type must be calculated.
  - This is accomplished by multiplying the total WBC count by the percentage of each cell type.
- The morphology of RBCs and WBCs is then assessed and recorded.
- The presence of any abnormal cells or toxic changes is reported and semiquantified.
- Veterinary technicians are responsible for identifying normal and abnormal RBC morphology.
- Morphology is evaluated using the oil immersion objective ($1000\times$ magnification) in the monolayer portion of the smear.
- Changes in the appearance of erythrocytes fall into one or more of the following categories: (1) changes in size; (2) changes in shape; (3) changes in color; (4) changes in cell behavior; and (5) appearance of inclusions.
- A variety of blood parasites can also be seen on a peripheral blood film.
  - Most of these are found on or within erythrocytes.
  - Parasites may also be found free of cells and within leukocytes and platelets.
- Leukocytes seen on blood smears from mammals include neutrophils, basophils, eosinophils, lymphocytes, and monocytes.
  - Segmented neutrophils, also known as segs or polymorphonuclear (PMN) cells, are mature WBCs that function mainly as phagocytes and are involved in inflammation.
  - Lymphocytes have functions within the immune system.
  - Monocytes are very large WBCs that are phagocytic and have immune system functions. Eosinophils are associated with allergic responses and are more numerous in patients with parasitic infections.
- Basophils are involved in the mediation of the immune system, and increased numbers are seen with a variety of inflammatory and infectious conditions.
- Changes in the appearance of leukocytes generally occur as a result of disease processes that affect the appearance and/or function of the cell.
- These changes can also occur as normal reactions to a disease process and may be nonpathologic.
- Leukocyte changes may affect the cell nucleus, cytoplasm, or both.
- Platelets are also referred to as thrombocytes.
  - In mammals, they are derived from the bone marrow cell called a megakaryocyte. Mammalian platelets are fragments of the cytoplasm of this bone marrow cell.
  - Platelets function to provide an initiating coagulation factor and are also capable of plugging small ruptures in small blood vessels.

Coagulation Testing

Hemostatic Defects

- The clinical presentation of patients with bleeding disorders includes petechia (pinpoint hemorrhage), ecchymoses (superficial hemorrhage $\approx$1 cm in diameter), purpura (bruising), epistaxis (bleeding from the nares), and prolonged bleeding after trauma or surgery.
- Patients may exhibit hematuria as a result of bleeding into the urinary bladder, melena as a result of bleeding into the digestive tract, or bleeding into joint cavities.
- Most bleeding disorders found in veterinary species are in canine species and are secondary to some other disease process.
- The most common inherited coagulation disorder of domestic animals is von Willebrand disease.
  - This disease results when the production of von Willebrand factor is decreased or deficient.
  - The disease occurs with relative frequency in Doberman dogs and has been reported in other canine breeds, as well as in rabbits and swine.
- Other coagulation disorders result from the decreased production or increased destruction of platelets as well as nutritional deficiencies, liver disease, and ingestion of certain medications or toxic substances.
- Thrombocytopenia refers to a decreased number of platelets and is the most common bleeding disorder of hemostasis in veterinary patients.
  - This can occur as a result of bone marrow depression that reduces the production of platelets or autoimmune disease that increases the rate of platelet destruction.
  - A large number of infectious agents, such as *Ehrlichia, Dirofilaria,* and parvovirus, can also affect thrombocyte production and destruction.
- Because the liver is the site of production of most coagulation factors, any condition that affects liver function can result in a coagulation disorder.

- Ingestion of toxic substances such as warfarin can also create bleeding disorders.
  - Warfarin is a common component of some rodenticides and acts to inhibit vitamin K function.
  - Because vitamin K is required for the synthesis of coagulation factors II, VII, IX, and X, this can create a deficiency in several necessary components of the coagulation cascade.
- Ingestion of medications such as aspirin can also cause bleeding disorders.

Disseminated Intravascular Coagulation
- Although not a disease entity on its own, disseminated intravascular coagulation (DIC) is associated with many pathologic conditions, including trauma cases and a large number of infectious diseases.
- The resulting hemostatic disorder may manifest as systemic hemorrhage or microvascular thrombosis.
- Because the triggering event and the resulting disorder are diverse, the laboratory findings are highly variable.
- Schistocytes may be seen on the blood film on DIC patients because of the intravascular destruction of erythrocytes.

Assessment of Coagulation and Hemostasis
- Coagulation tests are designed to evaluate specific portions of the hemostatic mechanisms.
- All patients should be evaluated for coagulation defects before undergoing surgery.
- Most coagulation tests can be completed with minimal time and equipment and are relatively inexpensive.
- Plasma samples for coagulation testing are collected into an appropriate anticoagulant.
- Tests to determine the concentration and/or function of specific coagulation factors are not routinely performed in veterinary practice.

Platelet Counts and Estimates
- Platelet counts are part of all coagulation profiles, as well as evaluation of the blood film for platelet morphology and clumping.
- A platelet estimate is performed when the veterinary technician completes the differential blood film evaluation.
- Most automated analyzers provide a platelet count.

Buccal Mucosal Bleeding Time
- This test detects abnormalities in platelet function.
- The test requires a standard spring-loaded bleeding time device, blotting paper or no. 1 Whatman filter paper, stopwatch, and tourniquet.
- The test is performed with the patient anesthetized and placed in lateral recumbency (Fig. 8.7).

Other Coagulation Tests
- The activated clotting time (ACT) test uses a preincubated tube that contains a diatomaceous earth material or is done with an automated analyzer.

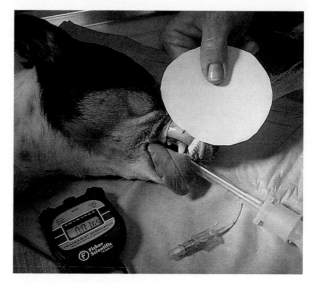

FIGURE 8.7 Buccal mucosa bleeding time test. (From Sirois M: *Principles and practice of veterinary technology*, ed 3, St Louis, 2011, Mosby; courtesy Dr. B. Mitzner.)

- The prothrombin time (PT) and activated partial thromboplastin time (aPTT) tests are usually determined with automated analyzers.
  - These analyzers use whole blood or plasma samples collected in citrate anticoagulant tubes.

CLINICAL CHEMISTRY
- Laboratory analysis of blood biochemical constituents is performed for a variety of reasons.
- A blood sample may be collected from a patient as part of a general wellness screening process, to confirm or rule out a specific disease, as part of management of a clinical case to evaluate the status of a previously diagnosed condition, or as part of emergency medical therapy.
- Biochemistry profiles, or groups of tests, are routinely performed using serum as the preferred sample type, although heparinized plasma may also be used with some analyzers.
- The chemicals being assayed are usually enzymes associated with particular organ functions or metabolites and metabolic by-products that are processed by certain organs.

Hepatobiliary Function Testing
- Hepatic (liver) cells exhibit extreme diversity of function and are capable of regeneration if damaged.
  - As a result, there are over 100 types of tests to evaluate liver and gallbladder function.
- In most cases, evaluation of several liver function test results is required to assess the overall status of the liver.
- Liver cells also compartmentalize the work, so damage to one zone of the liver may not affect all liver functions.
  - Usually, liver disease has greatly progressed before clinical signs appear.

- Liver function tests are designed to measure substances that are produced by the liver (primarily proteins), modified by the liver (e.g., bilirubin), or released when hepatocytes are damaged (primarily liver enzymes).
- The most commonly performed hepatobiliary tests in small animal practice are alanine aminotransferase (ALT), alkaline phosphatase (ALP), bilirubin, and total protein.

Protein

- In the small veterinary practice, total protein is usually measured with a refractometer.
- Total serum protein concentrations include all plasma proteins except fibrinogen and other coagulation proteins that have been removed during the coagulation process.
- Most serum proteins are produced by hepatocytes.
- Chemical analyzers also measure total protein concentration.
- Serum protein levels are affected by the rate of protein synthesis in the liver, the rate of protein catabolism in the animal, hydration status, and alterations in the distribution of proteins in the body.
- Dehydrated animals usually have elevated total protein values; overhydrated animals usually have decreased total protein values.
- Marked hemolysis falsely increases total protein levels.
- Do not use lipemic samples, especially if the refractometric method is used.
- Moderate icterus has no effect on the refractometric method.
- Heat, ultraviolet light, surfactant detergents, and chemicals can break down proteins, leading to artificially low results.
  Albumin
- Albumin is one of the most important proteins in plasma or serum and makes up approximately 35% to 50% of the total serum protein concentration.
- Albumin is synthesized by the liver.
- Albumin levels are also influenced by dietary intake, renal disease, and intestinal protein absorption.
- Albumin functions as a transport and binding protein of the blood and is responsible for maintaining osmotic pressure of plasma.
  Globulin
- Globulins are a complex group of proteins that include all the proteins (plasma or serum) other than albumin and coagulation proteins.
- The globulins are separated into three major classes by electrophoresis: alpha, beta, and gamma globulins.
- Most alpha and beta globulins are synthesized by the liver.
- The gamma globulins (immunoglobulins) are synthesized by plasma cells and are responsible for the body's immunity provided by antibodies.
- Immunoglobulins identified in animals include immunoglobulin G (IgG), IgD, IgE, IgA, and IgM.

- Globulin concentration is calculated by subtracting the albumin concentration from the total serum protein.

Bilirubin

- Bilirubin is assayed to determine the cause of jaundice (icterus), evaluate liver function, and check the patency of bile ducts.
- Bilirubin is an insoluble molecule derived from the breakdown of hemoglobin in the spleen.
- Two types of bilirubin, conjugated and unconjugated, are present in the plasma.
- Alterations in the ratios of the various bilirubin compounds help determine whether liver damage is present or if other conditions (e.g., bile duct obstruction) are contributing to disease.

Bile Acids

- Bile acids are produced from cholesterol in the liver and serve many functions, including aiding in fat absorption and modulating cholesterol levels.
- The gallbladder stores bile acids, which are then released into the intestinal tract.
- Most bile acids are actively resorbed in the ileum and carried to the liver, where they are reconjugated and excreted as part of the enterohepatic circulation of bile acids.
- Blood levels of bile acids in normal animals are very low, especially in fasted animals.

Enzyme Analyses

- Enzymes are specialized proteins that catalyze various chemical reactions.
- Most enzymes work intracellularly at a specific pH.
- Enzymes are usually not present in high concentrations in serum.
- Increased concentrations of enzymes in serum often indicate cellular damage.
- Enzyme assays usually involve measurement of the outcome of enzyme activity rather than specific measurement of the enzyme itself.
- Enzymes related to liver function in most mammals include the phosphatases and transaminases.
  Phosphatases
- The primary phosphatases in dogs and cats are the alkaline phosphatses (ALPs) and acid phosphatases (ACPs).
- Determinations of ACP levels are not usually carried out but may help in the diagnosis of certain types of hemolytic anemia.
- ALPs have multiple organ sources, including the liver, kidney, bone, and intestine.
- The extent of the increase aids in determining whether the patient has intrahepatic or extrahepatic damage.
- The ALP assay is most often used to detect cholestasis in dogs and cats.
- ALP levels can be increased in young, growing animals because of bone remodeling and increases in the bone isoenzyme level.

Transferases

- This group of enzymes is found primarily in tissues that have high rates of protein metabolism, especially the kidney, liver, and muscle.
- In small animal veterinary medicine, the transferases of clinical significance are alanine aminotransferase (ALT) and aspartate aminotransferase (AST).
- ALT is a liver-specific enzyme and a good indicator of hepatocellular damage in dogs, cats, and primates because the primary or major source of serum ALT is the hepatocyte.
- AST assays are used primarily to evaluate the extent of skeletal muscle damage in the equine and may also be used to evaluate cardiac muscle damage in some species.

Kidney Function Testing

- The primary chemical tests of kidney function are determination of urea nitrogen and creatinine levels.

Urea Nitrogen

- Blood urea nitrogen (BUN) is the principal product of protein catabolism.
- Normally, all urea passes through the glomerulus, and approximately 50% is resorbed by passive diffusion.
- Azotemia, an increase in levels of BUN and other nonprotein nitrogenous wastes, can occur when blood flow through the kidneys alters the glomerular filtration rate or when the urinary tract is obstructed.
- Dehydration will also result in azotemia because urea must be excreted in a large amount of water.
- Differences in rates of protein catabolism between male and female animals, young and adult animals, different species, and nutritional status will also affect BUN levels.

Creatinine

- Serum creatinine is produced from the metabolic breakdown of phosphocreatine in muscle tissue.
- The daily rate of creatinine production is relatively constant in any animal and is dependent on muscle mass.
- Creatinine is also primarily cleared by the kidney via glomerular filtration.
- Creatinine is used to evaluate renal function based on the ability of the glomeruli to filter creatinine from the blood and eliminate it in urine.
- Similar to BUN, if serum creatinine values are increased because of decreased renal function, this indicates that approximately 75% of the nephrons are nonfunctional.

Uric Acid

- Uric acid is an end product of the catabolism of nucleic acids.
- It is the primary end product of nitrogen metabolism in avian species and is actively secreted by the renal tubules.
- In most animals, uric acid is bound to albumin, passes through the glomerulus, and then is resorbed.
- It is usually converted to allantoin and excreted in the urine.

- In Dalmatian dogs, the liver is unable to convert uric acid, so these animals excrete uric acid rather than allantoin.
  - This also predisposes the breed to urate urolithiasis.
- Photometric analysis of uric acid is a complex procedure not commonly performed in veterinary clinical practice.
  - Newer methods of chemical analysis using liquid-stable reagents can enable uric acid testing in the veterinary practice laboratory.

Pancreatic Function Testing

- The pancreas functions as an endocrine and exocrine organ.
- The endocrine part of the pancreas contains small nodules of endocrine cells, the islets of Langerhans.
- Two primary hormones are produced within the islets: insulin and glucagon.
- Insulin prevents abnormally high blood glucose levels and allows glucose to enter the cells for use.
- A defect in insulin secretion or action leads to diabetes mellitus, characterized by abnormally high blood glucose levels and many metabolic difficulties.
- The other pancreatic hormone, glucagon, has the opposite effect and tends to increase the blood glucose level.
- The exocrine portion of the pancreas secretes enzymes necessary for digestion.
  - The primary enzymes are trypsin, amylase, and lipase.
- Serum feline pancreatic lipase immunoreactivity (fPLI) and canine pancreatic lipase immunoreactivity (cPLI) are immunologic tests that are specific for pancreatitis, and their use is now preferred as a serum test to diagnose patients with symptoms of pancreatitis.

Amylase

- Amylase is produced in a variety of tissues, including the salivary glands, small intestine, and pancreas, and functions in the breakdown of starch to glucose.
- Serial determinations of amylase in conjunction with lipase provide an indication of pancreatic function.
- Increased levels of amylase can occur with acute pancreatitis, flare-ups of chronic pancreatitis, and obstruction of the pancreatic ducts.

Lipase

- Lipase functions to break down the fatty acids of lipids.
- Not all animals with pancreatitis have elevated lipase levels.
- Lipase activity may also be elevated by nonpancreatic factors such as chronic renal failure, exploratory surgery, and corticosteroid use.
- Almost all serum lipase is derived from the pancreas.
- Excess lipase is easily filtered through the kidneys, so lipase levels tend to remain normal in the early stages of pancreatic disease.

Glucose

- A small portion of the pancreas is involved in the production of insulin.

- Insulin is required to facilitate the uptake of glucose by body cells.
- Blood glucose measurements provide an indicator of the status of pancreatic endocrine activity.
  - These can also be affected by a variety of factors, including diet and stress.
- The blood glucose level reflects the net balance between glucose production (dietary intake, conversion from other carbohydrates) and glucose use (energy expended, conversion to other products).
- Glucose use depends on the amount of insulin and glucagon being produced by the pancreas.
- As the blood insulin level increases, so does the rate of glucose use, resulting in decreased blood glucose levels.
- Glucagon acts as a stabilizer to prevent blood glucose levels from becoming too low.
- As the insulin level decreases, so does glucose use, resulting in increased blood glucose concentration.
- Although excess serum glucose can result from a variety of disease conditions, the highest blood glucose values are seen in diabetes mellitus.
  - This condition results from decreased or defective production of insulin.
- Without sufficient insulin, the body cells are unable to take up glucose.
- A variety of methods are available to evaluate blood glucose levels.
- Dedicated instruments for blood glucose testing are also readily available.
  - Most of these were initially designed for use in human medicine to allow diabetic patients to monitor their own blood glucose levels.
- It is vital that the blood serum or plasma be removed from contact with the erythrocytes immediately after blood collection.
  - If the sample is left in contact with the erythrocytes, the blood glucose levels can drop up to 10% per hour at room temperature.
  - If the blood sample cannot be centrifuged and the serum or plasma is not separated from the erythrocytes, collect the sample in a sodium fluoride tube.
  - Sodium fluoride inhibits the use of glucose by erythrocytes and therefore stabilizes glucose levels for up to 12 hours at room temperature, and for 48 hours if the sample is refrigerated. Refrigeration slows glucose use by erythrocytes.
- Because eating raises the blood glucose level and fasting decreases it, a 12-hour fast is recommended when possible for all animals, except for mature ruminants, before the blood sample is collected.

Fructosamine
- Fructosamine is a more specific indicator of pancreatic endocrine activity than glucose. It results from a reaction between glucose and serum protein.

- Fructosamine levels provide an indication of the average glucose levels over the life span of the protein ($\approx$1 to 3 weeks).

Other Serum Assays
Enzymes and Lactate
- Creatine kinase (CK), also referred to as creatine phosphokinase (CPK), is a cytoplasmic enzyme that appears in the serum in increased concentrations after cellular injury.
- Lactate dehydrogenase (LD) is a serum enzyme present in almost all tissues, although liver, muscle, and erythrocytes are the major sources of increased blood LD levels.
- Lactate, also referred to as lactic acid, is an indication of tissue hypoxia.
- Lactate values are frequently used to monitor and develop prognostic indicators for critically ill patients.
  - Handheld meters for in-house use are available for lactate testing.

Electrolytes
- Electrolytes are minerals that exist as positively charged or negatively charged particles in an aqueous solution.
- Positively charged particles are called cations, and negatively charged particles are called anions.
  - These particles function primarily in the regulation of acid–base and osmotic balance of the body.
- The primary method for electrolyte evaluation involves the use of ion-specific electrodes.
- The electrolytes that are most commonly measured are sodium (Na^+), potassium (K^+), chloride (Cl^-), calcium (Ca^{2+}), inorganic phosphorus (P), and magnesium (Mg^{2+}).
- Electrolytes can be measured using serum or heparinized plasma.
- It is important to remember that different salts of heparin are available: sodium heparin, potassium heparin, ammonium heparin, and lithium heparin.
  - When selecting an anticoagulant, do not choose a form of heparin that contains the substance that is being measured.

BASIC PRINCIPLES OF IMMUNOLOGY

- The term immune system refers to a variety of cells, tissues, organs, and organ systems that are involved in the body's defense mechanisms.
- Some components are present and active in the body at all times; others are created or activated in response to a foreign substance.
- Immunity can generally be divided into two types: passive and active.
- Passive immunity includes maternal antibodies from colostrum and physicochemical barriers, such as the skin and mucous membranes.
- Active immunity is developed or acquired and is classified as humoral or cell-mediated immunity.

- Humoral immunity is mediated by the production of unique proteins (antibodies), which are responsible for the specific recognition and elimination of antigens.
- Foreign substances that are capable of generating a response from the immune system are referred to as antigens.
- Antigens include bacteria, viruses, parasites, or even the body's own tissues (autoimmunity).
- Specific substances on the surface of the antigen are responsible for the recognition of an antigen by the body's immune system.
  - These substances are usually proteins and act as markers for the immune system.
- Recognition of these markers often results in the formation of antibody by the immune system.
- When antibodies are produced, the immune system retains a memory of the antigen and can respond more quickly to future attacks by the same antigen.
- Cell-mediated immunity is dependent on cells, in particular lymphocytes.
  - These lymphocytes recognize specific antigens, such as those of fungi, parasites, intracellular bacteria, or tumor cells, and help remove them from the animal by lysing the infected or cancerous cell or organism.

Immunologic Tests

- Dysfunction of the immune system can lead to an overactive immune system that produces immune-mediated disease or an underactive immune system that produces immunodeficiency disorders.
- These disorders can involve any component of the immune system (e.g., passive, humoral, cell mediated).
- Serologic testing is based on the ability to detect antibody–antigen interactions.
- Immunoassays usually contain monoclonal antibodies to an antigen or part of an antigen, such as a viral capsule or surface protein of a parasite.
- A few tests detect circulating antibody, rather than antigen, but these are used only when the antigen is not readily available for testing.

Enzyme-Linked Immunosorbent Assay

- Enzyme-linked immunosorbent assay (ELISA) tests are the most common types of immunologic tests performed in veterinary clinics (Fig. 8.8).
  - Every ELISA test has the same basic components: solid phase, conjugate, and chromogen.
- The solid phase may be a microwell, wand, flow-through membrane, or chromatographic strip.
- Conjugate reagents are embedded on the solid phase and usually consist of monoclonal antibodies bound to an enzyme.
- The chromogen is a photosensitive reagent that produces a color change in the test system.
- Adding patient sample to the solid phase is the first step in the test.
  - The sample is then allowed to incubate.

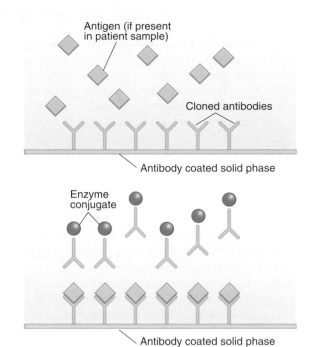

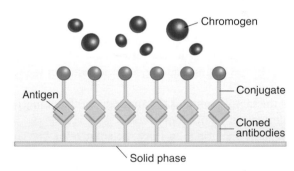

FIGURE 8.8 Principle of ELISA reaction. (From Sirois M: *Principles and practice of veterinary technology*, ed 3, St Louis, 2011, Mosby.)

- If specific antigen is present in the sample, it will bind to the antibody on the test surface.
- After the appropriate incubation time, the patient sample is washed away.
- If antigen has bound to the solid phase, it will not be washed away.
- Chromogen is then added that can react with the bound enzyme–antigen–antibody complex, if present, and produce a color change in the test system.

Rapid Immunomigration Assay

- The rapid immunomigration (RIM) assay, also known as immunochromatography, is similar to the ELISA method except that gold staining is used to replace the chromogen.
  - In these test formats, also known as lateral flow assays, the conjugate is an antibody bound to colloidal gold or latex instead of to an enzyme.

- The solid phase of a RIM test is a chromatographic strip.
- Most RIM tests require a flow solution, usually a buffered saline, to aid in the movement of the sample across the chromatographic strip.
- The RIM test is performed by adding the patient sample to the absorptive pad on the solid phase.
  - The conjugate is released as the sample flows onto the solid phase.
  - The sample and conjugate then pass across two test areas.
  - The first test area, known as the patient line, contains antibodies to the antigen that the test is designed to detect.
  - If the antigen is present in the sample, it will bind to the antibodies on the patient line and produce a color change on the patient line.
  - The sample and conjugate continue to flow to the second test area. The second area is a control line that contains antibodies to the conjugate.
  - A color change is produced on this line and indicates that the test is functioning correctly.

Agglutination Test
- Agglutination tests are used for the detection of antibodies to large particulate antigens.
  - The test requires adding a specific antigen to the test sample.
- If the sample contains the antibody for that antigen, agglutination (clumping) occurs.
- In some agglutination tests, the antigen may be coated with latex beads to induce agglutination reactions.
- Agglutination tests are usually performed on a slide or card.
- Agglutination tests are commonly used to diagnose brucellosis in dogs and determine blood types (Fig. 8.9).

Other Tests
- There are three major types of precipitation tests: immunodiffusion, radioimmunodiffusion, and immunoelectrophoresis.
- Several types of electrophoresis procedures are performed, primarily in reference or referral laboratories, rather than in clinical practice.
- The Coombs test is used to detect autoantibodies (antibodies to one's own tissues).
  - Although the Coombs test is fairly simple to perform, the expense of stocking the species-specific Coombs reagent for only occasional tests makes it impractical to run in-house.
- Although not commonly performed in veterinary practices, fluorescent testing is available at most veterinary reference laboratories.
  - These test procedures are frequently used to verify a tentative diagnosis made by the veterinarian.

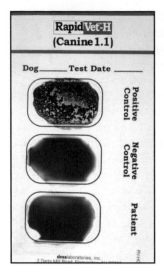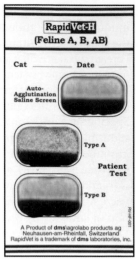

FIGURE 8.9 RapidVet-H blood typing card (DMS Laboratories, Flemington, NJ). (From Sirois M: *Principles and practice of veterinary technology*, ed 3, St Louis, 2011, Mosby.)

Immunology Analyzers
- Automated analyzers are available for use in the veterinary practice laboratory.
- Large reference laboratories often have automated analyzers for the performance of immunoassays.
  - These analyzers are capable of performing tests on numerous patients simultaneously.
- Most are completely automated and require only the patient information entered in the analyzer's computer and the patient sample loaded.
- Small in-house immunology analyzers are generally of the type that only read test results.
  - The technician prepares the sample and the test device and places the device on the analyzer.
  - The results are read by the analyzer at the appropriate time.

Chemiluminescence
- Many automated analyzers utilize the principles of chemiluminescence to detect and quantify specific antigens.
- The principle is similar to the ELISA method except that the test uses a substrate that reacts to produce light rather than an enzyme that reacts to produce color.
- The light produced can be detected by a photomultiplier, and the amount of light produced can be quantified.
- In addition to immunology testing, chemiluminescence has been used for detection and quantification of other substances, including thyroid hormones, cortisol, pancreatic lipase, progesterone, and testosterone.

Intradermal Skin Testing
- Patients with allergic skin diseases may be diagnosed with a combination of clinical signs and exclusion of suspected allergens or may require immunologic intradermal testing.

- Common causes of allergic skin disease include food allergy, contact dermatitis, insect bites and stings, inhalant allergy (e.g., pollen, mold), and atopy.
- Allergies are mediated by IgE antibody molecules and can be detected by using allergenic extracts of grasses, trees, weed pollens, molds, dust, insects, and other possibly offending antigens.
- The extracts are injected intradermally, and the injection sites are monitored for allergic reactions.
- A positive reaction appears as a raised welt, meaning that the animal is allergic to that antigen.

Antibody Titers

- Results of some antibody tests may be reported as positive or negative.
- Results of other antibody tests may be reported as antibody titers, or levels.
- The patient's serum is serially diluted to different concentrations, such as 1:10, 1:40, and 1:160.
- A test to detect antibodies is done on each of these dilutions, and the greatest dilution that tests positive is reported. For example, if 1:10 and 1:40 are positive and 1:160 is negative, the titer is reported as 1:40.
- If none of the dilutions is positive, the titer may be reported as negative, or the test may be repeated at lesser dilutions, such as 1:2, 1:4, or 1:8.
- A higher titer (positive at greater dilutions) indicates that more antibody is present.
- An antibody titer in a single sample may indicate only that the animal has been previously exposed to an infectious agent; the animal may not currently have an active infection.
- A rising titer in two or more samples indicates an active infection.

Common Errors and Artifacts

- The proper performance of these tests is vital to ensure accurate results.
- A number of other factors can produce false-positive or false-negative results.
- A false-positive result is a positive test result on a sample from a patient that is, in fact, negative for the antigen.
- A false-negative result is a negative test result on a sample from a patient that is, in fact, positive for the antigen.
- Many immunoassays incorporate controls that help determine the accuracy of the test results. A visible positive control indicates that the test kit is functional.
- The most common causes of false results are poor sample quality, inadequate washing (ELISA tests), improper incubation, cross-reacting proteins, or expired or improperly stored kits.

MICROBIOLOGY

- The term microbiology refers to the study of microbes, specifically bacteria.

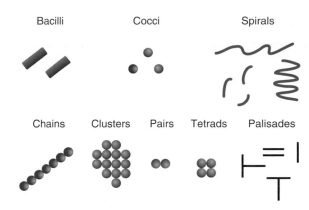

FIGURE 8.10 Bacterial cell shapes and arrangements. (From Hendrix CM, Sirois M: *Laboratory procedures for veterinary technicians*, ed 5, St Louis, 2007, Mosby.)

- Bacteria are small prokaryotic cells that have no nucleus, have few cellular organelles, and are variable in size, ranging from 0.2 to 2.0 μm.
- Bacteria can be classified into one of four general categories (cocci, bacilli, spirals, palisades) and can have a variety of arrangements (Fig. 8.10).
- Although most cellular organelles are absent, bacteria contain cell walls, plasma membranes, and ribosomes.
- Some contain capsules and flagella and can develop endospores.
  - These characteristics are often used in the differentiation of specific bacterial pathogens.
- Most bacteria are chemoheterotrophic; they obtain nutrients from nonliving components of their environment.
- Growth factors such as vitamins, amino acids, and nucleotides are also essential.
- Oxygen and temperature requirements vary among different species.
- Most species require a pH in the range of 6.5 to 7.5.
- Bacteria reproduce primarily by binary fission, and their numbers grow exponentially until essential nutrients are depleted, toxic waste products accumulate, and/or space becomes limiting.
- Microbiologic evaluations of tissues and body fluids can be used to determine the presence of specific disease-causing organisms and to aid in managing patient therapy.
- Table 8.1 summarizes bacterial pathogens of veterinary importance.
- Samples for microbiologic evaluation can be collected quickly by various methods, including swabbing, scraping, and aspiration.
- The specific techniques used depend on the type of lesion and its location on the animal's body.
- Careful attention to aseptic technique is critical to achieving diagnostic-quality results.

TABLE 8.1 Bacterial Pathogens of Veterinary Importance

Group	Genera
Spirochetes	*Leptospira* *Borrelia* *Treponema* *Brachyspira*
Spiral and curved bacteria	*Campylobacter* *Helicobacter*
Gram-negative aerobic bacilli	*Pseudomonas* *Francisella* *Brucella* *Neisseria* *Bordetella*
Gram-negative facultative bacilli	*Escherichia* *Proteus* *Shigella* *Yersinia* *Salmonella* *Citrobacter* *Klebsiella* *Aeromonas* *Enterobacter* *Actinobacillus* *Serratia* *Haemophilus* *Pasteurella*
Gram-negative anaerobic bacilli	*Bacteroides* *Fusobacterium*
Gram-positive bacilli	*Bacillus* *Listeria* *Clostridium* *Erysipelothrix* *Lactobacillus*
Gram-negative pleomorphic	*Rickettsia* Haemobartonella Ehrlichia Eperythrozoon Anaplasma Chlamydia *Mycoplasma*
Gram-positive cocci	*Staphylococcus* *Streptococcus* *Enterococcus*

From Sirois M: Principles and practice of veterinary technology, ed 3, St Louis, 2011, Mosby.

Mycology

- The study of fungi is referred to as mycology.
- Fungi are groups of organisms that are characterized by vegetative structures known as hyphae.
- Hyphae can grow into matted structures known as mycelia.
- Fungi contain eukaryotic cells with cell walls composed of chitin.
- The organisms are heterotrophic and may be parasitic or saprophytic.

- Fungi can be differentiated based on the structure of the hyphae and on the presence of spores. Different groups of fungi produce different types of spores.
- Various fungal organisms can affect veterinary species and cause superficial mycosis or deep mycosis (Table 8.2).

Sample Collection

- The specific choice of collection method depends on the location of the lesion on the animal's body, as well as the specific type of testing desired.
- Samples that are to be processed immediately can usually be collected using sterile cotton swabs.
  - However, this is the least suitable method of collection because contamination risk is high and cotton can inhibit microbial growth.
  - Oxygen can also be trapped in the fibers, making recovery of anaerobic bacteria less likely.
- Should delays in processing the sample be expected, a rayon swab in a transport medium must be used to preserve the quality of the sample.
- Aspirated samples and tissue samples can be collected in a fashion similar to that described later in this chapter for cytology samples.
- The following guidelines should be kept in mind for proper specimen collection and handling:
  - Collect the specimen aseptically as soon as possible after the onset of clinical signs and before the initiation of any treatment.
  - Keep multiple specimens separate from each other to avoid cross-contamination. This is essential for intestinal specimens because of the normal flora found there.
  - Samples that contain formalin should be stored and/or shipped to outside laboratories in containers that are separate from prepared slides and nonformalinized specimens.
  - Keep the specimen cool during transport. Swabs must be sent in transport medium. Bacteriologic, virologic, and *Mycoplasma* tests require separate swabs for each. Samples for anaerobic culture must be submitted cool or frozen.
  - If shipping involves dry ice, seal the container or swab to prevent entry of CO_2 into the container. Carbon dioxide released by dry ice may kill bacteria and viruses.
  - Swabs placed in a viral transport medium cannot be used for bacterial culture. Use duplicate bacterial transport media.

Sample Processing Materials

- Inoculating loops or wires for transfer of specimens to culture media are needed.
- A propane (Bunsen) burner or alcohol lamp is required to sterilize the inoculating loops and to flame the mouth of culture tubes before inoculation.
- When anaerobic or microaerophilic microbes are suspected pathogens, a candle jar or anaerobe jar will be required to provide the appropriate environment for microbial growth.

TABLE 8.2 Summary of Pathogenic Fungi, Species Affected, Disease or Lesions Caused, and Specimens for Diagnosis

Organism	Species Affected	Disease or Lesion	Specimens
Microsporum			
M. canis	Dogs, cats	Ringworm	Fresh plucked hair and skin scrapings from edges of lesions
M. distortum	Dogs, cats, horses, pigs	Ringworm	
M. gypseum	Horses, cats, dogs, other species	Ringworm	
M. persicolor	Voles, bats, dogs	Ringworm	
Trichophyton			
T. erinacei	Hedgehogs, dogs, people	Ringworm	
T. mentagrophytes	Most animal species	Ringworm	
T. rubrum	Primarily humans, but also dogs, cats	Ringworm	
Candida			
Candida spp. (e.g., C. tropicalis) can cause lesions	Dogs Cats	Mycotic stomatitis Enteritis of kittens	Fixed affected tissue or scrapings from affected tissue
Malassezia pachydermatis	Dogs	Chronic otitis externa	Fresh ear swabs
Cryptococcus neoformans	Humans, dogs, cats (infection frequently affects nervous systems)	Subacute or chronic affected tissue	Fresh nasal discharge, milk
Coccidioides immitis (southwest United States and South America; occurs in soil)	Humans, horses, cattle, sheep, dogs, cats, captive feral animals	Disease characterized by granulomas, often in bronchial and mediastinal lymph nodes and lungs; can cause lesions in brain, liver, spleen, kidneys	Fresh and fixed lesions and affected tissue
Histoplasma capsulatum (northeast, central, and southcentral United States; occurs in soil)	Humans, dogs, cats, sheep, pigs, horses	Disease that generally affects reticuloendothelial system; dogs, cats—ulcerations of intestinal canal; enlargement of liver, spleen, lymph nodes; tuberculosis-like lesions	Fresh and fixed lesions or affected tissue
Blastomyces dermatitidis (United States, Canada, and Africa; occurs in soil)	Humans, dogs, cats, sea lions	Granulomatous lesions in lungs and/or skin and subcutis	Fresh and fixed lesions and affected tissue
Sporothrix schenckii	Humans, horses, dogs, pigs, cattle, fowl, rodents	Subcutaneous nodules or granulomas that eventually discharge pus; can include involvement of bones and visceral organs	Fresh and fixed pus, granulomas
Rhinosporidium seeberi (not yet cultured in vitro)	Horses, dogs, cattle, humans	Characterized by polyps on the nasal and ocular mucous membranes	Fresh nasal discharge and polyps; fixed polyps
Aspergillus			
A. fumigatus main pathogen; potentially pathogenic	Many animal species and birds	Dogs—infection of nasal chambers	Fresh deep scrapings or affected tissue
Abortions			
A. nidulans			
A. niger			
A. flavus	Ducklings, domestic birds, pigs, dogs	Aflatoxicosis; affects liver and sometimes kidneys	Suspect food product

From Sirois M: Principles and practice of veterinary technology, ed 3, St Louis, 2011, Mosby.

Culture Media

- Culture media are available in dozens of formulations.
- General-purpose nutrient media provide basic requirements for bacterial growth.
- Selective media contain additives that allow certain microorganisms to grow while inhibiting the growth of others.
- Enriched media also promote the growth of certain microbes by providing specific growth factors for bacteria with strict nutrient requirements (fastidious bacteria).
- Differential media contain additives that detect certain biochemical reactions of the bacteria. Media are also available that incorporate the features of more than one type.
- Most small animal practice microbiology laboratories will require just a few of these.
- Media are also supplied as a solid form on culture plates or in tubes, liquid form in tubes, or dehydrated form.
- Dehydrated media are the least expensive.
  - However, they require additional preparation time and must be autoclaved before use and may not be financially justifiable unless the practice is performing very large numbers of microbiology tests.
- In veterinary practice, the most commonly used solid media in culture plates are Mueller-Hinton, trypticase soy agar with 5% sheep blood (commonly called blood agar), and MacConkey or eosin–methylene blue (EMB).
- Mueller-Hinton is the recommended medium for culture and sensitivity testing.
- MacConkey and EMB are both selective media that support the growth of gram-negative bacteria and incorporate an additional indicator to allow differentiation among gram-negative enteric bacteria based on their ability to ferment lactose.
- Blood agar is an enriched medium that allows differentiation among specific hemolytic organisms.
  - Pathogenic bacteria exhibit beta hemolysis on blood agar.
- Solid media in culture tubes are used primarily for the growth of fungi and yeasts.
- Additional media available in this form include those used for biochemical testing of microbes.
- The most common types of slant media tubes are Sabouraud dextrose or bismuth–glucose–glycine yeast (commonly referred to as "biggy").
  - Either type is suitable for the growth of **dermatophytes** and is usually described as dermatophyte test medium (DTM), regardless of which specific medium is present.
- Fungal cultures of solid tissue samples may require the use of a 20% potassium hydroxide reagent for preparation of the sample.
- A variety of companies produce culture plates that incorporate several different media within individual compartments.
  - Items such as the Bullseye Veterinary Plate (Fig. 8.11) provide five different types of media that can simul-

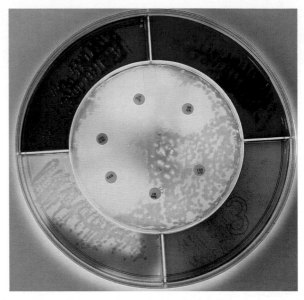

FIGURE 8.11 Bullseye culture medium (HealthLink, Jacksonville, FL). (From Hendrix CM, Sirois M: *Laboratory procedures for veterinary technicians*, ed 5, St Louis, 2007, Mosby.)

taneously select and differentiate microbes as well as provide antibiotic sensitivity data.
- Broth media in tubes is necessary for blood cultures and is also available in forms to provide differentiation of gram-negative enteric bacteria.
- Thioglycollate broth is a general-purpose medium that can be used for urine cultures.
- Specific blood culture tubes are available as evacuated tubes used for blood collection that contain both anticoagulant and culture media.
- Bacteria may often be partially differentiated based on their growth patterns on agar plates.
- Evaluation of colony characteristics should include form, elevation, margin, texture, and pigmentation (Fig. 8.12).
- The specific configuration made by a bacterial colony depends on the type of culture medium used as well as environmental conditions.

Stains

- Gram stain is an essential component of the microbiology laboratory.
- Acid-fast stains are useful in the identification of *Mycobacterium*.
  - These involve the addition of an agent such as dimethyl sulfoxide (DMSO) before addition of the primary stain.
  - The agent allows the stain to penetrate the stain-resistant cells of *Mycobacterium*.
  - The subsequent addition of acidic alcohol or dilute alcohol removes the stain. If the stain is not removed, the organism is said to be acid-fast.

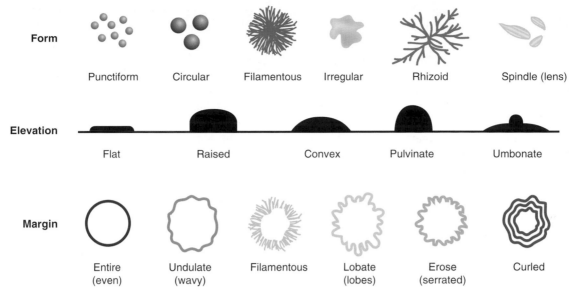

FIGURE 8.12 Bacterial colonies may be described on the basis of their form, elevation, and margins. (From Hendrix CM, Sirois M: *Laboratory procedures for veterinary technicians*, ed 5, St Louis, 2007, Mosby.)

- Flagella stains, capsule stains, endospore stains, and fluorescent stains are also available but have limited application in the average veterinary microbiology laboratory.
- Simple stains, such as crystal violet or methylene blue, are usually used for yeasts. Lactophenol cotton blue stain is often needed to prepare fungal culture samples for analysis and can also be used for cellophane tape preparations of external lesions.

Procedures

Inoculating Culture Media

- Aseptic technique is crucial to achieving diagnostic-quality results in microbiology.
- There are several methods for the inoculation of culture media, depending on the characteristics of the sample and type of testing needed.
- Because many samples contain multiple types of bacteria, most bacterial tests involve an initial step designed to isolate the bacterium of interest.

Inoculating Dermatophyte Test Media

- The procedures used for dermatophyte testing are slightly different from those used for general bacteriology testing.
- Either a DTM or plain Sabouraud dextrose agar can be used.
- DTM usually incorporates an additional reagent that causes a color change in the medium when *Microsporum canis* is present.
- It is important to note that some common contaminants can also induce this color change, and some cultures of *M. canis* do not produce color change on the medium.

- Suspect lesions may be gently cleaned with soap and water, and clean thumb forceps can be used to remove a few hairs and a small amount of epidermal scales from the periphery of the lesion.
- The hair and scale samples are then placed onto the surface of the culture medium, and a portion of the sample is pressed down into the medium.
- The culture is loosely covered and placed in a cabinet or drawer at room temperature.
- Starting at 48 hours after incubation, the inoculated medium must be inspected each day for evidence of color change.
- A flocculent growth accompanied by color change suggests *M. canis* infection.
- If no growth occurs after 7 days, the specimen should be redistributed over the medium and the culture procedure repeated.
- If growth is evident, the material should be stained and examined microscopically.
- A drop of lactophenol cotton blue stain is placed in the center of a microscope slide.
- A 2-inch piece of clear (not frosted) cellophane tape or Fungi-Tape is pressed against flocculent material observed growing on the plate.
- The tape is lifted and then pressed down into the drop of stain previously placed on the slide.
- The sample is evaluated microscopically for the characteristics of the organisms used to verify the species present.

Biochemical Test Materials

- Biochemical tests are often necessary to differentiate specific types of microbes.

- Biochemical testing may involve the use of specific liquid reagents or use media that contain the necessary reagents.
- The most commonly performed tests in the small veterinary practice laboratory are the oxidase and catalase tests.

Quality Control Concerns

- An effective quality control program is vital to achieving accurate and reliable results in any laboratory.
- Samples for microbiologic analysis are greatly affected by inappropriate or improperly performed collection methods.
- The timing of sample collection and processing must also be considered.
- Samples collected after medical treatment has begun or that are held for long periods before processing will yield unreliable results.
- Staining supplies and reagents must be stored and used correctly for maintenance of the integrity of these items.
- In addition to maintaining the sterility of collection and processing supplies, equipment used in the microbiology laboratory requires regular verification of performance.
  - This includes verification of temperatures in autoclaves and incubators.

CYTOLOGY

- The primary goal of the cytology evaluation is the differentiation of inflammation and neoplasia.
- Samples for cytology evaluation can be collected quickly and do not generally require specialized materials or equipment for proper evaluation.
- With careful attention to appropriate collection, preparation, and staining technique, a high-quality cytology sample can be obtained that may preclude the need for more invasive procedures to determine diagnosis, treatment, and prognosis for a patient.
- Several different preparations are often made from each sample.
  - This allows for additional diagnostic testing without additional collection.
- Samples may be processed as compression or modified compression preparations, impression smears, line smears, starfish smears, or simple smears.
- The exact type of preparation depends on the characteristics of the sample.
- Some samples may also require concentration by centrifugation.
- Fluid samples often require the addition of an anticoagulant and/or preservatives.
- A variety of staining techniques are also available for cytology specimens.
  - Some samples will require processing with more than one staining procedure.

- Collected and processed correctly, a cytology specimen is characterized as inflammatory, neoplastic, or mixed.
- The specimen is then described according to the presence of specific cell types.
- Fluid samples are classified as transudates, modified transudates, or exudates based on their gross appearance, total protein, and total nucleated cell count.
- In general, samples that are inflammatory are characterized by a predominance of neutrophils and macrophages (tissue monocytes).
- Inflammatory processes are characterized as suppurative, pyogranulomatous, or eosinophilic when specific cell types and numbers of cells are evident on the cytology preparation.
- Neoplastic samples are characterized by large numbers of tissue cells.
- Neoplastic cells are further evaluated for malignant changes.
- A combination of cell types may be present, which may indicate a neoplastic disease with secondary inflammation.

Collection and Preparation of Samples from Tissues and Masses

Impression Smears

- Impression smears are prepared from active lesions on an animal's body or from tissues removed during surgical procedures.
- For impression smears from active lesions, an initial impression is made before cleaning the lesion or initiating treatment.
  - Additional smears are prepared after cleaning the lesion.
- To prepare the smear, gently touch a clean glass slide to several areas of the lesion.
- Although this type of sample can be prepared quickly and easily, it tends to yield the fewest number of cells and can also be contaminated by bacteria that may be present because of secondary bacterial infection.
- Impression smears of tissue samples are made in a similar manner except that a fresh section of the tissue is made; the tissue is then blotted to remove excess blood and tissue fluid.

Scrapings

- Scrapings can be prepared from external lesions or from tissues removed during surgical procedures.
- To prepare a scraping, the lesion or tissue must be cleaned and blotted dry.
- If using tissue samples, a fresh section is cut before obtaining the sample.
- A dull scalpel blade is held at a 90-degree angle to the lesion or tissue and is gently pulled across the surface.
- A compression smear is then prepared from the material on the edge of the scalpel blade.
- The sample can also be smeared across a slide directly from the scalpel blade.

Swabbings

- Swab smears are most useful for fistulated lesions or collections from the vaginal canal.
- A sterile cotton swab is moistened with 0.9% saline and lightly swabbed along the surface of the tissue.
- The swab is then gently rolled across the surface of a clean glass slide.

Fine-Needle Biopsy

- A fine-needle biopsy sample can often provide much information to the clinician and may preclude the need for biopsy of lesions of internal organs.
- This type of sample preparation may also be preferred for the collection of samples from superficial lesions because bacterial contamination can be kept to a minimum.
- If microbiologic tests are to be performed on a portion of the sample collected or a body cavity (e.g., peritoneal and thoracic cavities, joints) is to be penetrated, the area of aspiration is surgically prepared.
- The procedure may be performed using an aspirate or nonaspirate technique.
- For the aspiration biopsy, equipment needed includes a 3- to 20-mL syringe and a 21- to 25-gauge needle.
  - Samples collected from softer tissue require smaller syringes and needles.
  - Firmer tissues require larger syringes and large-bore needles.
- The nonaspirate procedure can be used to collect samples from solid masses.

Preparation Techniques for Cytology Samples

- Samples collected from organs and masses can be prepared in several ways.
- The veterinary assistant is responsible for preparing the supplies needed.
- Regardless of the preparation method chosen, the smear must be made quickly to avoid deterioration of the sample.
- Several smears should be made and rapidly air-dried.
- Centesis refers to fluid samples collected from body cavities.
- Fluid removed from the abdominal, thoracic, and pericardial cavities should be well mixed with an appropriate anticoagulant (e.g., EDTA) and the specimen prepared as quickly as possible to prevent cellular deterioration.
- Slides can be prepared directly from the nonconcentrated fluid or from concentrated sediment after centrifugation of the sample.

Concentration Techniques

- Fluid samples may be centrifuged to concentrate the solid material before preparing smears. The technique is similar to that used for the preparation of urine sediment for microscopic analysis.
- The anticoagulated fluid is placed in a standard clinical centrifuge and spun for 5 minutes at 1000 to 2000 rpm (165 to 400 g).
- The supernatant is poured off, leaving a few drops in the tube, and sediment is gently resuspended in the remaining supernatant.

Vaginal Cytology

- Cytologic evaluation of vaginal tissues is used to determine the stage of estrus in the dog and cat and as an aid in timing of mating or artificial insemination.
- Samples are collected with the animal in a standing position, with the tail elevated.
- The external genitalia should be cleaned and rinsed.
- The veterinary assistant should prepare the necessary supplies, which include lubricant, vaginal speculum, and sterile moistened swabs.
- The veterinary technician will insert the lubricated vaginal speculum into the vagina, followed by a sterile moistened swab.
- The presence of specific types of epithelial cells, blood cells, and bacteria in a vaginal cytology sample is combined with behavioral history and clinical signs to determine estrous stage.

HISTOLOGY

- Many samples collected for cytology analysis will also require histologic evaluation. Histology samples are usually collected by biopsy and require special preparation to preserve the cells for detailed evaluation.
- Fixation of tissues is a critical first step.
- The fixative must rapidly denature cellular proteins to avoid autolysis of the sample.
- Fixatives are chosen based on their speed and penetrating ability.
- They must not excessively harden or soften tissues and, ideally, be nontoxic to the user and inexpensive.
- Common fixatives include acetic acid, isopropyl or isobutyl alcohol, chromic acid, and formalin.
- The size of the tissue sample also affects the rate of fixation.
- Samples must be sectioned so that the fixative can penetrate the entire tissue within 24 to 48 hours.
- For large tissue samples, several cuts should be made into the tissue to allow the fixative to penetrate rapidly.
- Most fixatives are capable of penetrating approximately 2 to 4 mm/24 hours.
- The amount of solution needed is generally 10 to 20 times the volume of the sample.
- Once adequately fixed, the sample can be transferred into a smaller container.

URINALYSIS

- Abnormalities in the urine may reflect a variety of disease processes involving several different organs.

- The basic equipment needed to perform a urinalysis is minimal and readily available in most veterinary clinics.

Sample Collection

- Collect urine samples in clean glass or plastic containers.
- Sterile containers are not necessary unless you are performing a urine culture.
- Urine samples are collected using one of the following methods.
  - Free-flow or clean catch: Collecting a specimen as the animal urinates
  - Expressing the bladder: Manual compression of the bladder using gentle, steady pressure applied through the abdominal wall
  - Catheterization: Placing a urinary catheter through the urethra into the bladder
  - Cystocentesis: Inserting a needle into the bladder through the ventral abdominal wall
- Bladder expression and cystocentesis require the bladder to be full enough to palpate and hold in position.
- Cystocentesis requires sterile collection equipment and aseptic technique.
  - Only specimens collected by cystocentesis are suitable for urine culture.
- Cystocentesis and catheterization are also performed to relieve bladder distention in animals unable to urinate.
- Manual compression cannot be performed on an obstructed animal because this could rupture the bladder.
- Bladder expression, catheterization, and cystocentesis all cause some degree of trauma.
- A first-morning urine sample is the preferred specimen because this sample is the most concentrated.
- The first few drops from a free-catch sample should be discarded because there is a high incidence of contamination by the debris normally present at the urethral opening in the first few drops.
- In females, the first drops of urine may also be contaminated with material from the genital tract, such as blood from an intact bitch in proestrus.
- Because physical, chemical, and microscopic characteristics of a urine specimen begin to change as soon as urine is voided, urine specimens should be analyzed immediately after collection.
- Samples left at room temperature for 1 hour or longer will have increases in pH, turbidity, and bacteria and decreases in glucose, bilirubin, and ketone levels.
- If specimens are left at room temperature for longer than 1 hour, cells and casts may also disintegrate, especially in dilute alkaline urine, or urine color may change because of oxidation or reduction of metabolites.
  - If analysis cannot be done immediately, refrigeration will minimize deterioration of the specimen.
  - The specimen should be brought to room temperature before testing.
- Chemical preservatives can also be added to urine.

- However, preservatives usually act as antimicrobial agents, so chemically preserved urine cannot be used for culture and may interfere with biochemical testing.

Complete Urinalysis

- A complete urinalysis has the following four parts:
  - Gross examination
  - Specific gravity measurement
  - Biochemical analysis
  - Sediment examination
- A systematic approach is vital to achieving high-quality, reproducible results.
- The gross examination includes an evaluation of color, clarity, odor, and volume.
- Normal canine and feline urine is light amber colored, clear, and has a characteristic odor. Normal urine output for canine and feline patients is 10 to 20 mL/pound in a 24-hour period.

Specific Gravity

- Specific gravity (SG) is a measure of the ratio of a volume of urine to the weight of the same volume of distilled water at a constant temperature.
- SG is an indicator of the concentration of dissolved materials in the urine and provides an indication of kidney function.
- The preferred method for determining SG is with the use of a refractometer.
- SG indicator pads on urinalysis dipstick tests may be unreliable in veterinary species.
- SG can be measured before or after centrifugation, as long as the procedure is always performed consistently in the clinic.

Biochemical Testing

- The chemical evaluation of urine is used to detect substances that may have passed into the urine as a result of damage to the nephron or overproduction of specific analytes.
- Most in-house urinalysis chemical tests use the dipstick format (Fig. 8.13). Dipsticks can be used to perform an individual test or multiple tests.
- Each reagent pad on the dipstick contains reagent for one specific chemical test.
- The reagent pad changes color during the reaction, and the color is visually compared with a color chart.
- Before using the dipstick, always note the expiration date and general condition of the strips.
- Containers of dipsticks should be stored at room temperature with the lid tightly capped. Avoid placing containers or color charts in direct sunlight.
- Always use well-mixed, room-temperature urine samples and perform chemical testing before adding any chemical preservatives.
- Read the instructions carefully, and evaluate color changes at the correct time interval. Because dipsticks are not configured for veterinary species, some tests

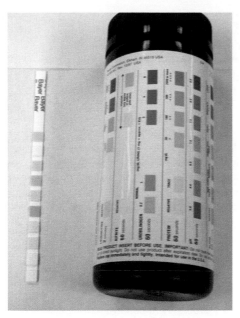

FIGURE 8.13 Reagent strip test container and combination dipstick strip. (From Hendrix CM, Sirois M: *Laboratory procedures for veterinary technicians*, ed 5, St Louis, 2007, Mosby.)

(e.g., SG, nitrite, leukocyte) may be unreliable with some species.

- Most urinalysis dipstick tests provide indicator pads for protein, glucose, ketones, pH, bilirubin, and blood.

Microscopic Examination of Urine Sediment

- The primary purpose of microscopic examination of urine is to determine the presence of abnormally formed elements (e.g., cells, casts, crystals) in the sample (Fig. 8.14).
- The presence of specific formed elements usually provides detailed diagnostic information to the clinician.
- The examination requires 5 to 10 mL of fresh urine.
- The sample should be centrifuged at low speed for approximately 5 minutes and then the supernatant poured off, leaving approximately 1 mL of supernatant with the sediment.
- The remaining sediment is resuspended in the supernatant and mixed gently.
- A drop of this suspension is then placed on a microscope slide, a coverslip is added, and the specimen is examined microscopically.

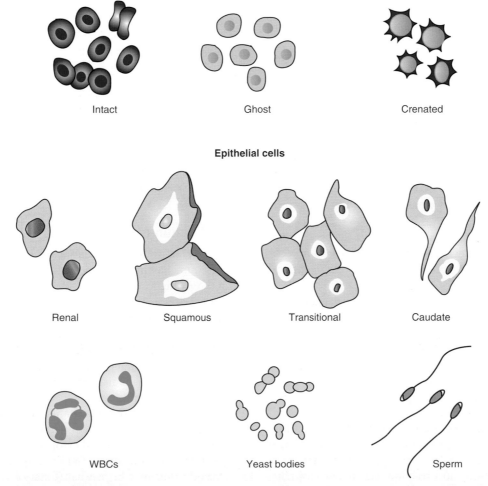

FIGURE 8.14 Cell types that may be found in urine. (From Hendrix CM, Sirois M: *Laboratory procedures for veterinary technicians*, ed 5, St Louis, 2007, Mosby.)

- Although stain may be added to the sample, this often creates artifacts and can add bacteria to the sample.
- When a stain is needed to classify cell types, it should be added after the initial evaluation of the specimen.

PARASITOLOGY

- Parasitology is the study of organisms that live in (internal parasites, endoparasites) or on (external parasites, ectoparasites) another organism—the host—from which they derive their nourishment.
- The host may be a definitive host, sheltering the sexual adult stages of the parasite, or an intermediate host, harboring asexual (immature) or larval stages of the parasite.
- Paratenic or transport hosts for some parasites are those in which the parasite survives without multiplying or developing.
- Parasite life cycles can be simple, with direct transmission, or complex and involve one or more vectors.
- A vector can be mechanical or biologic.
  - Mechanical vectors transmit the parasite, but the parasite does not develop in the vector.
  - Biologic vectors serve as intermediate hosts for the parasite.
- The term life cycle refers to the maturation of a parasite through various developmental stages in one or more hosts.
- For a parasite to survive, it must have a dependable means of transfer from one host to another and the ability to develop and reproduce in the host, ideally without producing serious harm to the host, which requires the following:
  - Mode of entry into a host (infective stage)
  - Availability of a susceptible host (definitive host)
  - Accommodating location and environment in the host for maturation and reproduction (e.g., gastrointestinal, respiratory, circulatory, urinary, or reproductive system)
  - Mode of exit from the host (e.g., feces, sputum, blood, urine, smegma), with dispersal into an ecologically suitable environment for development and survival
- For parasites that have one or more intermediate hosts, the definitive host is the one in which sexual maturity takes place.
- Parasites have a wide distribution within host animals.
- Parasites can have a negative impact in a number of ways, including the following:
  - Injury on entry (e.g., creeping eruption)
  - Injury by migration (e.g., sarcoptic mange)
  - Injury by residence (e.g., heartworms)
  - Chemical and/or physiologic injury (e.g., digestive disturbances)
  - Injury caused by host reaction (e.g., hypersensitivity, scar tissue)

BOX 8.2 Taxonomic Classifications of Parasites of Animals

Kingdom: Animalia (animals)
Phylum: Platyhelminthes (flatworms)
  Class: Trematoda (flukes)
    Subclass: Monogenea (monogenetic flukes)
    Subclass: Digenea (digenetic flukes)
  Class: Cotyloda (pseudotapeworms)
Phylum: Nematoda (roundworms)
Phylum: Acanthocephala (thorny-headed worms)
Phylum: Arthropoda (animals with jointed legs)
  Subphylum: Mandibulata (possess mandibulate mouthparts)
  Class: Crustacea (aquatic crustaceans)
  Class: Insecta
    Order: Dictyoptera (cockroaches)
    Order: Coleoptera (beetles)
    Order: Lepidoptera (butterflies and moths)
    Order: Hymenoptera (ants, bees, and wasps)
    Order: Hemiptera (true bugs)
    Order: Mallophaga (chewing or biting lice)
    Order: Anoplura (sucking lice)
    Order: Diptera (two-winged flies)
    Order: Siphonaptera (fleas)
Phylum: Sarcomastigophora
  Subphylum: Mastigophora (flagellates)
Phylum: Sarcomastigophora
  Superclass: Sarcodina (amoebae)
Phylum: Ciliophora (ciliates)
Phylum: Apicomplexa (apicomplexans)
Phylum: Proteobacteria
  Class: Alpha Proteobacteria
    Order: Rickettsiales
      Family: Rickettsiaceae
      Family: Anaplasmataceae

From Sirois M: Principles and practice of veterinary technology, ed 3, St Louis, 2011, Mosby.

Classification of Parasites

- Parasites of domestic animals are found in the Protista and Animalia kingdoms and in a large number of phyla in those kingdoms.
- Box 8.2 contains a summary of the taxonomic classifications of common parasites of domestic animals.

Kingdom Protista, Subkingdom Protozoa

- There are approximately 65,000 known protozoans in a wide variety of habitats, but only a small percentage of protozoans are parasitic.
- Protozoa are single-celled organisms with one or more membrane-bound nuclei containing deoxyribonucleic acid (DNA) and specialized cytoplasmic organelles.
- The life cycles of protozoa can be simple or complex.
- Reproduction may be asexual (binary fission, schizogony, budding) or sexual (syngamy, conjugation).

- The trophozoite (also known as the vegetative form) is the stage of the protozoal life cycle that is capable of feeding, movement, and reproduction.
- The trophozoite is often too fragile to survive transfer to a new host and generally is not infective.
- Transmission to a host often occurs when the protozoan is in the cyst stage.
- The phylum Sarcomastigophora (Sarcodina) includes the amoebas and flagellates.
  - The most common parasitic organism of dogs and cats in this phylum is *Giardia*.
- The phylum Apicomplexa contains the sporozoans.
- Sporozoal parasites are found within the host cells and commonly occur in the intestinal tract cells and blood cells.
- Oocyst is the name given to the cyst stage of this group of intestinal protozoa.
- The most common genera of veterinary importance include *Cystoisospora* (formerly *Isospora*) and *Toxoplasma*.

Kingdom Animalia

- Three of the phyla in this kingdom contain hundreds of species that are of veterinary significance.
- These include (1) Platyhelminthes: the flatworms; (2) Nematoda: the roundworms; and (3) Arthropoda: ticks, mites, and lice.

- The phylum Acanthocephala contains just a few species of veterinary significance.

Phylum Platyhelminthes

- Organisms in the phylum Platyhelminthes are commonly called flatworms because of the dorsoventral flattening of their body tissues.
- The two groups of veterinary importance are the cestodes (tapeworms) and trematodes (flukes).

Cestodes

- Two major groups of tapeworms are important in veterinary medicine: the cyclophyllidean tapeworms and the pseudophyllidean tapeworms.
- The cyclophyllidean tapeworms typically have one intermediate host (Fig. 8.15).
  - Organisms in this group include *Dipylidium caninum*, *Taenia* spp., and *Echinococcus* spp.
- The pseudophyllidean tapeworms have two intermediate hosts (e.g., *Diphyllobothrium latum*).
- Table 8.3 summarizes the cestode parasites of veterinary species.
- Typically, the larval stages of cestodes in domestic animals are more harmful (pathogenic) than the adult stages in the intestinal tract.
- The adult stages are the source of eggs, especially for cestodes, which can use humans as an intermediate host and pose a risk to human health (zoonotic).

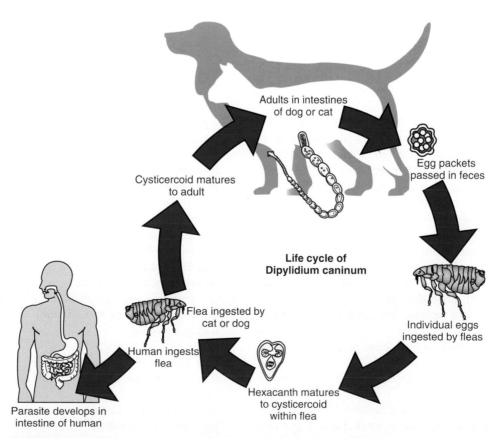

Life cycle of Dipylidium caninum

Adults in intestines of dog or cat

Egg packets passed in feces

Individual eggs ingested by fleas

Hexacanth matures to cysticercoid within flea

Human ingests flea

Flea ingested by cat or dog

Cysticercoid matures to adult

Parasite develops in intestine of human

FIGURE 8.15 Life cycle of *Dipylidium caninum*. (From Hendrix CM, Robinson E: *Diagnostic parasitology for veterinary technicians*, ed 4, St Louis, 2012, Mosby.)

TABLE 8.3 Selected Cestode (Tapeworm) Parasites of Dogs and Cats

Scientific Name	Common Name
Dogs	
Diphyllobothrium spp.	Broad fish tapeworm
Dipylidium caninum	Cucumber seed tapeworm
Spirometra spp.	Zipper tapeworm
Echinococcus granulosus	Hydatid disease tapeworm
Cats	
Echinococcus multilocularis	Hydatid disease tapeworm
Taenia taeniaeformis or Hydatigera taeniaeformis	Feline tapeworm
Diphyllobothrium spp.	Broad fish tapeworm
Dipylidium caninum	Cucumber seed tapeworm
Spirometra spp.	Zipper tapeworm

Adapted from Sirois M: Principles and practice of veterinary technology, ed 3, St Louis, 2011, Mosby.

- Cestodes are multicellular organisms that lack a body cavity.
- The body of tapeworms is long and dorsoventrally flattened and consists of three regions.
- The head (scolex) is modified into an attachment organ and bears two to four muscular suckers, or bothria, that may be armed with hooks.
- There may also be a snout (rostellum) on the head, which can be fixed or retractable; the rostellum can also be armed with hooks.
- Caudal to the head is a short neck of undifferentiated tissue, followed by the body (strobila), which is composed of segments (proglottids) in different stages of maturity.
- Proglottids near the neck are immature, followed by sexually mature proglottids, terminating with gravid segments containing eggs.
- Gravid proglottids break off and pass out of the body of the definitive host in the feces.
- New proglottids are continually formed from the undifferentiated tissue of the neck.
- Cestodes lack a digestive tract, and nutrients are absorbed directly through the body wall.
- The most prominent organs in cestodes are the organs of the reproductive system.
- Both male and female reproductive organs occur in an individual tapeworm.
- Cestodes also have a nervous system and an excretory system.
- The cestode egg contains a fully developed embryo, which has six hooks in three pairs (hexacanth embryo, or oncosphere), or a zygote that develops into a ciliated embryo (coracidium).

- The life cycle of tapeworms is always indirect and involves one or two intermediate hosts.
  - The intermediate hosts may be **arthropods**, fish, or mammals.
- Domestic animals can be definitive and/or intermediate hosts for tapeworms.
- The larval stages of some tapeworms found in domestic animals are called bladder worms because they resemble fluid-filled sacks, with one or multiple scoleces.
- When ingested by a definitive host, the bladder worms are released from the tissue of the intermediate host and develop into adult tapeworms within the digestive tract of the definitive host.
- Some cestodes have larval forms that are solid bodies (e.g., procercoid, plerocercoid, tetrathyridium).
- Domestic animals become infected with the larval stages of tapeworms by ingestion of the cestode egg or procercoid.

Trematodes

- The trematodes (flukes) are flatworms that, like cestodes, lack a body cavity.
- Trematodes are unsegmented and leaflike, with organs embedded in loose tissue (parenchyma).
- Trematodes also possess two muscular attachment organs, or suckers.
  - One sucker, the anterior sucker, is located at the mouth.
  - The other sucker, the ventral sucker or acetabulum, is located on the ventral surface of the worm near the middle of the body or at the caudal end.
- There are three main groups of trematodes, but only the digenetic trematodes are parasites of domestic animals.
- The life cycle of digenetic trematodes is complicated.
- They pass through several different larval stages (e.g., miracidium, sporocyst, redia, cercaria, metacercaria) and typically require one or more intermediate hosts, one of which is almost always a mollusk (e.g., snail, slug).
- The primary digenetic trematodes of concern in dogs is *Nanophyetus salmincola*.

Phylum Nematoda

- Organisms in the phylum Nematoda are commonly called roundworms because of their cylindrical body shape.
- The life cycle of nematodes follows a standard pattern consisting of several developmental stages—the egg, four larval stages that are also wormlike in appearance, and sexually mature adults.
- The infective stage may be an egg containing a larva, free-living larva, or larva within an intermediate or transport host.
- A life cycle is considered direct if no intermediate host is necessary for development to the infective stage.
- If an intermediate host is required for development to the infective stage, the life cycle is considered indirect.
- Transmission to a new definitive host can occur through ingestion, skin penetration of infective larvae, ingestion of an intermediate host, or deposition of infective larvae into or on the skin by an intermediate host.

- Once a nematode enters a new host, development to the adult stages may occur in the area of their final location or may occur after extensive migration through the body of the definitive host.
- The diagnostic stages of parasitic nematodes are typically found in feces, blood, sputum, or urine.
- Most parasitic nematodes are found in the intestinal tracts of their respective definitive hosts, but some are found in the lungs, kidney, urinary bladder, or heart.
- Table 8.4 summarizes the nematode parasites of dogs and cats.
- Nematodes of dogs and cats include *Toxocara* spp., *Toxascaris* spp., and *Ancylostoma* spp. *Trichuris vulpis*, the canine whipworm, derives its common name from the fact that adults possess a thin, filamentous anterior end (lash of the whip) and thick posterior end (handle of the whip).
- The egg of the whipworm is described as trichuroid or trichinelloid; it has a thick, yellow-brown, symmetrical shell with polar plugs at both ends.
- *D. immitis* (Fig. 8.16) is the heartworm of dogs.
- The life cycle of *D. immitis* requires an intermediate host to be transmitted from animal to animal.
- *D. immitis* adults live in the right ventricle and pulmonary artery.
- The male and female *D. immitis* adults mate, and the female produces microfilariae.
  - The microfilariae are released into the host's bloodstream, where they are ingested by feeding female mosquitoes.
  - The microfilariae grow and molt in the mosquito until they reach the infective stage.
  - Once they become infective, they enter a new host the next time the mosquito feeds (Fig. 8.17).
- Once in the new host, the larvae migrate and molt through various body tissues on their way to the heart.
- It is at this time that the larvae may grow and molt to become adults in sites other than the heart.

Phylum Acanthocephala

- Acanthocephalans are commonly referred to as thornyheaded worms.
- Acanthocephalans are rarely encountered but are occasionally found in pigs and dogs.
- The life cycle of an acanthocephalan is complex and involves an intermediate host, usually a crustacean or an insect.
- The main acanthocephalan of concern is *Oncicola canis*, an acanthocephalan found in dogs.

Rickettsial Parasites

- The rickettsia are a group of obligate, intracellular, gram-negative bacteria.
- The major taxonomic families are the Rickettsiaceae (Table 8.5), which include the genera *Rickettsia*, *Orientia*, and *Coxiella*, and the Anaplasmataceae, which include the genera *Anaplasma* and *Ehrlichia*.
- The organisms are transmitted by arthropod or helminth vectors.

TABLE 8.4 Selected Nematodes (Roundworms) of Veterinary Species

Scientific Name	Common Name
Dogs	
Acanthocheilonema reconditum (formerly *Dipetalonema reconditum*)	Skin filariid
Ancylostoma braziliense	Hookworm
Ancylostoma caninum	Hookworm
Capillaria plica	Bladder worm
Dioctophyma renale	Giant kidney worm
Dirofilaria immitis	Canine heartworm
Dracunculus insignis	Guinea worm
Eucoleus aerophilus (formerly *Capillaria aerophila*)	Lungworm
Filaroides spp.	Canine lungworm
Physaloptera spp.	Stomach worm
Spirocerca lupi	Esophageal worm
Strongyloides spp.	Threadworms
Thelazia californiensis	Eyeworm
Toxocara canis	Roundworm, ascarid
Trichuris vulpis	Whipworm
Uncinaria stenocephala	Northern canine hookworm
Cats	
Aelurostrongylus abstrusus	Lungworm
Ancylostoma braziliense	Hookworm
Ancylostoma tubaeforme	Hookworm
Aonchotheca putorii (formerly *Capillaria putorii*)	Gastrid capillarid of cats
Capillaria feliscati	Bladder worm
Eucoleus aerophilus (formerly *Capillaria aerophila*)	Lungworm
Physaloptera spp.	Stomach worm
Spirocerca lupi	Esophageal worm
Thelazia californiensis	Eyeworm
Toxascaris leonina	Roundworm, ascarid
Toxocara cati	Roundworm, ascarid
Trichuris campanula	Whipworm
Trichuris serrata	Whipworm

From Sirois M: Principles and practice of veterinary technology, ed 3, St Louis, 2011, Mosby.

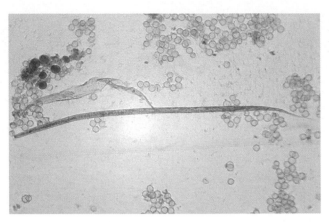

FIGURE 8.16 Microfilaria of *Dirofilaria immitis* found by the modified Knott technique. (From Hendrix CM, Robinson E: *Diagnostic parasitology for veterinary technicians*, ed 4, St Louis, 2012, Mosby.)

Phylum Arthropoda

- Organisms in the phylum Arthropoda are characterized by the presence of jointed legs and a chitinous exoskeleton composed of segments.
- Only certain groups of arthropods are parasitic. Members of other groups may act as intermediate hosts for the other parasites discussed earlier.
- When a parasite resides on the surface of its host, it is called an ectoparasite.
- Most ectoparasites are insects (e.g., fleas, lice, flies) or arachnids (e.g., ticks, mites).
- The following general characteristics differentiate the two major classes of arthropods of veterinary importance.
  - Insects have three pairs of legs, three distinct body regions (head, thorax, and abdomen), and a single pair of antennae.

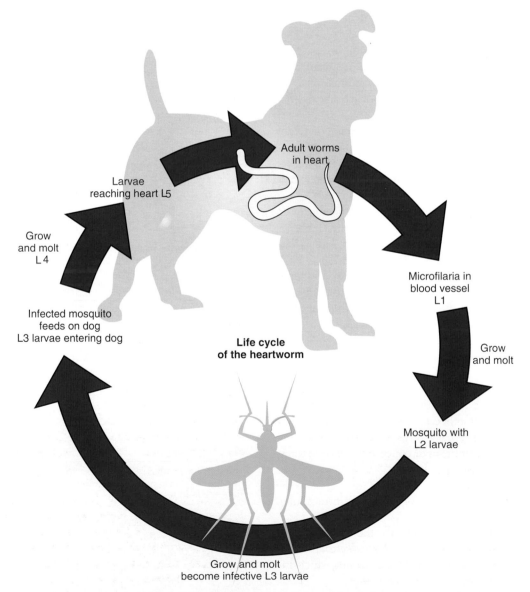

FIGURE 8.17 Life cycle of the canine *Dirofilaria immitis*. (From Hendrix CM, Robinson E: *Diagnostic parasitology for veterinary technicians*, ed 4, St Louis, 2012, Mosby.)

TABLE 8.5 Pathogenic Rickettsiaceae That Affect Animals

Agent	Disease	Vector	Geographic Distribution
Rickettsia rickettsii	Rocky Mountain spotted fever	*Dermacentor* spp., ticks, *Amblyomma cajennense*– *Rhipicephalus sanguineus*	Western Hemisphere
R. felis	Cat flea typhus	*Ctenocephalides felis* (cat flea)	Western Hemisphere, Europe
R. typhi	Murine typhus	*Xenopsylla cheopis* (rat flea)	Worldwide
R. prowazekii	Epidemic typhus	Human body louse, flying squirrel louse, squirrel flea	Worldwide

Adapted from Songer JG, Post KW: Veterinary microbiology: Bacterial and fungal agents of animal disease, St Louis, 2005, Saunders.

- Arachnids (adults) have four pairs of legs, a body divided into two regions (cephalothorax, abdomen), and no antennae.
- The mouth parts of insects vary in structure, depending on feeding habits, with adaptations for chewing and biting, sponging, or piercing and sucking.
- The sexes are separate, and reproduction results in the production of eggs or larvae. Development often involves three or more larvae followed by the formation of a pupa and a change in form or transformation (complete metamorphosis) to the adult stage.
- In other insects, development occurs from the egg through several immature stages (nymphs), which resemble the adult in form but are smaller (incomplete metamorphosis).
- Fleas and flies demonstrate complete metamorphosis, and lice demonstrate incomplete metamorphosis.
- Insects may produce harm to their definitive host as adults and/or larvae.
- Ticks and mites are the more important groups of arachnids in veterinary medicine, although some spiders and scorpions can harm domestic animals via toxic venoms.
- Arachnids are generally small—often microscopic.
- Life cycle stages consist of the egg, larva, nymph, and adult.

Fleas

- Fleas are blood-sucking parasites of dogs, cats, rodents, birds, and people.
- Fleas are vectors of several diseases, such as bubonic plague and tularemia.
- Cat and dog fleas, *Ctenocephalides felis* and *C. canis*, respectively, can act as intermediate hosts for the common tapeworm, *D. caninum.*
- Heavy infestations with fleas, especially in young animals, produce anemia.
- Flea saliva is antigenic and irritating, causing intense pruritus (itching) and hypersensitivity, known as flea bite dermatitis or miliary dermatitis.
- Fleas are laterally compressed, wingless insects with legs adapted for jumping.

- Flea infestations are encountered most frequently on dogs and cats and can be detected around the tail or head, on the ventral abdomen, and under the chin.
- Fleas demonstrate complete metamorphosis (Fig. 8.18).
- Flea eggs deposited on the host fall off and develop to larvae in the environment.
- Flea larvae can occasionally be found in the animal's bedding, on furniture, or in cracks and crevices of the animal's environment.
- Flea larvae are maggot-like, with a head capsule and bristles.
- Flea larvae feed on organic debris, including the excrement of adult fleas.
- Flea droppings are reddish brown, comma-shaped casts of dehydrated blood.
- Flea droppings in the animal's hair or coat indicate flea infestation.
- Fleas have preferred hosts, but they attack any source of blood if the preferred host is not available.

Lice

- Lice are dorsoventrally flattened, wingless insects with clawed appendages for clasping to the host's hairs.
- Lice are separated into two orders, based on whether their mouth parts are modified for chewing (Mallophaga) or sucking (Anoplura).
- Sucking lice have a long, narrow head; feed on blood; and move slowly on the host.
- Biting lice have a broad, rounded head; feed on epithelial debris; and can move rapidly over the host.
- Lice are host-specific, remain in close association with the host, and have preferred locations on the host.
- Lice glue their eggs or nits (Fig. 8.19) to the hairs or feathers of the host.
- Transmission is usually by direct contact but can occur through equipment contaminated with eggs, nymphs, or adults.
- Louse infestations (pediculosis) tend to be more severe in young, old, or poorly nourished animals, especially in overcrowded conditions and during the colder months.
- Sucking lice produce anemia, whereas biting lice are irritating and disturbing to the animal.

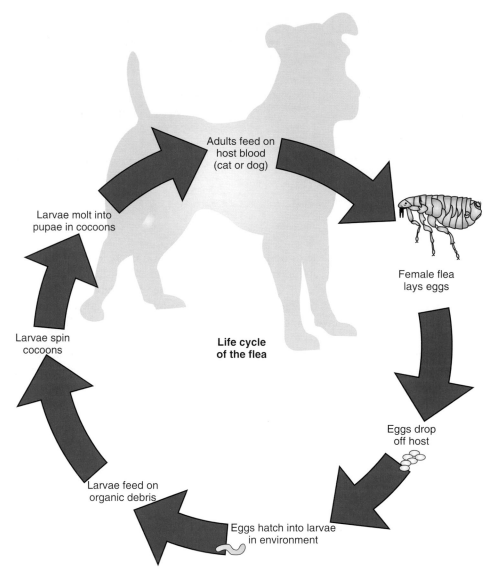

Adults feed on host blood (cat or dog)

Larvae molt into pupae in cocoons

Larvae spin cocoons

Life cycle of the flea

Female flea lays eggs

Larvae feed on organic debris

Eggs drop off host

Eggs hatch into larvae in environment

FIGURE 8.18 Life cycle of the flea. (From Hendrix CM, Robinson E: *Diagnostic parasitology for veterinary technicians*, ed 4, St Louis, 2012, Mosby.)

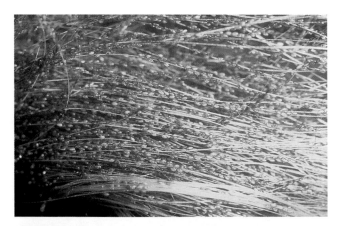

FIGURE 8.19 Thousands of nits cemented by female lice to the hair. (From Hendrix CM, Robinson E: *Diagnostic parasitology for veterinary technicians*, ed 4, St Louis, 2012, Mosby.)

- Common biting lice of domestic animals include *Trichodectes canis* and *Felicola subrostratus* (cat). *Linognathus setosus* is a common sucking louse of the dog.

Flies
- Flies are a diverse group of insects that undergo complete metamorphosis.
- Flies have one pair of wings, which may be scaled or membranous, and a pair of balancing structures, called halters.
- The mouth parts of flies may be adapted for sponging or piercing and sucking.
- Flies produce harm by inflicting painful bites, sucking blood, producing hypersensitive reactions, depositing eggs in sores, migration of larval stages through tissues of the host with escape through holes in the skin

(warbles), causing annoyance, and acting as vectors and intermediate hosts to other pathogenic agents.

- Biting midges (known as no-see-ums), *Culicoides* spp., are small flies.
- The females are blood suckers that inflict a painful bite.
- Black flies (buffalo gnats) are small flies with a characteristic humped back.
- They produce harm similar to that of no-see-ums and in great numbers can exsanguinate a host.
- Sand flies (*Phlebotomus* spp.) are mothlike flies, known primarily for their role in the transmission of leishmaniasis and viral diseases.
- The females suck blood.
- Mosquitoes are a large and important group of flies known for the annoying bites of the females, which suck blood, and also for their role in the transmission of numerous protozoal, viral, and nematode diseases to animals and humans.
- Botflies include *Cuterebra* spp., beelike flies, the adults of which do not feed.
- Adult botflies glue their eggs to the hairs of the host or deposit them at the entrance of animal burrows.
- The larvae hatch and penetrate the skin of the host (myiasis).
- Some migrate extensively through the host's body, and others develop locally.
- They produce large pockets in the subcutaneous tissues of the host with air holes in the skin known as warbles (Fig. 8.20).

Ticks

- Ticks are blood-sucking arachnids that are dorsoventrally flattened in the unengorged state. There are two types of ticks: hard ticks (Ixodidae) and soft ticks (Argasidae).
- Hard ticks are important vectors of protozoal, bacterial, viral, and rickettsial diseases.

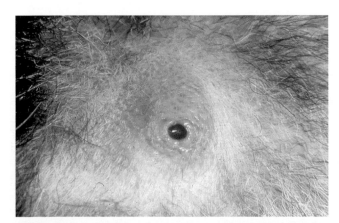

FIGURE 8.20 Larval *Cuterebra* spp. in a subcutaneous fistula. (From Hendrix CM, Robinson E: *Diagnostic parasitology for veterinary technicians*, ed 4, St Louis, 2012, Mosby.)

- The saliva of female ticks of some species is toxic and produces flaccid ascending paralysis in animals and humans (tick paralysis).
- The adults, larvae, and nymphs attach to the host and feed on blood; eggs are deposited in the environment (Fig. 8.21).
- Hard ticks are dorsoventrally flattened, with well-defined lateral margins in the unengorged state.
- Hard ticks have a hard, chitinous covering (scutum) on the dorsal surface of the body and may have grooves, margins, and notches (festoons), which are useful for identification purposes.
- Ticks may attach to and feed on one to three different hosts during a life cycle and are referred to as one-host, two-host, or three-host ticks.
- Important hard ticks in North America include *Rhipicephalus sanguineus*, *Dermacentor* spp., *Ixodes* spp., and *Amblyomma* spp.
- Soft ticks lack a scutum, and their mouth parts are not visible from the dorsal surface.
- The females feed often, and eggs are laid off the host.
- There are three genera of veterinary importance: *Argas* spp., *Otobius megnini*, and *Ornithodoros* spp.

Mites

- Mites are arachnids that occur as parasitic and free-living forms, some of which act as intermediate hosts for cestodes.
- Most parasitic mites are obligate parasites, which spend their entire life cycle on the host and produce the dermatologic condition referred to as mange.
- Most mite infestations (acariasis) are transmitted through direct contact with an infested animal.
- Burrowing mite infestations are diagnosed with deep skin scrapings at the periphery of lesions.
- Mites can be divided into two main groups: burrowing mites and nonburrowing mites.
- Another group of mites is parasitic only as larvae, the trombiculid mites, or chiggers.
- The burrowing mites include *Sarcoptes scabiei* and *Notoedres cati*.
  - These mites tunnel into the superficial layers of the epidermis and feed on tissue fluids. Sarcoptic mange caused by *S. scabiei* can affect most animal species, including humans, but is most commonly seen on dogs and pigs.
- *Demodex* spp. are also burrowing mites that live in the hair follicles and sebaceous glands of the skin.
  - They are considered part of the normal skin fauna of most mammals.
- Demodectic mange is most common in dogs and can be localized or generalized. Immunodeficiency, both genetic and induced by the mites, is necessary for an infestation to become clinically apparent.
- Deep skin scrapings are used to recover the cigar-shaped mites for diagnosis.

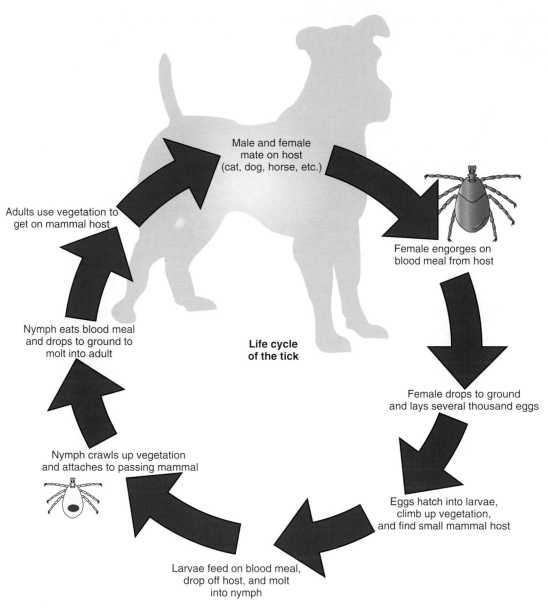

Life cycle of the tick

Male and female mate on host (cat, dog, horse, etc.)

Female engorges on blood meal from host

Female drops to ground and lays several thousand eggs

Eggs hatch into larvae, climb up vegetation, and find small mammal host

Larvae feed on blood meal, drop off host, and molt into nymph

Nymph crawls up vegetation and attaches to passing mammal

Nymph eats blood meal and drops to ground to molt into adult

Adults use vegetation to get on mammal host

FIGURE 8.21 Life cycle of the tick. (From Hendrix CM, Robinson E: *Diagnostic parasitology for veterinary technicians*, ed 4, St Louis, 2012, Mosby.)

- Nonburrowing mites live on the surface of the skin and feed on keratinized scale, hair, and tissue fluids.
- *Otodectes cynotis* and *Cheyletiella* spp. are examples of nonburrowing mites that are parasites of dogs and cats.

Diagnostic Techniques

- Parasites may be located in the oral cavity, esophagus, stomach, small and large intestines, internal organs, and skin of animals.
- Diagnostic stages can be found in sputum, feces, blood, urine, secretions of the reproductive organs, and epidermal layers of the skin.
- Samples collected for examination should be as fresh as possible and examined as soon as possible, preferably within the first 24 hours after collection.

- Clients can collect fecal samples and store them in any clean, sealable container, or collection can occur at the clinic.
- Refrigeration or fixation may be necessary if prompt examination is not possible.
- A sample of 5 to 50 g (the size of a pecan or walnut) may be needed, depending on which procedures are necessary.
- Pooled samples from a herd or kennel can be used, but generally it is better to examine several samples from individual animals.
- It is vital to take proper precautions when working with samples to prevent contamination of the work environment and to ensure personal health when handling agents transmissible to humans.

TABLE 8.6 Zoonotic Internal Parasites

Parasite	Host	Reservoir	Disease
Toxocara spp.	Dogs, cats	Dogs, cats	Visceral larva migrans
Ancylostoma spp.	Dogs, cats	Dogs, cats	Cutaneous larva migrans
Uncinaria stenocephala	Dogs, cats	Dogs, cats	Cutaneous larva migrans
Toxoplasma gondii	Cats	Cats, raw meat	Toxoplasmosis
Strongyloides stercoralis	Dogs, cats, humans	Humans, dogs, cats	Strongyloidiasis
Dipylidium caninum	Dogs, cats, humans	Flea	Cestodiasis
Echinococcus granulosus	Dogs	Dogs	Hydatidosis
Echinococcus multilocularis	Dogs, cats	Dogs, cats	Hydatidosis
Spirometra mansonoides	Dogs, cats	Unknown	Sparganosis
Sarcocystis spp.	Dogs, cats	Dogs, cats	Sarcosporidiosis
Cryptosporidium	Mammals	Mammals	Cryptosporidiosis
Trichinella spiralis	Mammals	Porcine and bear muscle	Trichinellosis
Thelazia spp.	Mammals	Flies	Verminous conjunctivitis
Giardia spp.	Mammals	Mammals	Giardiasis
Babesia spp.	Rodents, humans	Hard ticks	Babesiosis
Trypanosoma	Mammals	Reduviids	Chagas' disease

Adapted from Sirois M: Principles and practice of veterinary technology, ed 3, St Louis, 2011, Mosby.

- Table 8.6 lists some zoonotic internal parasites.
- Parasitologic examination of feces begins with gross examination of the sample, noting consistency; color; and the presence of blood, mucus, odor, adult parasites, or foreign bodies, such as string.
- Normal feces should be formed yet soft.
- Diarrhea or constipation can occur with parasitic infections.
- Most secretions are clear and moderately cellular.
- A yellowish discoloration with excessive mucus could signal infection.
- Blood in a sample can be fresh and bright red or partially digested (hemolyzed), appearing dark reddish brown to black and tarry.
- Excessive mucus in a sample generally indicates irritation to a mucosal membrane, with a proliferation of mucus-producing cells.
- This is common in parasitic infections of the respiratory system and lower digestive tract.
- Adult parasites, such as roundworms and tapeworm proglottids, can be found in vomitus or feces and can be identified.
- Microscopic examination of samples is the most reliable method for detection of parasitic infections.
- A calibrated ocular micrometer may be necessary to determine sizes and specific differentiation of some parasitic stages, such as microfilariae.

Sample Collection and Handling
Fecal Samples
- For tests to be valid, the fecal sample must be fresh and stored properly if testing is to be delayed.
- With small animals, it is common to provide the client with a collection container.
- Instruct the client to witness the animal defecating and collect the sample immediately. Samples can also be collected directly from the rectum using a fecal loop.
- A sample collected with a fecal loop is the least desirable because only a small quantity of sample is obtained, and the quantity may not be sufficient to find evidence of parasites.
- The sample should be refrigerated until it is to be examined.

Blood Samples
- The specific collection procedure varies somewhat, depending on the tests to be performed. Whole blood in EDTA or serum may be required.
- Standard collection methods for these sample types will yield appropriate samples for parasitologic testing.

Miscellaneous Samples
- Skin scrapings, cellophane tape collections, transtracheal washes, urine sample collections, and swabbings are all performed in parasitology.

- Standard protocols for these collections will yield appropriate samples.

Evaluation of Fecal Specimens

- Depending on clinical signs and patient history, specific parasite infestations may likely be suspected.
- This information helps guide the choice of test to be performed.
- All parasitology samples should undergo gross evaluation for the presence of abnormalities such as blood, mucus, and parasites that are large enough to see with the unaided eye (e.g., tapeworm segments).

Direct Smear

- Fecal direct smears are the simplest of the evaluation procedures.
- The procedure involves placing a small amount of feces on a clean glass slide and examining it microscopically for the presence of eggs and larvae.
- This method will also allow visualization of the trophozoite stages of protozoal parasites such as *Giardia* spp.
- A direct smear alone is not an adequate examination for parasites because only a small quantity of sample is examined, and parasitic infections can be missed.
  - However, it should be incorporated as a routine part of any parasitology examination.

Fecal Flotation

- Flotation methods are based on differences in the specific gravity of the life cycle stages of parasites found in feces and fecal debris.
- Simple fecal flotation is an example of a flotation method.
- Specific gravity refers to the weight of an object compared with the weight of an equal volume of distilled water and is a function of the total amount of dissolved material in the solution.
- Most parasite eggs have a specific gravity between 1.10 and 1.20 g/mL.
- Flotation solutions are formulated with a specific gravity higher than that of common parasite ova so that the ova float to the surface of the solution.
- Saturated solutions of sugar and various salts are used as flotation solutions and have a specific gravity ranging from 1.18 to 1.40 g/mL.
- Fecal debris and eggs with a specific gravity greater than that of the flotation solution do not float.
- Fluke eggs are generally heavier than the specific gravity of most routinely used flotation solutions and are not usually recovered using this technique.
- Nematode larvae can be recovered but frequently are distorted from crenation, making identification difficult.
- Commonly used flotation solutions are sugar, sodium chloride, sodium nitrate, magnesium sulfate, and zinc sulfate.

- Each solution has its advantages and disadvantages, including cost, availability, efficiency, shelf life, crystallization, corrosion of equipment, and ease of use.
- Selection is often determined by the type of practice and common parasites encountered in the area.
- The specific gravity of flotation solutions can be checked using a hydrometer and adjusted by adding more salt or more water to the solution.
- Leaving extra crystals of salt on the bottom of the solution ensures that the solution is saturated.

Centrifugal Flotation

- This procedure is similar in principle to the flotation procedure except that once the sample and solution are mixed, the specimen is strained to remove excess debris.
- A coverslip is added, and the specimen is centrifuged at 400 to 650 g for 5 minutes.
- Centrifugal force holds the coverslips in place during spinning, provided that the tubes are balanced.
- A bacteriology loop is then used to remove a drop of liquid from the surface of the tube, and the drop is examined microscopically.
- Centrifugal flotation is more sensitive than simple flotation; it recovers more eggs and cysts in a sample in less time.

Fecal Sedimentation

- The sedimentation procedure is used when suspected parasites produce ova too large to be recovered with standard flotation (e.g., fluke ova).
- The fecal sample is mixed in a small volume of water and strained into a centrifuge tube.
- The sample can be centrifuged at 400 g for 5 minutes or allowed to remain undisturbed for 20 to 30 minutes.
- The supernatant is poured off, and a pipette is used to remove a drop of the sediment.
- A drop from the upper, middle, and lower portions of the sediment is removed and then examined microscopically.
- Sedimentation is used primarily when fluke infections are suspected.
- Most fluke eggs do not float or are distorted by flotation solutions with a higher specific gravity, making it difficult to recognize them.

Cellophane Tape Preparation

- The cellophane tape method is often used to aid in identification of tapeworms.
- To collect the sample, a piece of cellophane tape is wrapped around a tongue depressor, with the adhesive side out.
- The animal's tail is raised, and the tongue depressor firmly pressed against the anus.
- The tape is then removed, applied to a glass slide that has a small amount of water on it, and examined microscopically.

Miscellaneous Fecal Examinations

- The Baermann technique is sometimes used to recover nematode larvae from feces, fecal culture, soil, herbage, and animal tissues but is rarely performed in small animal practice.
- In dogs and cats, a Baermann technique should be used when *Strongyloides* spp. infections are suspected.
- The procedure requires construction of a Baermann apparatus, which consists of a large funnel supported in a ring stand.
- A piece of rubber tubing is attached to the end of the funnel and placed in a collection tube. The fecal sample is placed in the funnel on top of a piece of metal screen.
- Warm water or warmed physiologic saline is passed through the sample.
- The larvae are stimulated to move by the warm water and then sink to the bottom of the apparatus.
- A drop of the material in the collection container is examined microscopically for the presence of larvae.
- Some parasites produce intestinal bleeding that may be evident as frank blood in the fecal sample or as darkened feces.
- Some intestinal bleeding can only be identified with chemical testing, referred to as fecal occult blood testing.
- Several types of kits are available for this procedure that act primarily to identify the presence of hemoglobin in the sample.
- Examination of vomitus may also aid in the diagnosis of parasitism.
- Some parasites (e.g., *Toxocara canis*) are often present in the vomitus of infected patients.
- Fecal culture is used to differentiate parasites whose eggs or larvae are not easily distinguished by examination of a fresh fecal sample.
- First-stage hookworm larvae in a dog or cat sample and some free-living nematode larvae in soil or on grass cannot be easily distinguished from first-stage *Strongyloides* larvae.
- After fecal culture, the third-stage larvae of many of these parasites can be identified to the genus level.

Evaluation of Blood Samples

- Examination of blood samples may reveal adult parasites and/or their various life cycle stages free in the blood or intracellularly.
- A variety of methods can be used for this determination, including thin or thick blood smears or buffy coat smears.
- Thin or thick blood smears are prepared in the same way as smears for a WBC differential count (see earlier discussion).
- Most parasites are carried with the laminar flow to the feathered edge of the slide.
- Parasites may be located between cells, on the surface of cells, or in the cytoplasm of cells. Thin blood films are most effectively used to study the morphology of protozoan and rickettsial parasites.

- A thick blood film or a buffy coat smear is more effective because it concentrates a larger volume of cells.
- The buffy coat smear is a concentration technique for the detection of protozoa and rickettsiae in WBCs.
- A microhematocrit tube is centrifuged as for a PCV determination.
- Microfilariae and some protozoa may also be found at the top of the plasma column.
- The technique is quick but cannot be used to differentiate *D. immitis* from *Acanthocheilonema reconditum*.

Direct Drop Test

- This is the simplest of the blood evaluations, although it is the least accurate because of the small sample size.
- A drop of anticoagulated whole blood is examined microscopically.
- The movement of parasites that are extracellular can be detected with this method.

Filter Test

- The filter technique is a method designed to concentrate microfilariae in blood.
- The blood is passed through a filter, which collects the microfilariae.
- Commercial kits use a detergent lysing solution and a differential stain. This procedure is primarily used in locations in which animals are expected to have circulating microfilariae (e.g., stray, shelter animal).

Modified Knott Test

- This method is used to concentrate microfilaria and can help in the differentiation of *Dirofilaria* from *Acanthocheilonema*.
- The procedure requires a mixture of blood and formalin or acetic acid solution in a centrifuge tube.
- The mixture is incubated at room temperature for 1 to 2 minutes and then centrifuged for 5 minutes.
- The supernatant is poured off, and a drop of methylene blue is added to the sediment in the tube.
- A drop of this mixture is transferred to a glass slide for microscopic evaluation.
- The modified Knott technique cannot detect occult heartworm infections.

Immunologic Tests

- A variety of tests are available to identify antigen and/or antibody to specific parasites.
- Most tests are based on the ELISA principle (see earlier) and are highly accurate and precise.
- Canine heartworm infections and *Toxoplasma* infections are routinely diagnosed with these methods.
- Antigen detection methods are preferred to microfilariae concentration methods in cats because these aberrant hosts circulate microfilariae only for a short time.
  - Antigen levels in the blood of infected cats may also be too low to detect.

- Approximately 25% of heartworm-infected dogs have occult infections; these can be detected with antigen tests.
- Occult infections are characterized by a lack of circulating microfilaria and occur if the infection is not yet patent, if the population of adult heartworms consists of only one sex, or if immune reactions of the host to microfilariae eliminate this stage from the bloodstream.
- Occult infections can also occur if animals infected with adult heartworms are given heartworm prevention medications of the ivermectin group.
- These interfere with oogenesis and sterilize the worms.

RECOMMENDED READINGS

Abbas AK: *Basic immunology updated edition: functions and disorders of the immune system*, ed 3, Philadelphia, 2011, Saunders.

Bowman DD: *Georgis' parasitology for veterinarians*, ed 10, St Louis, 2013, Saunders.

Cowell R, Tyler R, Meinkoth J: *Diagnostic cytology and hematology of the dog and cat*, ed 3, St Louis, 2008, Mosby.

Hendrix CM, Robinson E: *Diagnostic parasitology for veterinarians*, ed 5, St Louis, 2016, Mosby.

Latimer KS, Prasse KW, Mahaffey EA: *Duncan and Prasse's veterinary laboratory medicine: clinical pathology*, ed 5, Ames, IA, 2011, Blackwell.

Meyer DJ, Harvey JW: *Veterinary laboratory medicine: interpretation and diagnosis*, ed. 3, St Louis, 2006, Saunders.

Raskin RE, Meyer DJ: *Canine and feline cytology: A color atlas and interpretation guide*, ed. 3, St Louis, 2015, Saunders.

Sirois M: *Laboratory procedures for veterinary technicians*, ed 6, St Louis, 2014, Mosby.

Sodikoff C: *Laboratory profiles of small animal diseases: a guide to laboratory diagnosis*, St Louis, 2001, Mosby.

Tizard IR: *Veterinary immunology: An introduction*, ed 9, St Louis, 2013, Saunders.

Willard MD, Tvedten H: *Small animal clinical diagnosis by laboratory methods*, ed 5, St Louis, 2011, Saunders.

Diagnostic Imaging

KEY TERMS

ALARA	Echoic	Kilovoltage peak (kVp)	Radiolucent
Anechoic	Film latitude	Latent image	Radiopaque
Annular array	Film–focal distance (FFD)	Maximum permissible dose (MPD)	Rem
Anode	Fluoroscopy	Milliamperage (mA)	Sievert (SV)
Bucky	Focused grids	Mirror image	Slice thickness
Cathode	Heel effect	Object-film distance (OFD)	Sonolucent
Collimators	Hyperechoic	Penumbra effect	Source-image distance (SID)
Contrast	Hypoechoic	Radiographic density	Ultrasonography
Direct exposure film	Isoechoic		
Distance enhancement	Intensifying screens		

LEARNING OBJECTIVES

After reviewing this chapter, the reader will be able to:

1. Describe the components of the x-ray machine and the function of each part.
2. Explain how x-rays are produced.
3. Discuss the factors that affect radiographic quality.
4. Describe techniques and devices used to optimize radiographic quality.
5. Discuss the dangers of radiation and methods to avoid radiation injury.
6. Describe the procedures used to develop radiographs.
7. Explain proper positioning of animals for various radiographic studies.
8. Describe the basic physics of ultrasound.
9. List the components of ultrasound machines and the function of each part.
10. List the non–x-ray imaging modalities and provide an overview of each.

X-RAY GENERATION

- X-rays are a form of electromagnetic radiation.
- X-rays are similar to visible light but have a shorter wavelength, higher frequency, and higher energy; it is the higher energy that makes x-rays dangerous.
- The x-rays are generated when fast-moving electrons (from the cathode) collide with the anode (positive end of the x-ray tube).
- Within the x-ray tube, at the time of exposure, a stream of electrons is accelerated toward a tungsten anode target.
- The energy of the electrons interacting with the atoms of the target is converted to heat (99%) and x-rays (1%).
- Heat generation in the x-ray tube is a limiting factor in the production of x-rays.

X-ray Tube Anatomy

- The x-ray tube consists of a cathode (−) that contains a tungsten filament at which the electrons are generated when heated.
  - The tungsten filament is housed within a focusing cup to focus the beam of electrons on the focal spot of the anode.
- The anode (+) contains a rotating tungsten target wherein x-rays are generated at the focal spot.
- Both the anode and cathode are enclosed in a vacuum glass or metal envelope.
- A beryllium window in the glass envelope allows x-rays to pass with minimal filtration.
- An aluminum filter is placed outside the window in the collimator housing, usually on top of the mirror, to absorb the low-energy (soft) x-rays while allowing the more energetic and useful x-rays to form the primary x-ray beam.
- By law, any x-ray tube that generates over 70 kilovoltage peak (kVp) must have a collimator because there has to be a total filtration of 2.5-mm Al equivalent.
- The entire x-ray tube is surrounded by oil that acts as an electrical barrier while absorbing heat generated by the tube.
- The tube and oil are encased in a lead housing to prevent damage to the glass envelope from the outside and to absorb stray radiation.

- The heel effect is the result of unequal distribution of the x-ray beam intensity emitted from the x-ray tube along the cathode–anode axis.
  - Some x-ray tubes have a distribution of the x-ray beam intensity that decreases rapidly on the anode side of the tube as a result of primary x-ray beam absorption by the anode material (Fig. 9.1).
  - This can be used as an advantage when taking x-rays of areas of unequal thickness, such as the thorax or abdomen.
  - By placing the patient's head toward the anode side, the part of the x-ray beam with the higher intensity

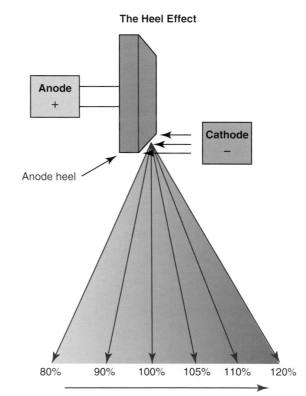

The Heel Effect

Percentage of central x-ray intensity increases

FIGURE 9.1 Anode heel effect. The x-ray beam intensity decreases toward the anode side because of absorption by the target and anode material. (In Sirois M: *Principles and practice of veterinary technology*, ed 3, St Louis, 2011, Mosby. Courtesy J. Johnson.)

(cathode side) is directed to the thickest area of the patient, as when radiographing a thorax.
- This produces a more even film density.
- The heel effect is most noticeable when using large film sizes, low kVp, and long focal–film distance.

Fluoroscopy

- **Fluoroscopy** is used for those patients for whom the visualization of dynamic structures is of importance.
  - Using an x-ray tube, a beam is directed through a patient onto a fluorescent screen or image intensifier to form an image.
  - This is commonly referred to as real-time imaging because it is a continuous stream of images.
  - The image is then transferred to a monitor and can be recorded on spot film or videotape, or digitized by computer.
  - Fluoroscopy is generally used for gastrointestinal (GI) studies (e.g., barium studies, gastrograms, upper GI studies), angiography (cardiac catheterizations), and myelography.
  - Fluoroscopy is not a commonly used modality in the general clinical setting because of economic limitations.

RADIOGRAPHIC IMAGE QUALITY

- **Radiographic density** is the degree of blackness on a radiograph.
  - The dark areas are made up of black metallic silver deposits on the finished radiograph.
  - These deposits occur in areas in which x-rays have penetrated the patient and exposed the emulsion of the film.
- Radiographic density can be intensified by increasing the mAs (a product of the milliamperage and time), which is a result of increasing the **milliamperage (mA)** or the exposure time in seconds (s).
  - This increases the mAs by increasing the number (quantity) of x-rays produced as a result of increasing the number of electrons in the electron cloud, or the time that the electrons are allowed to travel from the cathode to the anode.
- A higher kVp yields more radiographic density by increasing the penetrating power (quality) of the x-ray beam.

Radiographic Contrast

- Radiographic **contrast** is defined as the differences in radiographic density between adjacent areas on a radiographic image.
- Radiographs that show a long scale of contrast have a few black and white shades, with many shades of gray.
- A short scale of contrast has black and white shades, with only a few shades of gray in between.
- For most studies, a long scale of contrast is desirable.

- Obtaining a long scale of radiographic contrast depends on four factors: subject density, kVp level, film contrast, and film fogging.
- Subject density is the ability of the different tissue densities to absorb x-rays.
- The extent to which x-rays penetrate the various tissues depends on the differences in atomic number and thickness.
- On radiographs, air or lung tissue will appear **radiolucent**, or black, because it allows more of the radiation to pass through.
- With increasing density, the tissue will appear whiter, or more **radiopaque**, as it absorbs more of the radiation.
- Bone absorbs more x-rays than muscle and appears whiter (radiopaque) on the finished radiograph, whereas air in the thorax will appear more radiolucent in comparison.
- The thickness of the area also affects the number of x-rays absorbed.
- The scale of radiographic contrast can be lengthened or shortened by increasing or decreasing the kVp.
- Film contrast also affects radiographic contrast.
  - Long-latitude film allows for more variation in technique while still producing a diagnostic radiograph.
- The scale of contrast can be shortened by changing the exposure technique when using long-latitude film.
- Film fogging can greatly decrease radiographic contrast by decreasing the differences in densities between two adjacent shadows.
- Film can become fogged from low-grade light leaks in the darkroom, scatter radiation, heat, and improper processing.

Radiographic Detail

- A diagnostic radiograph is one with diagnostic radiographic detail.
- Radiographic detail is considered to be of diagnostic quality when the interfaces between tissues and organs are sharp.
- Patient motion and the **penumbra effect** have the greatest influence on radiographic detail.
- The penumbra effect causes a loss of detail and results in collimation (limitation) of the x-ray beam.
  - The fuzziness caused by stray x-rays is known as the penumbra effect.
  - The smallest focal spot size should be used whenever possible to prevent this effect.
- Another factor that affects the amount of penumbra is the source-image distance, which is the distance between the source of the x-ray and the film.
- The term **source-image distance (SID)** is preferred, but **film–focal distance (FFD)** and SID are used interchangeably.
- The penumbra effect can be decreased by increasing the SID (Fig. 9.2).
- There is a limit to how much the SID can be increased because of what is stated in the inverse square law.
  - According to this law, the intensity decreases at a rate inverse to the square of the distance.

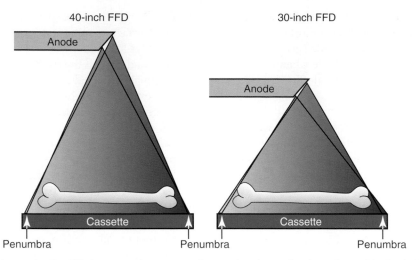

FIGURE 9.2 Increasing the SID decreases the amount of penumbra, increasing the radiographic detail. *FFD,* Film–focal distance. (From Sirois M: *Principles and practice of veterinary technology,* ed 3, St Louis, 2011, Mosby.)

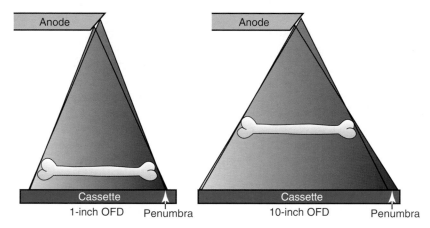

FIGURE 9.3 Increasing the OID increases the amount of penumbra, decreasing the radiographic detail. *OFD,* Object-film distance. (From Sirois M: *Principles and practice of veterinary technology,* ed 3, St Louis, 2011, Mosby.)

- In simpler terms, if the SID is doubled, the mAs must increase by a factor of 4 to maintain the same radiographic density.
- In most cases, this is not practical because the shortest possible exposure times are necessary to counteract patient motion.
- An SID of 36 to 40 inches is sufficient to minimize the penumbra effect.
- The third factor that affects penumbra is the object-image distance (OID).
  - This is the distance from the object being imaged to the film or image receptor.
  - The penumbra is decreased by keeping the OID as short as possible (Fig. 9.3).
- Using a combination of these factors, the penumbra can be minimized and good radiographic detail achieved.
- Patient motion causes loss of detail because of blurred interfaces.

- A blurred image is generally a result of long exposure time combined with motion of the patient.
  - This can be controlled by using the shortest possible exposure.
  - If the image remains blurred, the patient should be sedated.

Distortion
- Distortion occurs when the x-ray beam is not perpendicular to the recording surface.
- Foreshortening occurs when the object is not parallel to the recording surface.
  - This distorts size by shortening the length of the object.
  - This occurs mainly when imaging the long bones, such as the humerus or femur.
  - If one end of the bone is farther from the recording surface than the other, the bone appears shorter.

- The object being radiographed must be parallel to the recording surface and the OID kept as short as possible.
- Increasing the OID increases the penumbra and greatly magnifies the size of the object.
- The degree of magnification increases as the distance to the recording surface becomes greater.
- It is important to project areas between a series of radiodense and radiolucent objects accurately.
  - The vertebral column is a good example.
  - The vertebrae must be parallel to the recording surface.
  - When radiographing the cervical vertebrae in lateral recumbency, if the patient is allowed to lie naturally, the midcervical vertebrae tend to sag.
  - This produces false narrowing of the intervertebral spaces.
  - A small amount of padding beneath the patient brings the vertebral column parallel to the recording surface.
- Distortion can also occur when the x-ray beam is not perpendicular to the recording surface.
- X-rays in the center of the primary beam penetrate perpendicular to the intervertebral spaces.
- As the distance from the center of the primary beam increases, the x-rays strike the intervertebral spaces at an increasing angle.
  - False narrowing of the intervertebral space occurs because of this increase in distance from the center of the primary beam.
  - To combat such distortion, it is sometimes necessary to make multiple images of the vertebral column, centering the primary beam over multiple areas.
  - This type of distortion is also apparent when radiographing complex joints, such as the stifle and elbow.
  - When imaging these areas, be sure the center of the primary beam is directly over the joint.

Scatter Radiation

- When an x-ray photon strikes an object, it can do one of three things: it can pass through the object, be absorbed by the object, or produce scatter radiation (secondary radiation).
- Scatter radiation fogs the film, greatly decreasing the contrast, and is a safety hazard to patients and personnel.
- Scatter radiation is projected in all directions.
- Exposure techniques that use a high kVp produce more scatter radiation.
- Body parts measuring 10 cm or larger produce enough scatter radiation to significantly decrease detail on the radiograph.
- Beam-limiting devices are commonly used to decrease scatter radiation by confining the primary beam to the area being examined.
- Several types of beam-limiting devices are available.
  - Diaphragms are sheets of lead with a rectangular, square, or circular opening that limits the size of the primary beam to the size of the diaphragm used.

- Collimators consist of adjustable lead shutters installed in the tube head of the x-ray machine.
- Finally, filters are used to absorb the less penetrating or soft x-rays as they leave the tube head. Filters are made of a thin sheet of aluminum and are placed over the tube window.

Grids

- Grids are used to decrease scatter radiation and increase the contrast on the radiograph.
- As the thickness of the area being imaged increases, the amount of kVp required also increases.
- As the kVp increases, more scatter radiation is produced.
- To minimize scatter radiation, grids are necessary when radiographing areas 10 cm or more in thickness.
- A grid is a series of thin, linear strips made of alternating radiodense and radiolucent material.
- The radiodense strips are made of lead, whereas the radiolucent spacers are plastic, aluminum, or fiber.
- The grid is placed within or under the table between the patient and imaging receptor.
- X-rays that penetrate the patient and pass in perfect alignment between the lead strips expose the film.
- Scatter radiation diverges in all directions and is more likely to be absorbed by one of the lead strips.
- The grid also absorbs a portion of the usable x-rays.
  - To compensate for this loss, the number of x-rays generated must be increased by increasing the mAs.
  - Depending on the type of grid used, the increase may be up to 6.6 times the mAs required for the tabletop exposure.
- Grids are manufactured with parallel or focused lead strips arranged in a crossed or linear configuration.
- Parallel grids have the lead strips placed perpendicular to the grid surface.
  - X-rays and scatter radiation that interact with the lead strips are absorbed, whereas those that interact with the spacers pass through to expose the film.
  - A disadvantage of a parallel grid is that the x-ray beam diverges at increasing angles and is absorbed at the periphery of the grid.
  - This decreases the number of x-rays reaching the film near the grid edges, commonly called grid cutoff.
- Focused grids have the lead strips placed at progressively increasing angles to match the divergence of the x-ray beam.
  - By angling the lead strips, cutoff of the primary beam is eliminated and radiographic density is uniform.
- The grid manufacturer supplies a list of distances called the grid focal distance; setting the SID out of the grid focal distance results in primary beam cutoff on the periphery of the radiograph.
- Cutoff of the primary beam also occurs if the grid is not perpendicular to or centered with the x-ray tube.
- Grids produce thin white lines on the finished radiograph.

- Visibility of the grid lines can be decreased in three ways.
  - First, the lead strips can be made as thin as possible while retaining the ability to absorb scatter radiation effectively.
    - The thinner the lead, the thinner the white line that it produces on the radiograph.
  - The second way is to increase the number of grid lines per inch, making the individual lines less visible.
    - To increase the grid lines per inch and keep the thickness of the lead the same, the width of the radiolucent strips must be decreased.
    - This produces a grid with more lead in it, which absorbs more of the primary beam and requires higher mAs.
    - A grid with 80 to 100 lines/inch is sufficient to make the grid lines less visible.
  - The third way is by using a Potter–Bucky diaphragm, also called a **Bucky**.
    - This device puts the grid in motion as the x-rays are generated, blurring the white grid lines on the radiograph.
    - The Bucky is placed in a cabinet beneath the x-ray table, with a tray to hold the cassette. When a grid is used in combination with a Bucky, fewer lines per inch are necessary.
    - This allows for the use of lower mAs.
    - One disadvantage of using a Bucky mechanism in veterinary medicine is the noise and vibration that it produces.
    - Some animals may object to this and struggle or move during the x-ray exposure.

Exposure Variables

- Four exposure factors control radiographic density, contrast, and detail: mAs, kVp, FFD, and OID.
- Changing one of these factors usually requires adjustments in another factor to maintain the same radiographic density.

Milliamperage and Exposure Time
- The mAs is a product of the milliamperage and exposure time.
- The milliamperage controls the number of electrons in the electron cloud generated at the filament of the cathode.
- When the mA is increased, the temperature of the filament is increased, producing more electrons to form the electron cloud.
- Increasing the mA increases the amount of radiographic density because more x-rays are generated.
- Exposure time refers to the time during which the electrons are allowed to flow from the cathode to the anode.
- By varying the exposure time, the number of x-rays generated is controlled.
- Using a longer exposure time allows the electrons more time to cross from the cathode to the anode, thus generating more x-rays.

- Exposure time and mA are inversely related.
- As mA increases, the exposure time required to maintain the desired number of x-rays generated decreases.
- Many different combinations of mA and time can be used to produce the same mAs. For example, consider the following:

$$300\,mA\,at\,\frac{1}{60}\,sec = 5mAs$$

$$200\,mA\,at\,\frac{1}{40}\,sec = 5mAs$$

$$100\,mA\,at\,\frac{1}{20}\,sec = 5mAs$$

- When faced with a choice of which mAs to use, always choose the one with the fastest exposure time to minimize effect of patient motion on the film.
- The mAs can be used to adjust the radiographic density by following these rules:
  - To double the radiographic density, double the mAs.
  - To halve the radiographic density, halve the mAs.

Kilovoltage Peak
- The kVp is the voltage applied between the cathode and the anode that is used to accelerate electrons flowing from the cathode toward the anode side.
- Increasing the kVp causes the electrons to move faster, increasing the force of the collision with the target, which produces an x-ray beam with a shorter wavelength and more penetrating power.
- The correct kVp setting is determined by the thickness of the part being imaged; thus the thicker the part, the higher the kVp setting, because more penetration is needed.
- As with mAs, there are rules when changing the radiographic density with kVp:
  - To double the radiographic density, increase the kVp by 20%.
  - To halve the radiographic density, decrease the kVp by 16%.

Source-Image Distance
- The SID is the distance from the target to the recording surface (film).
- For most radiographic procedures, this distance is held constant, at approximately 36 to 40 inches.
  - In some situations, the SID must be changed.
  - This requires changing one of the other factors to maintain radiographic density.
  - If the SID is doubled, the mAs must be increased by a factor of 4 to maintain radiographic density because the same number of x-rays must diverge to cover an area that is four times as large.
  - Changing the SID does not affect the penetrating power of the beam, so the kVp remains constant.

Object-Image Distance

- The OID (also called the object-film distance [OFD] if not using digital imaging) is the distance from the object being imaged to the recording surface (film or digital recording plate).
- OID should be as short as possible to minimize the penumbra effect and the magnification that occurs with a long OID.

RADIOGRAPHIC FILM

- X-ray film consists of three layers: a thin protective layer, an emulsion containing silver halide crystals, and a polyester film base.
- The first layer is a thin, clear gelatin that acts as a protective coating to protect the sensitive film emulsion.
- The second layer is the emulsion, which contains finely precipitated silver halide crystals in a gelatin base and coats both sides of the film base.
- When placed in the developing chemicals, the emulsion swells, allowing the chemicals to act on the exposed or sensitized crystals without losing the crystals.
  - Once the emulsion is dry, it hardens again, trapping the black metallic silver.
- The film base is in the center of the film, giving it support; it does not produce a visible light pattern or absorb the light.
- When the silver halide crystals are exposed to electromagnetic radiation, they become more sensitive to chemical change.
  - These sensitized crystals are what make up the latent image.
- When the film is placed into the developer, the latent image is reduced to black metallic silver.
  - The remaining silver halide crystals are removed in the fixer.
  - This produces varying shades of black metallic silver and the clear film base.
- Film is sensitive to all types of electromagnetic radiation.
  - These include gamma radiation, particulate radiation (alpha and beta), x-rays, heat, and light.
- Film is also sensitive to excessive pressure, so care must be taken when handling and storing radiographic film.
- The two types of film used in veterinary radiography are screen-type film and direct exposure film.
- Screen-type film is more sensitive to the light produced by intensifying screens.
- Two screen-type films are blue-sensitive and green-sensitive films.
- Blue-sensitive film is more sensitive to light emitted from screens containing blue light–emitting phosphors.
  - Calcium tungstate and some rare earth phosphors are the most common blue light–emitting phosphors.
  - They emit light in the ultraviolet, violet, and blue light range.

- Green-sensitive film is most sensitive to light from green light–emitting phosphors.
  - Rare earth phosphors are the most common green light–emitting phosphors.
- Direct exposure film is more sensitive to direct x-rays than it is to light.
  - Because it does not use the intensifying effect of the screens, it requires higher mAs than screen film.
  - General anesthesia or heavy sedation may be necessary to prevent patient motion and blurring on the radiograph because of the higher mAs.
  - Direct exposure film is mainly used to image the extremities or rostral mandible or maxilla, where good detail is needed.
  - It is often used for imaging exotic animals and in dental radiology studies.
  - It is packaged in a paper folder enclosed in a stout lightproof envelope.
  - Take care when handling this film because it is protected only by paper. Pressure artifacts can easily occur.
  - Some direct exposure film can only be processed manually because of the thickness of the emulsion.
- Film speeds are rated as high (regular or fast), average (par), and slow (detail).
- The faster the film, the more sensitive it is and the lower mAs it requires.
- Average-speed (par) film is used for most veterinary radiography applications.
- Another important feature in x-ray film is film latitude, which is the film's inherent ability to produce shades of gray.
- Film with a long or increased latitude can produce images with a long scale of contrast (many shades of gray).
- Longer-latitude film is desirable because it allows for greater exposure errors but still produces a diagnostic radiograph.
- Proper storage and handling of the film are important to ensure a good diagnostic radiograph.
- Unexposed film should be stored in a cool, dry place, away from strong chemical fumes.
- A base fog can develop if film is stored under adverse conditions over a long period.
- Film is pressure-sensitive, so it should be stored on end and not laid flat on its side.

Intensifying Screens

- Intensifying screens contain fluorescent crystals bound to a cardboard or plastic base.
  - When exposed to x-rays, the crystals emit foci of light.
- Placing radiographic film in direct contact with the screens accurately records any x-rays that penetrate the patient.
- Approximately 95% of the film's radiographic density results from fluorescence of the intensifying screens and only 5% is the result of direct x-ray exposure.

- For each x-ray photon the screen absorbs, it emits 1000 light photons, amplifying the photographic effect of the x-rays.
- The film is sandwiched between two screens mounted inside a lightproof cassette.
- The cassette holds the film in close, uniform contact with the screens.
- The screens are supported by a plastic or cardboard base and have a thin reflecting layer and a phosphor layer.
- The reflecting layer reflects the light back toward the film side or front of the screen.
- The most common phosphor used today consists of rare earth elements such as lanthanum oxybromide and gadolinium oxysulfide, which emit green light.
  - Rare earth screens allow shorter exposure time.
- A thin waterproof protective coating that prevents static during cassette loading and unloading is over the phosphor layer.
  - It also provides physical protection and is a surface that can be cleaned.
- Intensifying screens are available in three different speeds: high (regular), par (medium), and slow (detail or fine).
- High-speed screens require less exposure time compared with the par or slow speed, but detail is decreased.
  - When changing from a high-speed screen to a par-speed screen, the mAs must be increased two times.
  - When changing from high speed to slow speed, the mAs must be increased four times to maintain radiographic density.
- Routine cleaning is necessary to ensure that the screens are free from dirt and foreign materials that can block the light emitted from the screens, leaving parts of the film unexposed.
  - The result is a white area on the film that resembles the foreign material.
  - Processing chemicals can cause permanent damage if the screen surface is not cleaned promptly.
- The screens should be cleaned with a soft, lint-free cloth and screen-cleaning solution or warm water.
- Do not use denatured alcohol or abrasive products because they can damage the protective coating and phosphor layer.
  - Be sure to allow the screen to completely dry before reloading.
- Cassettes are precision instruments and should be handled that way.
- Do not drop them or set heavy objects on them.
  - This can result in poor film–screen contact and blurring of one area of the image.
- To check the film–screen contact of your screens, place paper clips over the surface of the cassette. Use enough to cover every area completely.
  - Expose the cassette using 50 to 60 kVp and half the mAs that you would use for a nongrid extremity.

- Process the film and view it dry.
- Any areas with poor film–screen contact are indicated by a blurred image of the paper clips.

X-RAY EQUIPMENT

- There are three basic types of x-ray equipment: portable, mobile, and stationary units.
- A portable unit can be carried to the animal.
  - These machines generally have a fixed mA set by the manufacturer at 15 to 30 mA, a variable kVp ranging from 40 to 90, and exposure times as short as $\frac{1}{120}$ second.
  - Because the mA is fixed, the exposure time is changed to increase the radiographic density.
  - For this reason, motion can be a problem with some animals because of the prolonged exposure times.

The mobile unit can be transported to the patient.
  - Because of its large size, it is limited to in-hospital use, such as in the treatment room or perhaps in a driveway (Fig. 9.4).
  - These units generally produce a maximum 300 mA, 125 kVp, and a $\frac{1}{120}$-second exposure.
  - The tube head on a mobile unit can be suspended above a table for small animal radiography.
- Stationary units are those that are installed in a room with proper leaded wall shielding for radiography.
  - These units have many different exposure capabilities, depending on the quality desired.
- A general small animal practice that does mainly routine radiographic examinations may be well served by a

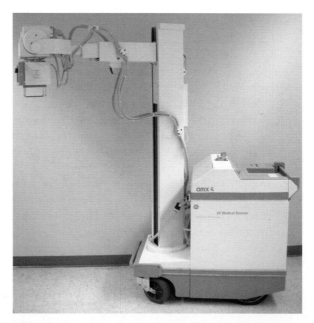

FIGURE 9.4 Mobile x-ray unit. (From Sirois M: *Principles and practice of veterinary technology*, ed 3, St Louis, 2011, Mosby.)

machine with 300 mA, 125 kVp, and at least a $\frac{1}{120}$-second output.

- Practices that provide specialty services, such as internal medicine or surgery referrals, will require higher-output equipment.

DIGITAL X-RAY IMAGING

- The increased availability and affordability of digital radiography have made replacing analog systems much easier, and digital systems are now common.
- Digital radiography refers to the process whereby images are obtained and displayed on appropriate computer monitors in a grayscale digital display.
- Three main types of digital systems are currently available: computed radiography (CR), digital radiography (DR), and charge-coupled device (CCD) technologies.
- An advantage of the use of digital systems is that the digitized image can then be enhanced and viewed by using computer software that enables contrast, brightness, zoom, and pan adjustments, as well as measurement of various anatomic structures.
- Other advantages of digital radiography include elimination of the need for film, processing chemicals, and screens.
- Existing x-ray machines can be retrofitted for DR use, or standard CR systems will be accepted without any changes being made to the grid cabinet or Bucky mechanism.
- With CCD systems, however, a brand-new radiology generator and table will need to be purchased.
- DR systems may reduce the number of repeat radiographs needed caused by inappropriate exposure settings or chemical processing errors.
- A hard-copy film can still be made from digital radiographs using dry laser printers for printing images, if necessary.

Computed Radiography

- CR uses a cassette system not unlike conventional film–screen systems.
- Instead of having two screens and a film within the cassette, there is an imaging plate (IP) that contains a photostimulable phosphor, which can store the radiation level received at each point on the plate.
  - This eliminates the need for film as a medium for viewing radiographs.
- Instead of chemical processing, the cassette is run through a computer scanner that uses a scanning laser beam.
  - This causes the electrons to relax to a lower energy level, which emits light.
  - These light measurements are proportional to the amount of radiation reaching and being absorbed by the IP in a given area.
  - This light is measured, and the digital image created.

- The imaging plate is then erased by fluorescent light in the reader, and the IP is reloaded into the cassette for reuse.
- The imaging plate can be reused thousands of times.

Digital Radiography

- DR also uses an imaging plate comprising an array of detectors.
  - The detectors translate or convert the x-rays into an electrical signal or pulse that is then digitalized by the computer to an image.
- This imaging plate is connected directly to a computer dedicated to that function, thereby eliminating the need for a cassette such as that used in a CR system.
- This plate can be permanently placed in an x-ray table or can be portable, depending on the user's needs.

Digital Radiography Storage

- Digital radiography (and other modalities, such as computed tomography [CT], magnetic resonance imaging [MRI], ultrasound, and NM) uses a DICOM (*d*igital *i*maging and *co*mmunications in *m*edicine) format, which is the universally accepted format for the dispersion and storing of medical information.
- Each DICOM file includes the pertinent information associated with the patient, such as modality, date and time of examination, and patient identification and number.
- DICOM files are encrypted so that patient and image data are kept secure and tamper-proof.
- Storage of these DICOM files can be as simple as archiving to a compact disc (CD), digital video disc (DVD), or magnetic optical disc (MOD), or it can be managed through a picture archiving and communication system (PACS).
- A PACS has the advantage of storing multiple patients and making images available to multiple computers within a hospital or network of hospitals.

RADIATION SAFETY

- Radiation ionizes intracellular water, which releases toxic products that can damage critical components of the cell, such as deoxyribonucleic acid (DNA).
- When radiation comes into contact with the cells of living tissue, it can do the following:
  - Pass through the cells with no effect.
  - Produce cell damage that is reparable.
  - Produce cell damage that is not reparable.
  - Kill the cells.
- Radiation damages the body in several ways.
  - It may have carcinogenic effects, which means that cancer may develop in body tissues.
  - Effects on the body may be genetic, occurring in future generations.

- Tissues that are most sensitive to ionizing radiation are those with rapidly growing or reproducing cells.
- The reproductive organs may suffer from temporary or permanent infertility, decreased hormone production, or mutations.
- The hematopoietic (blood-forming) cells are relatively sensitive to ionizing radiation.
- The lymphocytic blood cells are most sensitive.
- Damage to blood cells can reduce resistance to infection and cause clotting disorders.
- The thyroid gland, intestinal epithelium, and lens of the eye are also radiosensitive.
- There may be an increased incidence of squamous cell carcinoma with chronic, low-level skin exposure.
- Radiodermatitis (reddened, dry skin) can result from excessive, chronic, low-level radiation exposure.
- The developing fetus is sensitive to the effects of ionizing radiation.
  - The degree of sensitivity depends on the stage of pregnancy and the dose received.
  - The preimplantation period (0 to 9 days) is the most critical time for the embryo.
  - The period of organogenesis (10 days to 6 weeks) carries the greatest risk of congenital malformation in the fetus because this is the critical development period for fetal organs.
  - The fetus may have skeletal or dental malformations.
  - Other abnormalities include microphthalmia (small eyes) and overall growth retardation.
  - A fetal dose greater than 25 rad (0.25 gray [Gy]) is recognized as the threshold for significant damage to the fetus (for an explanation of these units of measure, see "Terminology" later).
  - The fetal period (6 weeks to term) is the least sensitive time for the fetus; however, growth may be affected and mental retardation may occur.
  - Irradiation after 30 weeks is less likely to cause abnormalities because the sensitivity of the fetus approaches that of the adult.

Terminology

- Rem stands for roentgen equivalent in man.
- Rem units are used to express the dose equivalent that results from exposure to ionizing radiation.
- Rem takes into account the quality of radiation, so doses of different types of radiation can be compared.
- The sievert (SV) is the current terminology used to define a rem (1 SV = 100 rem).
- A millirem (mrem) is equal to 0.001 rem or $\frac{1}{1000}$ rem.
- A rad is the radiation absorbed dose. Current terminology is Gy (1 Gy = 100 rad).
- MPD is the maximum permissible dose.
- The National Council on Radiation Protection and Measurements recommends that the dose for occupationally exposed persons not exceed 5 rem/year.

- An occupationally exposed individual is one who normally performs his or her work in a restricted access area and has duties that involve exposure to radiation.
- ALARA stands for *as low as reasonably attainable*.
- The MPD for nonoccupational persons is 10% of the MPD for occupationally exposed persons, or 0.5 rem/year.
  - This is known as the ALARA MPD.
- A fetus should not receive more than 0.5 rem during the entire gestation period.
- A pregnant employee who chooses to continue working around radiation-producing devices should wear an additional badge at waist level, underneath the lead gown, to monitor the fetal dose; this should not exceed 0.05 rem/month.
- Lead shielding should be a requirement for all personnel remaining in the room while an exposure is made.
- Lead gowns, gloves, and thyroid shields should all contain at least 0.5 mm of lead.
- Lead-based glasses can also be worn to protect the lens of the eye.
- Lead apparel is expensive, so it should be handled appropriately.
- Lead aprons should be draped over a rounded surface, without folds or wrinkles, to prevent cracks in the lead.
- Lead gloves can be stored with open-ended soup cans inserted to prevent cracks and provide air circulation to the liners.
- Lead gloves should be radiographed every 6 months to check for damaged areas.
- Lead gowns should be checked every 12 months to screen for holes and cracks in the lead.
- Check gloves and gowns for damage by radiographing them using 5 mAs and 80 kVp.
- Nonleaded protective aprons have recently become available and provide the same protection as standard lead apparel; nonleaded apparel is much lighter in weight.
- Lead mittens and hand shields are also available; these are not generally recommended because part of the hand may be exposed to scatter radiation.
- Another method for decreasing personnel exposure is by increasing the distance from the primary beam.
- If the animal cannot be sedated or anesthetized, personnel restraining the animal should try to remain as far as possible from the x-ray source during exposure.
- During exposure, if restraining an animal, one should use tape and sandbags and/or other types of mechanical restraints to extend the distance of the gloved hands from the collimated area.
- Employees should take care to wear protective apparel properly to obtain full protection.
- Placing a glove on top of a hand for protection does not protect the hand from scatter radiation.
- The scatter can come from any direction, including from under the tabletop.

- Using the fastest film–screen combinations allows reduced exposure time for the patient and personnel by using less mAs.
- Proper darkroom practices and technique charts allow for the consistent production of high-quality films, which reduces the number of repeat radiographs.
- It is important to collimate the primary beam down to the area of interest because this reduces the exposure of personnel to scatter (secondary) radiation.
- A 2-mm Al filter is used at the tube window to filter out soft rays that are too weak to penetrate the patient.
- If these rays are not filtered out, they scatter about the room, fogging the film and striking personnel.
- Each clinic should have a radiation protection supervisor.
  - Responsibilities include educating personnel on radiation safety, monitoring safety practices, and maintaining a radiologic badge system.
  - The supervisor also maintains x-ray equipment, darkroom facilities, and radiographic records.
- A good radiation control program consists of safe x-ray equipment, low-exposure techniques, use of positioning aids, proper measuring of patients, proper positioning methods, shielding, and monitoring personal radiation exposure (Box 9.1). The x-ray equipment is usually under the control of the state government (e.g., state board of health).
- Regulations vary among states, so check with your state government about their policy regarding radiation-producing devices.

> **BOX 9.1** General Radiation Safety Rules
>
> - Always wear lead gloves and apron as well as lead thyroid shield when remaining in the room during radiography or fluoroscopy. Lead protective shielding must be worn by all individuals involved in restraint of the animal.
> - Always wear a radiation-monitoring device on your collar outside the apron or on the edge of the glove when working around x-ray equipment. (Note: Badges should not be exposed to sunlight, dampness, or extreme temperatures. This could cause falsely high readings.)
> - Never allow any part of your body to be exposed to the primary beam. Lead clothing does not protect against primary beam exposure.
> - Wear lead-based glasses to protect the lens of the eye.
> - Use mechanical restraints such as tape and sandbags; distance will aid in minimizing exposure.
> - Use alternative methods of restraint (e.g., drugs, tape, sandbags) when using high-exposure radiographic techniques.
> - Pregnant women and persons <18 yr should not be involved in radiographic procedures. Use proper safety precautions.
> - Only those required for restraint should remain in the room when an exposure is made.

Adapted from Sirois M: Principles and practice of veterinary technology, ed 3, St Louis, 2011, Mosby.

DARKROOM TECHNIQUES

- Along with a good technique chart, proper darkroom techniques should be followed to ensure consistent production of high-quality radiographs.
- Properly exposed radiographs can quickly become nondiagnostic with poor film handling and darkroom techniques.

Darkroom Setup

- For most veterinary practices, the darkroom must be just large enough to provide a dry bench area away from the wet bench area.
- The dry bench area is for unloading and loading cassettes and film storage.
- The wet bench area is for film processing and drying.
- These areas must be separated to prevent processing chemical splashes from damaging the dry films or sensitive intensifying screens.
- Sufficient electrical outlets should be available to power the safelights, view boxes, and labeling equipment.
- The most important feature of a darkroom is that it be light-tight.
- White light that leaks around the door, through a blackened window, or around ventilation fans can fog the film.
- Film is more sensitive after it has been exposed to x-rays, so even low-grade light leaks decrease the quality of the finished radiograph.
- When checking for light leaks, stand in the darkroom for at least 5 minutes to allow your eyes to adjust to the darkness.
- Look around the door frame, ventilation fan, or blackened windows for any signs of white light.
- Because work in the darkroom is done with a limited amount of light, painting the walls and ceiling a light color that reflects the available light helps greatly.
- The darkroom should have adequate ventilation to prevent volatile chemical fumes from accumulating in the room.
- These fumes can cause fogging of the film, damage to electrical equipment, and health problems for personnel.
- A light-tight ventilation fan installed in the ceiling helps remove the fumes and also controls the temperature and humidity in the room.
- The exhaust from automatic processors and film dryers should also be vented away from the darkroom because they contain volatile chemical fumes.

- Cleanliness is important in the darkroom because intensifying screens and the film are handled in this area.
- Dirt and hair on countertops can fall into cassettes, causing white artifacts on subsequent radiographs from that cassette.
- Chemical spills also cause artifacts on the radiographs and damage the intensifying screens. Keeping wet and dry areas of the darkroom clean prevents these problems.

Film Identification

- Permanent labeling is necessary for all radiographs.
- Each film must be identified before the film is processed for legal purposes and for certification organizations.
- The labeling can be done during or after the exposure, but it must be done before the film is processed.
- The label should include the clinic name, date, owner's name, address, patient's name, and some patient data, such as age and breed.
- There are several methods for film identification.
  - One method is the photo labeler, which uses a cassette containing a leaded window that protects a small area of the film during exposure.
    - During identification, the window slides back from the protected area to expose the information on a card.
    - This forms a latent image of the information on the film.
    - Manual printers are similar to photo labelers, except that they use a flash of light through an information card to produce a latent image on the film.
    - The manual printer is placed in the darkroom, and the film is taken out of the cassette to be identified.
  - Another method uses lead letters or radiopaque tape.
    - These are placed on the cassette during exposure of the radiograph.

Safelights

- A safelight provides sufficient light to work in the room but does not cause fogging of the film.
- Safelights can be mounted to provide light directly or indirectly.
- With direct lighting, the safelight is mounted at least 48 inches above the workbench and directed toward the workbench.
- Indirect lighting has the safelight directed toward the ceiling and uses the reflected light to illuminate the room.
- With indirect lighting, the safelight can be mounted closer to the bench but should be as high as possible.
- Many types of safelight filters are available to filter out light in different areas of the light spectrum.
- Film that is blue light–sensitive requires a safelight that filters out blue and ultraviolet light.
- Film that is green light–sensitive requires a safelight to filter both green and blue light.
- Periodically check the safelight filter.
  - First, make a moderate exposure on a film using approximately 1 to 2 mAs and 40 to 50 kVp. Film that

has been exposed to x-rays is more sensitive to low-grade light, producing an overall fogged appearance.
  - Cover two-thirds of the film with black paper or cardboard, and allow the remaining third to be exposed to the safelight for 30 seconds.
  - After 30 seconds, uncover another third of the film and wait 30 more seconds.
  - Repeat the process for the final third and develop the film.
  - This test exposes portions of the film to the safelight for 30, 60, and 90 seconds and then it is processed.
  - When the film is dry, look for areas of increased film density.
  - If an increase in density is detected, a close check of the darkroom is necessary.
- Improper safelight distance, a cracked safelight filter, and light leaking around the filter can all cause film fogging.

Film Processing

Chemistry

Developer

- The developer's main function is to convert the sensitized silver halide crystals into black metallic silver.
- Sensitized silver halide crystals are those that have been exposed to electromagnetic radiation, making them susceptible to chemical change.
- The developer contains five ingredients: a solvent, reducing agents, restrainer, activator, and preservative.
- Water is used as the solvent to keep all the ingredients in solution.
- It also causes the film emulsion to swell so that the reducing agents can penetrate the sensitized crystals.
- Reducing agents change the sensitized silver halide crystals into black metallic silver.
- Restrainers are used to protect the unexposed silver halide crystals by preventing the reducing agents from affecting the unsensitized crystals.
- Activators help soften and swell the film's emulsion so that the reducing agents can work effectively.
- Preservatives prevent the solution from oxidizing rapidly.
- Developing chemicals are manufactured in two forms: liquid and powder.
- The liquid form may be a concentrate that requires dilution with water.
- Working-strength liquid solutions that do not require dilution are also available.
- The powder form should never be mixed in the darkroom because the chemical dust contaminates unprotected film, causing artifacts.

Fixer

- The fixer removes the unchanged silver halide crystals from the film emulsion, leaving the black metallic silver.
- It also hardens the film emulsion, decreasing the susceptibility to scratches.
- The fixer contains five ingredients: solvent, fixing agent, acidifier, hardener, and preservative.

- As with the developer, the solvent for the fixer is water.
- It keeps the ingredients in solution and causes the film emulsion to swell, allowing the fixing agents to reach the unexposed crystals.
- The fixing agent clears the remaining silver halide crystals from the film emulsion.
- The acidifier is used to neutralize any alkaline developer remaining on the film.
- The hardener prevents excessive swelling of the film emulsion, shortening the drying time. The final ingredient is the preservative, used to prevent decomposition of the fixing agents.
- Fixer chemicals are manufactured in two forms: liquid and powder.
- The liquid form may be a concentrate that requires dilution with water.
- Working-strength liquid solutions that do not require dilution are also available.
- The powder form requires dissolving and mixing to get it into solution.
- It should never be mixed in the darkroom because the chemical dust can contaminate unprotected film, causing artifacts.

Equipment
Manual Processing
- With the ready availability of reasonably priced automatic processors, few veterinary clinics now use manual methods.
- Manual processing is sometimes used for dental radiographs and other nonscreen films used for exotic animal radiography.
- Manual processing tanks are usually made from stainless steel and are large enough to accept 14- by 17-inch film hangers.
  - Tanks with a 5-gallon capacity are sufficient.
- Plastic or wooden lids are needed to cover the developer and fixer tanks, which reduces the rate of evaporation and oxidation of the chemicals.
- Separate stirring rods for the developer and fixer are used to mix the chemicals before processing.
- An accurate timer and floating thermometer should be available.
- Developing x-ray film is a chemical process that depends on the duration of immersion in the chemicals and the temperature of the chemicals.
- Manufacturers generally recommend a temperature for the chemicals they produce. Most use 68°F (20°C), with 5 minutes of developing time.
- The time can be decreased by 30 seconds for every 2°F increase in developer temperature, or the time can be increased by 30 seconds for every 2°F decrease in developer temperature.
- The rinse bath removes developer from the film, preventing carryover into the fixer tank. Agitating the film in the running water bath for 30 seconds removes the developer

adequately. The rinse water should be continually exchanged to prevent accumulation of developer.
- The fixing process is also dependent on immersion time and temperature of the chemicals.
- The standard temperature is 68°F (20°C), and the fixing time is double the developing time.
- The temperature affects the time that the film is left in the fixer; the warmer the chemicals, the shorter the fixing time.
- The film can be removed from the fixer after 30 seconds and viewed with white light.
  - However, it must be placed back into the fixer for the remainder of the time.
- Direct exposure film has a thicker emulsion and requires a longer time in the fixer.
- The final wash rinses away the processing chemicals.
- Failure to rinse the film completely results in a film that eventually becomes faded and brown due to oxidation of the chemicals remaining in the film emulsion.
- The wash tank should have fresh circulating water to decrease the time needed for the final wash.
- Generally, the wash time is at least 30 minutes.
Maintenance
- There are two methods for maintaining manual processing tanks.
- The first is the exhausted method.
  - With this method, allow the chemicals to drain back into their respective tanks and not into the wash tank.
  - This permits the exhausted chemicals to remain in the tank, maintaining the chemical levels.
- The second method is the replenishing method.
  - Do not allow the chemicals to drain back into their respective tanks, but place them in the wash tank.
  - The chemical levels are maintained by replenishing with chemicals that are more concentrated than those in the initial solution.
  - In this way, the potency and levels of the chemicals can be preserved.
- With either method, the chemicals should be changed every 3 months.
Automatic Processing
- Use of an automatic processor has some advantages over manual processing.
- Automatic processors can develop film more quickly; they can process and dry a film in 90 to 120 seconds.
- Automatic processors consistently provide high-quality radiographs that eliminate the need for repeat radiographs because of processing errors.
- Automatic processors move the film through the developer, fixer wash bath, and dryers at a uniform rate of speed.
- Chemicals and film are specially manufactured to withstand the high temperatures involved in automatic processing.
  - The chemicals are kept at temperatures of approximately 95°F (35°C), depending on the type of film and equipment used.

Maintenance

- Small tabletop automatic processors are easily maintained in most veterinary practices.
- The equipment should be completely cleaned every 3 months.
  - This includes draining and cleaning the tanks.
- A 1:32 solution of laundry bleach (e.g., Clorox) helps reduce algae and remove chemical buildup.
- The rollers can be cleaned with a mild detergent and soft sponge.
- When any cleaning solution is applied to the tanks or rollers, they should be rinsed thoroughly before replacing the chemicals.
- Check the springs and gears for signs of wear and replace if necessary.
- Wipe the feed tray and top rollers with a clean, soft sponge every day to remove dirt, debris, and chemical residue between episodes of routine maintenance.

Silver Recovery

- When an exposed film is placed in the developer, the exposed silver halide crystals are converted to black metallic silver.
  - The remaining silver halide crystals are removed from the film in the fixer.
  - Over time, the fixer solution becomes rich with silver that can be reclaimed.
- Silver recovery systems can be attached to automatic processors to filter and store the silver that would normally be discarded down the drain.
- The black metallic silver in the processed radiographs can also be recovered.
- The manual processing fixer solution, silver recovery systems, and old radiographs can be sold to companies that reclaim the silver.

RADIOGRAPHIC ARTIFACTS

- An artifact is any unwanted density in the form of blemishes caused by improper handling, exposure, processing, or housekeeping.
- Artifacts can mimic or mask a disease process or distract from the overall quality of the film.
- Before radiographing an animal, check for external debris, wet hair, or any lumps or bumps on the patient. Remove any dirt or mats from the coat. If the coat is wet, dry it as much as possible. Remove any collars, leashes, or halters. Bandage material is visible on radiographs, so remove it, if feasible. Boxes 9.2 and 9.3 list common artifact problems.

RADIOGRAPHIC POSITIONING AND TERMINOLOGY

- A basic knowledge of directional terminology is essential when describing radiographic projections.

BOX 9.2 Causes of Common Radiographic Artifacts That Occur Before Processing

Fogged Film
- Film exposed to excessive scatter radiation. A grid is necessary when radiographing areas ≥10 cm (overall gray appearance).
- Film exposed to radiation during storage.
- Film stored in an area that was too hot or humid.
- Film exposed to a safelight filter that was cracked or inappropriate for the type of film used.
- Film exposed to a low-grade light leak in darkroom.
- Film expired.

Black Crescents or Lines
- Rough handling of film before or after exposure.
- Static electricity caused by low humidity.
- Scratched film surface before or after exposure.
- Fingerprints from excessive pressure before or after exposure.

Black Areas
- Black, irregular border on one end of film caused by light exposure while still in the box or film bin.
- Black, irregular border on multiple sides of the film caused by felt damage in the cassette.

White Areas
- Foreign material between the film and screen.
- Chemical spill on the screen, causing permanent damage to the phosphor layer.
- Contrast medium on the patient, table, or cassette.
- White fingerprints on film from oil or fixer on fingers before processing.
- Visible grid lines.
- Grid lines on the entire film from FFD outside the range of the grid's focus.
- Grid lines more visible on one end of the film and overall decrease in radiographic density caused by the grid's not being centered in the primary beam.
- Grid lines on the entire film caused by the grid's not being perpendicular to the center of the primary beam.
- Grid lines more visible in some areas than others from grid damage.

Decreased Detail
- Patient motion.
- Poor film–screen contact.
- Increased object–film distance.
- Decreased FFD.

Adapted from Sirois M: Principles and practice of veterinary technology, ed 3, St Louis, 2011, Mosby.

BOX 9.3 Causes of Common Radiographic Artifacts That Occur During Manual or Automatic Processing

Increased Radiographic Density With Poor Contrast
- Film overdeveloped (longer than manufacturer recommendation)
- Film developed in hot chemicals; correct temperature for manual tanks is 68°F (20°C); for automatic processors, 95°F (35°C)
- Film overexposed

Decreased Radiographic Density With Poor Contrast
- Film underdeveloped (shorter than manufacturer recommendation)
- Film developed in cold chemicals; correct temperature for manual tanks is 68°F (20°C); for automatic processors, 95°F (35°C)
- Film processed in old or exhausted chemicals
- Film underexposed

Uneven Development
- Lack of stirring, allowing chemicals to settle to tank bottom
- Repeated withdrawal of film from tank to check on development results
- Uneven chemical levels

Black Areas, Spots, or Streaks
- Identical black areas on two films processed together from films stuck to one another in fixer and not cleared properly
- Black area on only one film from film sticking to side of tank
- Well-defined spots or streaks from developer splash before processing
- Black lines along full length of the film and equal distance apart from pressure of rollers in the processor

Defined Areas of Decreased Radiographic Density
- Identical light areas on two films processed together from sticking together in the developer
- Light area on one film from film sticking to the side of the tank during development
- Air bubbles clinging to the film during development
- Well-defined spots or streaks from fixer splash before processing

Clear Areas or Spots
- Streaks where emulsion scratched away
- Large clear areas from leaving film in final wash too long and emulsion sliding off film base

Entire Film Clear
- No exposure
- Film placed in fixer before developer

Film Turns Brown
- Improper final wash

Adapted from Sirois M: Principles and practice of veterinary technology, ed 3, St Louis, 2011, Mosby.

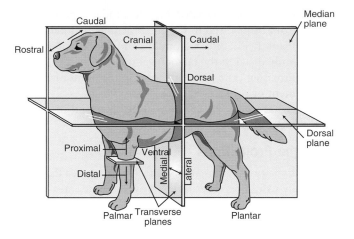

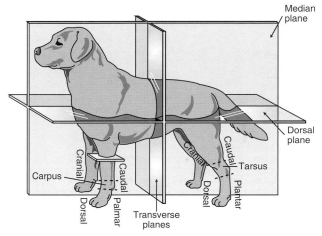

FIGURE 9.5 Anatomic planes of reference and directional terms. (From Colville TP, Bassert JM: *Clinical anatomy and physiology for veterinary technicians*, ed 2, St Louis, 2008, Mosby.)

- The American College of Veterinary Radiology (ACVR) has standardized the nomenclature for radiographic projections by using currently accepted veterinary anatomic terms.
- The projections are described by the direction at which the central ray enters and exits the part being imaged (Fig. 9.5):
  - Ventral (V): Body area situated toward the underside of quadrupeds
  - Dorsal (D): Body area situated toward the back or topline of quadrupeds; opposite of ventral
  - Medial (M): Body area situated toward the median plane or midline
  - Lateral (L): Body area situated away from the median plane or midline
  - Cranial (Cr): Structures or areas situated toward the head (formerly anterior)
  - Caudal (Cd): Structures or areas situated toward the tail (formerly posterior)
  - Rostral (R): Areas on the head situated toward the nose

- Palmar (Pa): Situated on the caudal aspect of the front limb, distal to the antebrachiocarpal joint
- Plantar (Pl): Situated on the caudal aspect of the rear limb, distal to the tarsocrural joint
- Proximal (Pr): Situated closer to the point of attachment or origin
- Distal (Di): Situated away from the point of attachment or origin

Oblique Projections

- Oblique projections are used to set off an area that normally would be superimposed over another area.

- Some rules should be followed when deciding which type of oblique projection is needed and how it is to be identified:
  - The area of interest should be as close to the cassette as possible. This decreases magnification and increases detail.
  - Place a marker on the cassette or near the anatomy within the primary beam during exposure to indicate the direction of entry and exit of the primary beam.
- Table 9.1 shows the landmarks used to produce radiographs of various body parts.

TABLE 9.1 Landmarks Used in Producing Radiographs of Various Body Areas

Body Part	Cranial or Proximal Landmark	Caudal or Distal Landmark	Center Landmark	Comments
Thorax	Manubrium sterni	Halfway between xiphoid and last rib	Caudal border of the scapula	Expose at peak inspiration.
Abdomen	Halfway between xiphoid and caudal border of the scapula	Greater trochanter	Last rib	Expose at peak expiration.
Shoulder	Midbody scapula	Midshaft humerus	Over joint space	
Humerus	Shoulder joint	Elbow joint	Midshaft	
Elbow	Midshaft humerus	Midshaft radius	Over joint space	
Radius, ulna	Elbow joint	Carpal joint	Midshaft	
Carpus	Midshaft radius	Midshaft metacarpus	Over joint space	
Metacarpus	Carpal joint	Include digits	Midshaft	
Pelvis	Wings of ilium	Ischium		
Pelvis ventrodorsal (VD), flexed	Wings of ilium	Ischium		Pushes stifles cranially
Pelvis VD, extended	Wings of ilium	Stifle joint		Femora parallel to each other and table
Femur	Coxofemoral joint	Stifle joint	Midshaft	
Stifle	Midshaft femur	Midshaft tibia	Over joint space	
Tibia, fibula	Stifle joint	Tarsal joint	Midshaft	
Tarsus	Midshaft tibia	Midshaft metatarsal	Over joint space	
Metatarsus	Tarsal joint	Include digits	Midshaft	
Cervical vertebrae	Base of skull	Spine of scapula		Extend front limbs caudally; collimate width of beam to increase detail.
Thoracic vertebrae	Spine of scapula		Halfway between xiphoid and last rib	Collimate width of beam to increase detail.
Thoracolumbar vertebrae			Halfway between to increase detail	Collimate width of beam xiphoid and last rib.
Lumbar vertebrae	Halfway between xiphoid and last rib	Wings of ilium		Collimate width of beam to increase detail.

Adapted from Sirois M: Principles and practice of veterinary technology, ed 3, St Louis, 2011, Mosby.

- For most small animal patients, abdominal and thoracic radiographs require a VD and lateral projection.

CONTRAST STUDIES

- The purpose of a contrast study is to delineate an organ or area against surrounding soft tissues.
- They are useful for determining the size, shape, position, location, and function of an organ. The information obtained from a contrast study complements or confirms findings of the survey radiographs.
- Positive contrast agents are radiopaque on a radiograph.
- Negative contrast agents produce radiolucent areas on a radiograph.
- Obtaining survey radiographs before doing a contrast study establishes proper exposure technique and proper patient preparation.
- Because most contrast studies require multiple images, it is important to label each film with the time and sequence.
- Always record the amount, type, and administration route of the contrast agent.

Positive Contrast Media

- Positive contrast media contain elements with a high atomic number; elements with a high atomic number absorb more x-rays.
  - Thus fewer x-rays penetrate the patient and expose the film, creating a white area on the radiograph.
- Two common types of positive contrast agents are barium sulfate and water-soluble organic iodides.
- Barium sulfate is commonly used for positive contrast studies of the GI tract.
  - It is insoluble and is not affected by gastric secretions.
  - Therefore it provides good mucosal detail on the radiograph.
  - Barium sulfate preparations are relatively inexpensive and are manufactured in the form of powders, colloid suspensions, or pastes.
  - A disadvantage of using barium sulfate is that it can take 3 hours or longer to travel from the stomach to the colon.
  - Also, it can be harmful to the peritoneum, so it should never be used when GI perforations are suspected.
  - While administering barium orally, take care to prevent the patient from aspirating barium into the lungs; aspiration of large amounts can be fatal.
- A product that consists of barium-impregnated polyethylene spheres is also available and may present less risk of peritonitis when GI perforation is present.
- Water-soluble organic iodides in ionic form are also used for positive contrast procedures.

- Different forms of the water-soluble organic iodides can be administered intravenously, orally, or by infusion into a hollow organ or into the subarachnoid space.
  - Because they are water soluble, they are absorbed into the bloodstream and excreted by the kidneys.
  - These agents may be used to perform contrast studies of the GI tract when perforation is suspected.
- Ionic water-soluble organic iodides for intravenous (IV) use are prepared in various combinations of meglumine and sodium diatrizoate.
  - Diatrizoate can also be infused into hollow organs, such as the urinary bladder, or into fistulous tracts.
- Ionic water-soluble organic iodides cannot be used for myelography because they are irritating to the brain and spinal cord.
- Nonionic water-soluble organic iodides are used for myelography and can be used intravenously.
  - Because of their low osmolarity and chemical nature, they cause fewer adverse effects when placed in the subarachnoid space.

Negative Contrast Media

- Negative contrast agents include air, oxygen, and carbon dioxide.
- They all have a low atomic number, appearing radiolucent on the finished radiograph.

Double-Contrast Procedure

- Double-contrast procedures use both positive and negative contrast media to image an organ or area.
- The most common organs imaged with double contrast are the urinary bladder, stomach, and colon.
- In most cases, the negative contrast medium is added first and then the positive contrast medium.
- Mixing a negative contrast medium with a positive contrast medium can cause air bubbles to form, which might be misinterpreted as lesions.

ORAL RADIOLOGY

- Many abnormalities, diseases, and traumatic events may affect the tooth subgingivally.
- Dental radiography is now considered the standard of care and should be included as part of the diagnostic and treatment plan for every patient.

Radiographic Equipment

- Although it is possible to do oral radiography using standard equipment with intraoral films and rapid developer/fixer solutions, a variety of digital systems are available that are dedicated for use in dentistry.
- Extraoral films and oblique projections can be used for survey films, but these generally produce some degree

of superimposition of other oral structures over the area to be viewed.

- Small, flexible intraoral films can be used with the standard radiographic unit with few variations.
- Intraoral films provide excellent detail, and superimposition of other oral structures is rarely a problem, unless positioning was incorrect.
- The unit can be used with the radiographic head positioned at a 36- to 40-inch focal distance for two-thirds to three-fifths of a second at 100 mA.
- It is preferable if the radiographic head is mobile, however, to decrease the focal distance to 12 inches and the exposure time to one-tenth to one-fifteenth of a second to minimize distortion and exposure.
- Depending on the equipment, the kVp may vary from 65 for a small dog or cat up to 85 for a large breed.
- The intraoral films come in a variety of small sizes (0, 1, 2, 3, 4); No. 2 film (periapical) is most commonly used. No. 4 film (occlusal) measures 2 by 3 inches and can be used to view a larger area of the incisors and canines or the nasal cavity (also for small rodents, birds, and cat feet).
- Intraoral film is nonscreened, double-emulsion film encased in a black paper sleeve with a lead foil back sheet that helps prevent back scatter produced by x-rays bouncing back off the table.
- Dental films can be developed in standard tanks or automatic processors (taped to the lead end of a larger film).
- Rapid dental developer and fixer solutions can be used in individual containers, either in the existing darkroom or in a chairside developer at the dental station.
  - After rehydrating the emulsification of the film in water for 3 to 5 seconds, developing time ranges from 15 to 30 seconds, using fresh developing solutions.
  - After a water rinse, fixing time is in the same range, so a film can be developed in less than 1 minute.

Radiographic Techniques

- The difficulty of oral radiography lies in positioning the film and the patient to obtain an image with the least distortion.
- A **parallel technique** is used only with the mandibular premolars/molars, when the film can be placed parallel to the teeth, with a corner pressing down into the intermandibular space.
  - With the film so positioned, the x-ray head can then be aimed perpendicular to the parallel items.
- Elsewhere in the oral cavity, the film cannot be positioned directly against the object to be viewed, particularly in the maxilla, because of the shape of the palate.
- To accommodate for this obstacle, the **bisecting angle technique** can be used to minimize distortion that is inherent when the film cannot be placed parallel to the tooth.
  - If the x-ray beam is aimed perpendicular to the film, the tooth image will be shortened; if it is aimed perpendicular to the long axis of the tooth, the image will be elongated.

- Therefore if the beam is aimed midway between the two positions, the image should approximate the size of the tooth itself.
- One way to visualize this is to imagine an angle formed by the line of the film and the line of the long axis of the tooth or its root.
- Once this angle is assessed, a line that would bisect this angle is determined.
- Certain corrections must be made when taking x-rays of the maxillary premolars and molars in the cat.
- Because of its prominent zygomatic arch, if one followed the standard bisecting angle rule, there would be superimposition of the arch over these teeth.
- To avoid this, the operator must come in at a steeper angle, thus creating elongated teeth but no interference from the cat's zygomatic arch.

Patient Positioning and Film Placement

- Although dental radiographs may be taken from a variety of positions, for consistency, all the patients should have their hard palates or nose parallel to the table.
- Positioning devices such as wedges, fluid bags, and towels can be helpful in maintaining the patient's position.
- When placing the film in the mouth, always center the film under the area of interest.
- To hold the film into position, gauze and tape rolls are commonly used.
- Patient positioning for maxillary incisors and canines of the dog and cat will be placed in ventral recumbency; for mandibular incisors and canines of the dog and cat, the patient will be in dorsal recumbency.
  - Place the film centered below incisors and canines and over the endotracheal tube.
  - If the canines are too large to be included in the same film as the incisors, the film will be centered under the desired canine tooth and parallel to the hard palate.
  - If the film is placed as far back as the third premolar, the roots of the canines will be included in the x-ray.
- Patient positioning for maxillary premolars and molars of the dog and cat will be in ventral recumbency.
  - The film is placed along the hard palate near the tongue side of the opposite teeth (film will be mostly over the hard palate).
  - The long end of the film is parallel to the muzzle.
- Patient positioning for the mandibular premolars and molars will be in lateral recumbency.
  - The film is placed in the vestibule (space) between the tongue and teeth with the long end of the film parallel to the muzzle.
  - Center the film under the area of interest.
- The dimple on the film is a permanent marker. It will be useful in determining which side of the mouth you are viewing once the film is developed (Fig. 9.6).
  - The up side of the dimple points toward the cone of the x-ray machine.

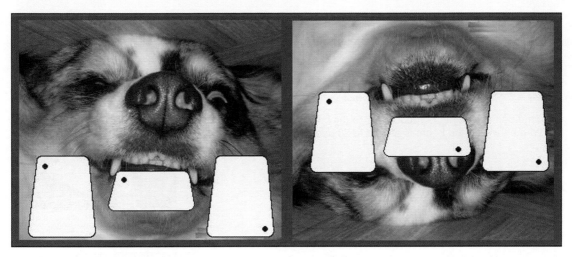

FIGURE 9.6 Dimple placement in the mouth. (From Sirois M: *Principles and practice of veterinary technology*, ed 4, St Louis, 2017, Mosby.)

- When the film is placed lengthwise in the patient's mouth, the dimple remains on the outside of the mouth.
- When the film is placed parallel to the canines, the dimple is positioned to match the right side of the mouth.

Cone Placement

- Cone position is the angle in which you place the cone of the x-ray machine to acquire the view you desire.
- To set the cone, you will need to position two angles: the perpendicular (up and down) angle and the lateral (side to side) angle (Table 9.2).
- This can be the most difficult part of dental radiology because the shape and position of the patient's head will affect the position of the cone.

DIAGNOSTIC ULTRASOUND

- Diagnostic ultrasound (ultrasonography) is a noninvasive method of imaging soft tissues.
- A transducer sends low-intensity, high-frequency sound waves into the soft tissues, where they interact with tissue interfaces.
  - Some of the sound waves are reflected back to the transducer, and some are transmitted into deeper tissues.
  - The sound waves that are reflected back to the transducer (echoes) are then analyzed by the computer to produce a grayscale image.
- Use of ultrasound in conjunction with radiography gives the veterinarian an excellent diagnostic tool.
  - Radiographs demonstrate the size, shape, and position of the organs.
  - Ultrasound displays the findings found on the radiographs as well as the soft tissue textures and dynamics of some organs (e.g., motility of the bowel).

Transducers

- Ultrasound transducers emit a series of sound pulses and receive the returning echoes.
- A weak electrical current applied to the piezoelectric crystals incorporated in the transducer causes the crystals to vibrate and produce sound waves.
- After sending a series of pulses, the crystals are dampened to stop further vibrations.
- When struck by the returning echoes, the crystals vibrate again, and these echoes are converted into electrical energy.
- Transducers are available in different configurations, mechanical or electronic.
- The scan plane can be a sector scan (pie-shaped image) or a linear array scan (rectangular image).
  - A mechanically driven sector scan can be produced by a belt and pulley used to wobble a single crystal or rotate multiple crystals across a scan plane.
  - Another method of producing a sector scan is with the use of a phased array or annular array configuration.
  - With a phased array configuration, the crystals are pulsed sequentially with a built-in delay to create a so-called pseudosector scan plane.
  - An annular array arranges the crystals in concentric rings.
  - By using electronic phasing of the many crystals, annular array transducers produce a two-dimensional image by steering the entire array through a sector arc.
- The frequency of the transducer determines the amount of detail or resolution of the image.
  - As frequency increases, the wavelength gets shorter.
  - The shorter the wavelength, the better the resolution of the image.

Terminology Describing Echotexture

- Echogenic or echoic means that most of the sound is reflected back to the transducer.
  - Echogenic areas appear white on the screen.

TABLE 9.2 Cone Placement for Dental Radiographs

CANINE MAXILLARY INCISORS

Center beam over the nose. Aim cone downward at a 50- to 60-degree angle to hard palate.
OR
Aim beam at the dorsal midline, perpendicular to the bridge of the nose. Then tip the tube so the beam is angled at 20 degrees caudally.

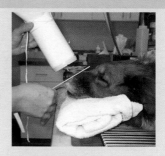

CANINE MAXILLARY CANINES

Lateral: Cone is centered over canine and adjacent to PM2. Aim cone about 80 to 90 degrees to the midline and tipped down at a 45-degree angle to the hard palate.
Beam directed canine to canine.
OR
Aim beam dorsally over the top canine, similar to the upper incisor view. Then tip the tube so the beam is angled at 20 to 30 degrees caudally and 20 to 30 degrees toward the midline.

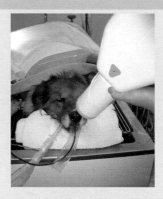

CANINE MAXILLARY PREMOLARS

PM1-3: Position cone over desired premolars. Aim cone from a lateral direction at a 45-degree angle to hard palate.
OR
Aim cone dorsally over the top of the target teeth. Tip the tube so the beam is angled ≈45 degrees toward the midline.

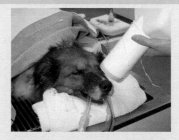

CANINE MAXILLARY 4TH UPPER PREMOLAR

Lateral: Cone is positioned over premolars and molars. Aim cone (perpendicular to the head) at lateral canthus of the eye at a 45-degree angle to the hard palate.

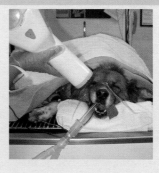

TABLE 9.2 Cone Placement for Dental Radiographs—cont'd

CANINE MAXILLARY 4TH UPPER PREMOLAR

Mesiolateral: Cone is positioned over premolars and molars. Aim cone vertically at lateral canthus of the eye at a 45-degree angle to the hard palate.

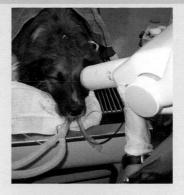

Distolateral: Cone is positioned over premolars and molars. Aim cone distally at lateral canthus of the eye at a 45-degree angle to the hard palate.

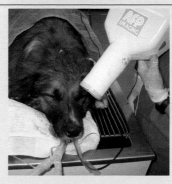

CANINE MAXILLARY MOLARS

Cone is positioned over premolars and molars. Aim cone (perpendicular to the head) at lateral canthus of the eye at a 45-degree angle to the hard palate.
OR
Aim cone dorsally over the top of the target teeth. Tip the tube so the beam is angled ≈45 degrees toward the midline.

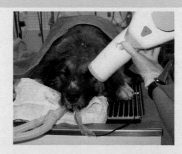

CANINE MANDIBULAR INCISORS

Center beam over the lower incisors. Aim cone downward at ≈60-degree angle to hard palate.
OR
Aim beam on the ventral midline, perpendicular to the mandible. Then tip the tube so the beam is angled at 20 degrees caudally.

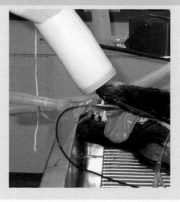

Continued

TABLE 9.2 Cone Placement for Dental Radiographs—cont'd

CANINE MANDIBULAR CANINES

Center over lower canines to PM2. Aim cone laterally at interproximal space between canine and I3. Tip down at 45- to 60-degree angle to hard palate. Beam directed canine to PM3-4.

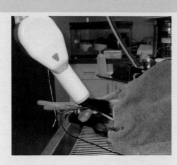

CANINE MANDIBULAR PREMOLARS AND MOLARS

PM1-2: Same as PM3-4. Can be viewed in canine x-ray also.
PM3-4: Center beam over target tooth at a 90-degree angle (perpendicular) to the film.
And a 60-degree angle to table top. Use gauze to stabilize film in mouth.
M1-3: Same as PM3-4.

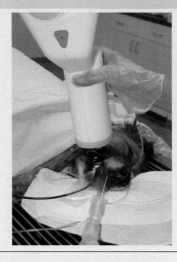

From Sirois M: Principles and practice of veterinary technology, ed 4, St Louis, 2017, Mosby.

- Sonolucent means that most of the sound is transmitted to the deeper tissues, with only a few echoes reflected back to the transducer.
  - Sonolucent areas appear dark on the screen.
- Anechoic is used to describe tissue that transmits all the sound through to deeper tissues, reflecting none of the sound back to the transducer.
  - Anechoic areas appear black on the screen and are generally fluid-filled structures.
- Soft tissues are represented not only as black or white but also as many shades of gray.
  - Hyperechoic is used to describe tissues that reflect more sound back to the transducer than surrounding tissues.
  - Hyperechoic areas appear brighter than surrounding tissues.
  - Hypoechoic is used to describe tissues that reflect less sound back to the transducer than surrounding tissues.

- Hypoechoic areas appear darker than surrounding tissues.
- Isoechoic is used to describe tissue that appears to have the same echotexture on the screen as surrounding tissues.

Patient Preparation
- To achieve an optimal acoustic window and produce the best-quality image, the transducer head must be placed into close contact with the skin.
- The animal's hair must be clipped and, in some cases, shaved before the study.
- An acoustic coupling gel is used on the patient's skin to eliminate the air interface and improve the acoustic window.
- Before applying the acoustic coupling gel, wipe the area with alcohol or generous amounts of soapy water to remove any loose hairs, dirt, and skin oils.
- Fasting of small animals before abdominal ultrasound examination is recommended.

- Ingesta and gas in the bowel decrease the amount of the abdomen that can be visualized.

Instrument Controls

- Ultrasound equipment has many controls for adjusting the quality of the image.
- Controls include those for brightness and contrast, depth, gain and power, and time gain compensation.

Artifacts

- Proper identification of artifacts is important to prevent confusion or misinterpretation.
- Some artifacts are beneficial when making a diagnosis.
  - Two such artifacts include acoustic shadowing and distance enhancement.
  - Acoustic shadowing occurs when the sound is attenuated or reflected at an acoustic interface. This prevents the sound from being transmitted to the deeper tissues, resulting in no echoes or fewer echoes returning from those areas.
  - Structures that can cause acoustic shadowing include bone, calculi, mineralized tissues and, occasionally, fat.
  - Distance enhancement occurs when the sound beam traverses a cystic structure.
  - Tissues deep to the cystic structure appear brighter than surrounding tissues.
  - The enhancement occurs because the sound that travels through the fluid-filled areas is less attenuated than the sound in surrounding tissues.
  - This artifact is useful in establishing that an anechoic or hypoechoic structure is actually fluid filled.
- Many artifacts have no diagnostic use, although if not identified as artifacts, they can lead to confusion.
  - One of these is the slice thickness artifact, which occurs when the transducer receives echoes with different amplitudes from the same area at the same depth.
  - Reverberation occurs when sound is reflected off a highly reflective interface (e.g., soft tissues to air or soft tissues to bone or metal) and then reflected back into the tissues by the surface of the transducer.
  - This bouncing back and forth can continue until the sound energy has completely attenuated. Each time the sound returns to the transducer, it produces an image at a location on the screen proportional to the time of travel between the transducer and reflective interface.
  - This creates a series of lines that are of equal distance apart on the screen.
  - The mirror image artifact creates the illusion of the liver on the thoracic side of the diaphragm or the appearance of a second heart beyond the lung interface.
  - This artifact can be produced in areas with strongly reflective interfaces.
  - Sound transmitted into the liver is reflected off the diaphragm.

- Some of these echoes are not reflected directly toward the transducer but back into the liver. In the liver, some of the misdirected echoes are reflected back to the diaphragm and then to the transducer.
- The computer sees the misdirected echoes as being reflected from the other side of the diaphragm.
- One way that this artifact can be minimized is by decreasing the depth to include only the area of interest.

ENDOSCOPY

- Endoscopic imaging can be used to diagnose disease as well as collect tissue samples for analysis.
- The opportunity to examine and obtain tissue samples without the invasiveness of surgery makes endoscopy one of the best methods for evaluating the digestive system.
- Responsibilities of veterinary staff members assisting with endoscopy include selection, care, and maintenance of the endoscopes and care and positioning of the patient.

Types of Endoscopes

- Rigid endoscopes are commonly used for rhinoscopy, female cystoscopy, laparoscopy, arthroscopy, vaginoscopy, and thoracoscopy.
- Flexible endoscopes are used for GI endoscopy, male cystoscopy, and bronchoscopy examinations.
- Flexible endoscopes are also used for percutaneous placement of gastrostomy tubes in small animals.

Rigid Endoscopes

- Rigid endoscopes are composed of a metal tube, lenses, and glass rods.
- They vary in size and characteristics; however, all are composed of a hollow tube containing no fiber bundles.
- Rigid endoscopes should be held by the eyepiece and not by the rod.
- Even slight bending of the rod section could change the angle of deflection, decreasing the degree of visualization.
- Rigid endoscopes should never be handled in bunches or piled on top of one another.

Flexible Endoscopes

- There are two types of flexible endoscopes: fiber-optic and video.
- Fiber-optic endoscopes use glass fiber bundles for the transmission of images.
  - These bundles transmit light from the light source to the distal tip of the endoscope.
- Fiber-optic glass fiber bundles are fragile and can be damaged easily.
- Broken fibers show up on the monitor screen as black dots.

- Too many of these black dots (many broken fiber bundles) can significantly reduce the field of view.
- Video endoscopes contain a microchip located at the distal end that records and transmits the image to a computer and then to a monitor screen.
- The image can be recorded; pictures can be recorded to show the owner and can be included in the patient's record.

Endoscopy Room

- In an ideal situation, all endoscopic examinations are performed in the same room.
- Because the lights are usually dimmed during endoscopic examination to reduce glare on the viewing monitor, a room with curtains or shades is ideal.
- A sturdy cart with three or four shelves can conveniently store the light source, suction unit, endoscope, and any accessory equipment until ready for use.
- All necessary equipment should be located near this endoscopy unit so that it can be reached quickly if needed during endoscopy.
- All anesthetic equipment must be ready before the procedure begins.

Accessory Instruments

- Accessory instruments can be passed through the working channel of the flexible endoscope and directed to a specific area.
- The most basic instruments include biopsy forceps, foreign body removal forceps, and a cytology brush.
- All personnel involved with endoscopic procedures should wear examination gloves.
- The endoscope should not be allowed to contact the video accessories or any other potentially conductive object directly; wearing latex gloves offers added protection against electrical shock.

Care of Endoscopes

Cleaning a Flexible Endoscope

- All endoscopy equipment should be thoroughly cleaned as soon as possible after the procedure.
- Necessary cleaning supplies include:
  - Examination gloves
  - Cleaning solution
  - Two large basins for cleaning solution and distilled water
  - Distilled water
  - Methyl alcohol
  - Lint-free gauze pads
  - Cotton-tipped applicators
  - Channel-cleaning brush
- Immediately after the procedure, flush water and then air through the air–water channel of the flexible endoscope.
- Gently wipe off the insertion tube with soft gauze or a cloth that has been soaked in an approved detergent solution.

- Place the distal end of the endoscope in detergent–water mixture and suction a small amount through.
  - Alternatively, suction water and then air a few times.
- Remove the air–water valve, suction valve, and biopsy cap and place them in a small amount of cleaning solution to soak.
- Pass the channel-cleaning brush through the biopsy channel and suction the channel repeatedly until the brush comes out clean.
- Clean the brush each time it is passed through the channel.
- If the endoscope has a suction cleaning tube, it should then be placed on the biopsy port.
- Place the end of the suction cleaning tube and the end of the endoscope into a mixture of detergent and water.
- Cover the suction valve hole with your finger and suction soapy water, distilled water, and then air to dry the endoscope.
- Remove the suction cleaning tube and carefully clean the valve holes with a cotton-tipped swab.
- Clean and rinse the air–water valve, suction valve, and biopsy cap and replace them on the endoscope.
- It is a good preventive measure to lubricate the air–water and suction valves lightly periodically to prevent cracking.
- Wipe off the outside of the endoscope with an alcohol-soaked gauze pad.
- Clean the lenses with an approved lens cleaner by applying some lens cleaner onto a soft gauze pad and rubbing the lens; then rub with a clean gauze pad.
- Replace any lens caps, light source insertion bar covers, and venting caps before placing the endoscope back into the cabinet.
- For proper drying of the biopsy channel, leave the biopsy port in an open position.
- Biopsy instruments should be immersed in soapy water, brushed carefully with a cleaning brush, and then rinsed.
- Check to be sure that the jaws of biopsy instruments are not sticking by opening and closing them carefully.

Storing an Endoscope

- The ideal way to store a flexible endoscope is in a hanging position in a well-ventilated cabinet.
  - This allows the endoscope to drain completely after cleaning and permits better air movement through the channels.
- The padded case in which the endoscope was supplied by the manufacturer is another possible storage area; however, little air circulates in these containers and moisture in the channels of the endoscope offers an environment for bacterial growth.
- Rigid endoscopes are best stored in their original carrying case.

Gastrointestinal Endoscopy

Patient Preparation

- For GI endoscopy, the patient should be fasted for 12 to 24 hours.
  - A longer period of fasting may be required in patients with delayed gastric emptying.

- An IV catheter should be placed and fluid administration started.
- Endotracheal intubation and proper endotracheal tube cuff inflation are needed to avoid aspiration of gastric contents in the event of regurgitation.
- For colonoscopy, all feces should be removed from the colon before endoscopic examination; however, this is not always possible.
  - Food should be withheld from the patient for at least 36 hours.
- For rigid colonoscopy, a warm water enema (10 to 20 mL/kg) the evening before the procedure, another enema the following morning, and a final enema 1 hour before the examination usually provide enough cleansing.

COMPUTED TOMOGRAPHY

- Using x-rays and a bank of detectors, a CT scan provides a cross-sectional image of all tissue types of the body region scanned based on the physical density of the tissue compared with water.
- Within the CT scanner, there are an x-ray tube and multiple detectors on a slip ring device that allows the tube to move freely in a circular motion around a patient.
- The patient is stationary on a table that is passed through the rotating x-ray beam.
- The images are then reconstructed into thin slices through the patient, similar to a slice from a loaf of bread.
- The raw data from the image acquisition can be reprocessed using a dedicated computer for soft tissue or edge-enhanced display or reformatted into other imaging planes, such as dorsal and sagittal planes, from the original data that were acquired in a transverse plane.
- CT is frequently used for imaging many disease processes, such as cancer, fractures, lung disease, and vascular anomalies.
- CT also provides invaluable information for surgical and radiation treatment planning.
- Unlike radiography and ultrasound, tomographic imaging frequently requires the patient to be anesthetized.

MAGNETIC RESONANCE IMAGING

- MRI uses a high-strength external magnetic field, a variety of radiofrequency excitation pulses, and the natural resonance (normal circular motion of the atom) of protons (hydrogen ions) in the body to visualize the structure and function of organs.
- MRI is primarily used to examine the internal organs; it is noninvasive and superior to other modalities for imaging soft tissue.
- The primary examinations performed using MRI include imaging of the brain, spinal cord and intervertebral disc areas, tumor localization and extension within soft tissues, tendon and muscle injury, vascular and arterial anomalies or disease, and thoracic and abdominal organs.
- The principles of MRI imaging are complex.
  - Many types of magnets are used, but they can be summarized as being low- and high-field strengths depending on the strength of the magnetic field, which is measured in tesla (T).
  - Low-strength field magnets are 0.3 T or less, and high-strength field magnets are 0.6 T and higher.
  - The patient is placed in this external, strong magnetic field, and the magnetic field is then manipulated by small increments as a specific radiofrequency (RF) is transmitted into the patient to cause certain changes in the orientation and speed with which the protons resonate.
  - All the protons then relax, based on the immediate interactions of the protons and the type of tissue of which the protons are a part.
  - This relaxation produces weak RF signals, which are detected by coils surrounding the area of interest in the patient.
  - These signals are then processed through a computer and converted into images of the patient.
- Depending on the MRI scan performed, contrast medium may or may not be administered. Gadolinium is the most common contrast medium used for enhancement of tissues in MRI. Given IV, it enhances or brightens tissues such as vessels and tumors.
- Serious safety concerns apply when housing and operating an MRI unit.
  - It is prudent to remember that for superconducting magnets of high-field strength, the magnet is always on.
  - No ferromagnetic object can be taken into the room in which the magnet is kept.
  - The magnet will forcibly pull any ferromagnetic objects into the magnet.
  - This could cause serious damage to the MRI machine, patient, or operator who might be within its path.
  - A few examples of ferrous objects include gas anesthesia machines, collars, watches, glasses, hairpins, ink pens, clipboards, IV poles, and cell phones.
  - MRI-compatible gas anesthetic machines and monitoring equipment are available.
  - Certain metallic surgical implants may also be of concern.
  - It is necessary to know the type of implant and manufacturer of the implant to make sure that it contains no ferromagnetic component.
  - Microchips do not seem to cause any issues other than magnetic susceptibility artifacts in the image.
  - Keep a small magnet outside the room and test objects for their magnetism when there is any doubt.
- Although MRI units are uncommon in general veterinary practices, most university veterinary hospitals and referral hospitals have MRI units or access to one for diagnostic imaging.

NUCLEAR MEDICINE

- Nuclear medicine, also called scintigraphy, is an imaging modality that uses radionuclides and a gamma camera to detect the decay of gamma radiation emitted from the radionuclide within the patient.
  - This allows for imaging of anatomic, physiologic, or metabolic processes that occur within the patient.
- The most common radionuclide used for imaging is technetium-99m (^{99m}Tc).
  - ^{99m}Tc has a low-energy gamma ray (140 keV), with a short physical half-life of 6 hours.
  - ^{99m}Tc is typically bound to a specific pharmaceutical that then targets the organ of interest after IV administration.
- The most common nuclear medicine studies performed in veterinary medicine are thyroid scans, bone scans, renal function testing with calculation of the glomerular filtration rate (GFR), and hepatobiliary scans.
- The most common therapeutic nuclear medicine application in veterinary medicine is radioactive iodine (^{131}I). ^{131}I is used for the treatment of hyperthyroidism and thyroid tumors.
- Because of the potential for radioactive contamination, examination gloves and laboratory coats are worn at all times when handling any radionuclide or radioactive patient.
- Special housing considerations are a factor for the radioactive patient after the study because technetium is primarily excreted in the urine and feces.
- Each state or locality has strict release criteria for patients that are imaged with radionuclides.
- Special holding areas are required to isolate the radioactive patient to prevent contamination of other areas of the hospital and personnel.
- Patients treated with ^{131}I require an isolated and well-ventilated area because of the potential for the aerosolization of iodine.
- Radioactive iodine may be excreted in saliva, feces, and urine.
- Because ^{131}I has a longer physical half-life (2.82 days) than ^{99m}Tc (6 hours), patients are required to stay in the isolation area longer than patients undergoing a ^{99m}Tc radiopharmaceutical study.

RECOMMENDED READINGS

Brearley MJ, Cooper JE: *A colour atlas of small animal endoscopy*, St Louis, 1991, Mosby.

Brown M, Brown L: *Lavin's radiography in veterinary technology*, ed 5, St Louis, 2014, Saunders.

Burk RL, Ackerman N: *Small animal radiology and ultrasonography*, ed 3, St Louis, 2003, Saunders.

Curry TS, Dowdey JE, Murry RC: *Christensen's physics of diagnostic radiology*, ed 4, Philadelphia, 1990, Lea & Febiger.

Han CM, Hurd CD: *Practical diagnostic imaging for the veterinary technician*, ed 3, St Louis, 2000, Mosby.

Nyland TG, Mattoon JS: *Small animal diagnostic ultrasound*, ed 2, St Louis, 2003, Saunders.

Sirois M, Anthony E, Mauragis D: *Handbook of radiographic positioning for veterinary technicians*, Clifton Park, NY, 2010, Delmar Cengage.

Sirois, M. Schlote, J. *Diagnostic Imaging for Veterinary Technicians*, Minneapolis, MN. 2016, bluedoor Publishing,

Thrall DE: *Textbook of veterinary diagnostic radiology*, ed 5, St Louis, 2007, Saunders.

Traub-Dargatz JL, Brown CM: *Equine endoscopy*, ed 2, St Louis, 1997, Mosby.

Large Animal Nursing and Husbandry

KEY TERMS

Agammaglobulinemic
Body condition score
Boluses
By-product feeds
Chain twitch

Colostrometer
Commissure
Concentrates
Cross tying
Crutched

Decubital ulcers
Diastema
Drenching
Ensiling
Farrowing

Feed analysis
Feedstuff
Forages
Frick speculum
Gestation

KEY TERMS

Gilts

Hay

Hog snare

Humane twitch

Laminitis

Needle teeth

Nonnutritive feed additives

Orogastric administration

Perivascular

Proximate analysis

Silage

Spoilage

Squeeze chute

Thrush

Wether

Withdrawal time

LEARNING OBJECTIVES

After reviewing this chapter, the reader will be able to:

1. Describe the general husbandry needs of large animals.
2. Describe restraint methods used with large animals.
3. Explain and demonstrate routine procedures used in grooming and foot care.
4. Discuss the techniques used in general nursing care of large animals.
5. Discuss the methods of sample collection for laboratory analysis.
6. Compare and contrast various routes of administration of medication in large animals.
7. Identify and describe various methods of sample collection for laboratory analysis.

INTRODUCTION

- The term large animal is used to describe animals generally found on farms and used for production or recreation.
- This includes the production of meat, wool, eggs, milk, and by-products used in making other products.

LIVESTOCK NUTRITION

- Livestock species (cattle, horses, pigs, sheep, goats) require certain essential nutrients to meet metabolic and physiologic needs.
- As a result of their pregastric fermentation system, nonprotein nitrogen (e.g., urea), in addition to rumen-degradable dietary protein, can be used by the resident microbes as a nitrogen source of synthesis of microbial proteins.
- Microbial protein then passes into the abomasum (true stomach) and is digested like any other dietary protein.
- Dietary fiber is required to maintain adequate gastrointestinal function in herbivores (plant-eating animals) with active microbial fermentation chambers.
  - These include ruminants and hind gut–fermenting animals (horses).
- Gastrointestinal anatomy has a very critical role in the animal's ability to derive essential nutrients from the feedstuffs available.
- The plant material consumed by livestock species contains cellulose, hemicellulose, pectin, and lignin compounds that are indigestible by people and carnivorous predators.
  - Microbes within the gut use these plant compounds, and the animal uses the end products of microbial fermentation.
- Animals have evolved in many ways to take advantage of microbial fermentation in their digestive process.
- The rumen of cattle, sheep, and goats functions as a pregastric fermentation vat (Fig. 10.1). This allows ruminants to efficiently derive nutrients from plant material.

- In hind gut fermenters, such as horses, a greatly enlarged colon serves as a fermentation vat. These animals can also digest plant material, but not to the same extent as ruminants.
- As a result of differences in their anatomy, ruminants digest prefermented feed material, whereas hind gut herbivores ferment predigested feed material.
- Pigs are considered omnivores, which means that they can digest materials of both plant and animal origin, although they are primarily fed less bulky plant materials.
- Pigs have some microbial fermentation capacity in their enlarged, sacculated colon, but not to the extent of hind gut fermenters or ruminants.

Feedstuffs

- A feedstuff is any dietary component that provides some essential nutrient or serves some other function.
- Feedstuff types include forages (roughages), concentrates, by-products, mineral and vitamin supplements, and nonnutritive additives.
- Nonnutritive feedstuffs may provide bulk, flavor, odor, or color or act as an antioxidant to protect other dietary components.
- The variety of feedstuffs available for use in a given geographic area depends on the crops grown locally.
- Potential feedstuffs must be matched with the appropriate livestock species, based on nutrient requirements and gastrointestinal tract capabilities.
- Feedstuffs may be divided into a number of categories, based on their source and nutrient concentration.
- General categories include forages (roughages), concentrates, by-products, mineral and vitamin supplements, and nonnutritive additives.
- Forages are feeds made up of most or all of the plant.
- Forages generally have large amounts of fiber, low energy density, and high bulk (low weight per unit volume).

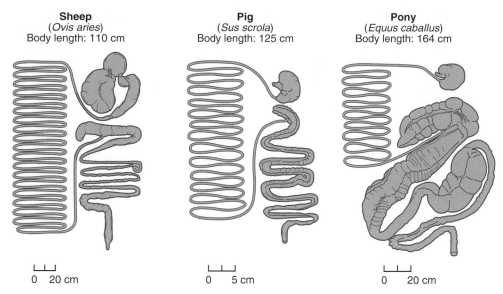

Sheep
(*Ovis aries*)
Body length: 110 cm

Pig
(*Sus scrola*)
Body length: 125 cm

Pony
(*Equus caballus*)
Body length: 164 cm

0 20 cm

0 5 cm

0 20 cm

FIGURE 10.1 Schematic diagrams comparing the gastrointestinal tract of ruminants (sheep), horses, and pigs. (From Sirois M: *Principles and practice of veterinary technology*, ed 3, St Louis, 2011, Mosby.)

- A forager's protein content depends on the type of plant and stage at harvesting.
  - For example, alfalfa hay has much higher protein levels than grass hays at a comparable stage of plant growth.
- Within plant species, there is an increase in fiber content and a decrease in protein content, energy content, and overall digestibility with advancing maturity of the plant.
  - The decrease in digestibility with maturity is because of increasing lignin content of the plant.
  - Lignin is an inert compound that increases rigidity of the plant cell wall.
- Straw represents the most mature and indigestible form of forages.
- Forages fed to livestock belong to either the legume or grass plant families.
- Legumes commonly used for forage production include alfalfa, red and white clover, bird's foot trefoil, and vetch.
  - Grasses offer more variety for forage production and include Bahia grass, Bermuda grass, bluegrass, bromegrass, fescue, timothy, orchard grass, reed canary grass, ryegrass, and Sudan grass.
  - Other grass forages that can be used for cereal grain production include corn, wheat, rye, oats, and sorghum.
  - Of these, corn is the most important forage and cereal grain product grown for livestock.
- Forage products are harvested and stored for livestock feeding purposes in a number of ways.
- Livestock may graze grasses, legumes, and other broadleaf vegetation (forbs and browse).
  - Allowing livestock to harvest forage avoids costs incurred in mechanical harvesting and storage.

- However, forage quality and quantity can be extremely variable, depending on plant maturity and environmental conditions.
- Intensive rotational grazing is a more controlled method.
  - In this method, animals are allowed to graze restricted areas of forage for limited periods and are then moved to another area; the forage in the grazed area is allowed to regrow until the animals are returned for grazing.
  - With highly managed rotational grazing, forage quality can be maintained at a very high level.
- Forage crops can also be mechanically harvested, stored, and fed using various methods.
- Green chop or spoilage represents forage harvested at a given stage of development and fed directly.
  - Green chop contains a high water content (75% to 85%) and available nutrients; however, it must be harvested daily to avoid rapid deterioration with storage.
- Ensiling is a harvesting process by which forage is chopped and placed into a storage unit (e.g., silo) that excludes oxygen.
  - As the forage ferments, lactic acid is produced and the pH decreases.
  - This effectively "pickles" the forage to a partially fermented state called silage.
- Good-quality silage can be stored indefinitely in upright silos, bunker silos, or plastic bags—the important feature being exclusion of oxygen.
- Silage has an intermediate water content (55% to 75%) and has the least loss of nutrients from harvesting and storage.
  - Grass, legume, and corn silages are the most common ensiled forages fed to livestock.

- Hay is forage that is cut and allowed to dry before being collected into bales for storage.
- Hay should have less than 15% water to be stable in storage. Harvesting losses are high in hay making, but storage losses are usually minimal if it is properly dried.
- Concentrates are generally low in fiber and high in energy and/or protein.
- Cereal grains, such as barley, corn, millet, oats, rye, sorghum, and wheat, are the seeds of many of the grass species.
- Cereal grains contain large amounts of energy in the form of starch and are added to diets to increase energy density.
- Other feed products used as energy concentrates include molasses, root crops (e.g., turnips, beets, carrots), and potatoes.
- Fats and oils of plant or animal origin contain 2.25 times the energy density of carbohydrates and are also used as energy concentrates.
- Concentrate feeds that contain more than 20% crude protein are subclassified as protein supplements.
- Protein supplements may be of plant or animal origin, including marine fish.
- Plant-based protein products are derived from oilseed crops such as soybean, canola, cottonseed, sunflower, and peanut seed meals.
  - Of these, soybean meal is by far the most common oilseed meal fed to livestock.
  - Oil from the seeds is harvested for a variety of industrial and nutritional uses; the remaining seed contains more than 40% crude protein.
- Animal-based protein supplements are derived from rendered animal or fish tissues or from dried-milk products.
  - Animal proteins generally range from more than 50% crude protein to 90% crude protein.
  - Compared with plant-based protein sources, animal protein sources have a better amino acid composition relative to requirements.
- By-product feeds are residues of the feed-processing industry and span a wide array of feedstuffs.
  - Examples of by-product feeds include sugar beet pulp, bakery waste, blood, bone meal, brewer's grains, tallow, and whey.
- Many by-product feeds contain substantial amounts of fermentable fiber, energy, and protein.
- Mineral and vitamin supplements are sources of individual minerals or a combination of minerals, with or without vitamins.
- Fat-soluble vitamins are supplemented primarily in the form of premixes.
- Fat-soluble vitamins are sensitive to oxidation, sunlight, heat, and fungal growth.
- Certain water-soluble vitamins may be supplemented in swine and horse diets; they are not routinely supplemented in ruminant diets.

- Yeast cultures are good sources of B complex vitamins and are commonly added to livestock diets.
- Nonnutritive feed additives can include buffers, hormones, binders, and medications.
- Feed medications may include antibiotics, antifungals, anthelmintics, antiparasitics, and ionophores (antibiotics with growth-promoting effects).
  - Their use is regulated by the Food and Drug Administration in an effort to prevent tissue residues.
- Nonnutritive additives are used to stimulate animal performance, improve feed efficiency, and improve animal health or metabolic status.

Feed Analysis

- Different classes of feedstuffs contribute variable amounts of the essential nutrients (Table 10.1).
- Feed analysis is a procedure by which chemical analysis determines the proportion of specific components of a feedstuff.
- The proximate analysis includes determinations of dry matter (DM), crude protein (CP), ether extract (EE, crude fat), crude fiber (CF), and ash.
- The nonfiber carbohydrate portion of the feed is termed nitrogen-free extract (NFE).

FEEDING MANAGEMENT OF LIVESTOCK

- The goal of any livestock feeding management program is to provide sufficient daily amounts of the essential nutrients for optimal (cost-effective) productivity.
- Because feed costs account for the greatest amount of total production costs in the livestock industry, minimizing feed costs helps ensure profitability.
- By-product feeds are widely used when available because they usually are of lower cost.

Dairy Cattle

- Dairy cattle are segregated and housed by production stages and fed according to specific nutrient requirements.
- Typical feeding groups on a dairy farm include milk-fed calves, growing replacement heifers, nonlactating pregnant cows (dry cows), and lactation groups.
- Lactation groups are usually based on level of milk production, parity (first lactation versus older cows), days in milk, or a combination of these factors.
- Feeding systems and housing facilities vary among dairy farms, depending on prevailing environmental conditions.
- Smaller family dairies with fewer than 100 cows generally have individual tie stalls, and cows are fed individually.
- The amounts of forage and concentrates are fed according to production level and body condition score (Table 10.2).
- In larger dairies cows are generally housed in free-stall barns or in open drylots, depending on environmental conditions.

TABLE 10.1 Relative Nutrient Content of Various Feedstuffs for Livestock

| | | | RELATIVE NUTRIENT CONTENT | | | | |
| | | | Minerals | | Vitamins | | Fiber |
Feedstuff Group	Protein	Energy	Macro	Micro	Fat-Sol	B-Complex	
High-quality roughage	+++	++	++	++	+++	+	+++
Low-quality roughage	+	+	+	+	−	−	++++
Cereal grains	++	+++	+	+	+	+	+
Grain mill feeds	++	++	++	++	+	++	++
Fats and oils	−	++++	−	−	−	−	−
Molasses	+	+++	++	++	−	+	−
Fermentation products	+++	++	+	++	−	++++	±
Oil seed proteins	++++	+++	++	++	+	++	+
Animal proteins	++++	+++	+++	+++	++	+++	+

From Sirois M: Principles and practice of veterinary technology, ed 3, St Louis, 2011, Mosby.
+ to ++++: low to very high content.
±: may or may not be present in significant amounts.
−: not present.

TABLE 10.2 Body Condition Scoring Classifications for Livestock

Body Condition Scoring Scale*		Generalized Animal Description†
1.0	1	*Emaciated.* All bones obviously protruding; no subcutaneous fat evident
1.5	2	*Very thin.* Bones visible and easily palpated; minimal subcutaneous fat
2.0	3	*Thin.* Thin, flat musculature; prominent ribs, pelvic bones, and spinal processes
2.5	4	*Moderately thin.* Minimal subcutaneous fat; individual ribs not obvious
3.0	5	*Moderate.* Smooth musculature; bones not visible but palpable
3.5	6	*Moderately fleshy.* Fat palpable; soft fat over ribs and covering pelvis
4.0	7	*Fleshy.* Fat visible; ribs barely visible; spinal processes buried in fat
4.5	8	*Fat.* Thick neck; ribs difficult to palpate; rounded appearance to pelvis
5.0	9	*Grossly obese.* Bulging fat all over; patchy fat pads around tailhead

From Sirois M: Principles and practice of veterinary technology, ed 3, St Louis, 2011, Mosby.
*The body condition scoring scale used depends on the species. Dairy cattle, sheep, pigs, and goats are typically scored on a scale of 1 to 5, whereas beef cattle and horses are scored on a scale of 1 to 9.
†When determining body condition score, evaluate for the presence or absence of fatty tissue over the neck, ribs, spine, and pelvis independent of animal body weight and frame size.

- Drylots are found primarily in the southern and western United States, whereas free-stall barns are found anywhere in the United States.
- In larger dairy management systems, cattle are fed in groups at a common feedbunk, rather than individually.
- Feedbunks may be located within the free-stall facility or along one side of the drylot.
- Although feeding management of dairy cattle depends on the type of facility available, there are some options as to how feed is delivered to the animals.
- Forage (hay, silage) may be fed separately from concentrates in any of the feeding management systems described.
- Concentrates may be fed separately in the milking parlor or from computerized feeders.

- Parlor grain feeding and computerized feeding are becoming more common with current interest in pasture-grazing management systems.
- In large dairies, the most common method of feed delivery is by total mixed ration (TMR).
  - In this system, all individual feed ingredients are mechanically mixed in a feed wagon and presented as a single mixture to the cows.
  - This allows cows to consume the same blend of nutrients in each bite and minimizes selectivity.
- Some dairies feed what might be termed a partial TMR in that dry hay is fed separate from the rest of the diet.

Beef Cattle

- Beef cattle management can be divided into cow–calf and cattle feeding (feedlot) operations. Cow–calf enterprises produce calves that enter the breeding herd or are sent to cattle-feeding operations (feedlots).
- Forage use is the basis of cow–calf enterprises.
- Feed costs account for more than 60% of production costs and therefore must be minimized.
- Cows are allowed to graze pasture or range land, depending on availability, and then are supplemented with energy, protein, and vitamin–mineral supplements as necessary to meet specific nutritional requirements.
- Depending on geographic location and season, pasture grazing may be replaced with feeding of dry hay or silage.
- Supplementation programs depend on prevailing forage quality relative to nutrient requirements of the various production units.
- Cow–calf operations may have feeding groups for bulls, replacement heifers, growing calves, maintenance, and pregnant or lactating cattle.
- Cattle-feeding enterprises involve feeding calves from weaning to slaughter and include backgrounding, stocker, and feedlot systems.
- In backgrounding and stocker feeding systems, weanling calves are placed on low-cost pasture and supplementation feeding programs to gain weight at a moderate rate and then sold to feedlot operations.
- The goal of a feedlot enterprise is to maximize rate of gain and feed conversion efficiency for the lowest cost.
- New arrivals at the feedlot are initially fed a high-forage, low-concentrate diet to acclimate the animal to the operation.
  - The proportion of forage is gradually reduced and concentrate increased to facilitate the desired rate of gain.
- To minimize feeding costs, a wide variety of by-product feeds and grain products is fed.
- To ensure animal health with high-grain feeding, ionophores, buffers, and antimicrobial agents are incorporated into the feedlot diet.
- Generally, the feedlot diet is fed as a TMR similar to the method for dairy cattle.

Nutrition in the Debilitated Calf
Feeding Colostrum

- Because calves are born essentially agammaglobulinemic (without immunoglobulins), provision of colostrum shortly after birth is critically important for the calf to obtain passive maternal antibodies.
- As a general rule, beef calves should be fed all of the dam's first-milking colostrum as soon as they develop a suckle reflex.
- If dairy cow colostrum is used, be sure that the colostrum is of sufficient quality.
- The quality of colostrum is a rough measure of the concentration of immunoglobulin.
  - This is most easily determined by use of a colostrometer, a simple tool that measures the specific gravity of the colostrum.
- Dairy cows produce much more colostrum than beef cows do, but generally the quality and the concentration of immunoglobulin are lower.
- If calves are provided with dairy cow colostrum, it can be administered orally at 10% of body weight over the first 24 hours of life.
- Absorption of maternal colostral immunoglobulin by the calf's intestine usually begins to decrease after the first feeding of colostrum or at about 8 hours of age.
  - Therefore it is important that the first feeding of colostrum is usually of fairly large magnitude.
- If the calf has a vigorous suckle reflex, allow the calf to nurse all of the dam's colostrum that it will consume.
- If more colostrum is available, continue to feed it throughout the first 24 hours, offering it at 2-hour intervals and allowing the calf to suckle.
- If the calf does not have a suckle reflex, continue to offer the colostrum frequently, looking for development of a suckle reflex up to about 6 hours of age.
- If the calf has not developed a suckle response at that time, intubate the calf and give all of the colostrum from a beef heifer or 5% of the calf's body weight in colostrum from a dairy cow.
- For administration of colostrum or milk, allowing the calf to suckle versus intubating is an important question.
- If the calf has already been nursing the dam and is presented for treatment beyond the first several days of age, it is common for the calf to refuse a rubber nipple feeder.
- It may be worthwhile to reintroduce the calf to the dam because it may then suckle the dam quite readily.
- If it is a newborn calf that has not yet suckled the dam, it will usually suckle from a nipple feeder as readily as from the dam's teats.
- Development of a suckle reflex is a very important indicator of the calf's status.
- Calves with a variety of problems, including hypoxemia, hypoglycemia, hypothermia, or acidosis resulting from

dystocia, frequently do not develop the reflex until these problems are corrected.

- Therefore lack of a suckle reflex is a good indicator of one or more of these problems.
- In some cases if these problems are present, the calf may not absorb immunoglobulin, even if colostrum is provided via intubation.

- Development of a suckle reflex usually suggests improvement in an underlying condition.
  - Further, when other problems are present, the calf's gastrointestinal tract may not be fully functional.
  - Therefore repeated intubation of newborn calves or calves of older ages suffering from similar problems may result in large accumulations of fluid in the forestomachs or abomasum.
- If you resort to intubation to supply the calf with oral fluids or milk, carefully monitor the calf for fecal production and palpate its abdomen, looking for evidence that the fluid administered is sequestering in the gastrointestinal tract, rather than proceeding on through and being absorbed.
- If the calf will not suckle and there is evidence that fluid has accumulated in the gastrointestinal tract, continue to offer fluids frequently via nipple feeder but discontinue orogastric intubation.
- Stimulation of the calf to develop a suckle reflex is another important function of the dam.
- Most calves are very responsive to stroking or rubbing along the back, especially near the tailhead.
- If the calf is not suckling well, such rubbing stimulation can often provide very rewarding results.
- If the calf has been sleeping or is compromised by one of the aforementioned problems, it may require several minutes before it begins to suckle.
  - Therefore it is worthwhile to repeatedly introduce the nipple into the calf's mouth and try to deliver a small amount of milk before giving up and assuming the calf does not have a suckle reflex.
- Newborn ruminants, such as calves and lambs, essentially function as monogastric animals while they are nursing.
- Fermentation of the swallowed milk in the rumen and reticulum would likely result in digestive upsets.
- Closure of a structure called the esophageal groove enables the swallowed milk to bypass the rumen and reticulum and pass directly into the omasum and abomasum.
  - Closure of the groove is stimulated by the act of nursing and by the presence of milk.
- When the maturing animal begins eating solid foods, the groove does not close, and the swallowed food enters the rumen and reticulum for microbial fermentation, as in adult animals.

Feeding Milk
- Beyond colostral feeding, provision of milk as nutrition is obviously of critical importance.

- Although dairy calves are often raised with the provision of only 10% of body weight per day as fluid milk, this practice should not be mistakenly construed as providing optimal nutrition.
- The strategy of providing 10% of body weight per day is geared to enhancing intake of solid feeds so that dairy calves can be weaned at an early age.
- Most calves, if given the opportunity, freely consume between 20% and 30% of their body weight in milk per day.
- Although sick calves may not have a very hearty appetite, a recovering calf or premature calf commonly has an exaggerated appetite.
- For these reasons provide a calf with up to 3% of its body weight per feeding and offer milk feedings at approximately 2-hour intervals.
- With this regimen some calves consume more than 30% of their body weight in milk per day.

Feeding Electrolytes
- For calves with fluid loss because of neonatal enteritis, oral electrolyte solutions are commonly offered as a means to provide additional fluid therapy.
- Calves with mild-to-moderate dehydration may respond adequately with only oral fluid supplementation, whereas calves with severe dehydration require intravenous fluid support.
- It has been a common practice to withhold milk from calves with enteritis.
  - You do not have to hold to that practice, but rather offer milk via nipple feeder if the calf will accept it.
- Because milk alone will not provide the electrolytes that have been lost through the gastrointestinal tract, provide oral electrolyte solutions at alternate feedings with the milk.
- The electrolyte fluids and milk or milk replacer should not be mixed because this adversely influences normal milk digestion.
- Offer milk at 2% to 3% of body weight maximum, alternating with oral fluid feedings offered at 5% of body weight per feeding, with the alternate feedings at 2-hour intervals.
- Many calves refuse the milk feedings but eagerly suckle the electrolyte.
  - With this regimen, even when calves do refuse the milk, they can be provided as much as 30% of body weight per day in additional oral electrolyte fluids.

Horses
- Horse feeding management is primarily designed to meet the nutritional requirements of individual horses.
- Although horses are not ruminants, they require a substantial amount of dietary fiber, in the form of forage, to maintain a healthy digestive tract.
- Forages fed to horses are primarily hay and pasture.
- Silage is not commonly fed to horses because of their sensitivity to the molds and mycotoxins potentially found in silage.

- Many varieties of grasses and legumes can be suitable forages for horses.
- The need for energy, protein, and mineral–vitamin supplementation depends on forage quality and nutrient requirements of the horse.
- Corn, barley, and oats are common grain supplements fed to horses for added energy.
- Fat supplementation has been advocated to provide energy for growing, lactating, and working horses.
- Protein sources such as linseed, canola, and soybean meal are commonly used.
- By-products containing fermentable fiber, such as rice bran and beet pulp, are becoming more popular.
- Commercial horse feeds available to horse owners range from complete feeds (no supplementation required) to specific vitamin–mineral supplements.
- Various grain supplements containing energy, protein, minerals, and vitamins are available.
- These commercial grain supplements may be formulated specifically for growing foals, lactating mares, or geriatric horses, or they may be more generic in purpose.
- Horse owners should match the concentrate to their forage relative to energy, protein, mineral, and vitamin requirements.
- A proper horse-feeding program would provide adequate amounts of water and provide sufficient energy to achieve and maintain proper body condition.
- The diet must then be balanced for protein, minerals, and vitamins according to the National Research Council recommendations.
- Appropriate dental care and parasite management programs should accompany all horse-feeding systems.

Feeding and Watering Hospitalized Horses
- Hospitalized horses often have special dietary needs, particularly when their diseases create a catabolic state.
- Horses that can chew and swallow normally should be fed their usual diet if their disease permits.
- Good-quality alfalfa or grass hay, such as timothy hay, can be fed.
  - Good-quality oat hay is also a suitable feed.
- Horses with gastrointestinal disturbances, such as colic or diarrhea, need special consideration.
- Horses recovering from impactions may need more laxative feeds, such as alfalfa hay, grass pasture, and even bran mashes.
- Horses with diarrhea or those that have been operated on for colic may benefit from a diet that is not so rich, such as timothy or oat hay.
- Hay pellets or cubes that contain alfalfa or a mixture of alfalfa and Bermuda or oat hay can also be used.
  - If added carbohydrate is needed, a pelleted feed that also contains grains may be fed.
  - Pelleted feed produces less dust and may be better for horses recovering from respiratory allergies or pneumonia.

- Horses recovering from gastrointestinal ulceration may also need to be fed a pelleted ration because the increased fiber and stem in hay may irritate and exacerbate certain kinds of ulcers.
- Pellets soaked to make gruel can be fed to horses with oral lesions, facial fractures, dental problems, or recurrent episodes of choke.
  - Feed softened in this manner is easier for the animal to chew and swallow.
- Horses with neuromuscular disorders such as botulism may be unable to chew and swallow normally.
- A pelleted ration that has been soaked may be the only feed the animal can eat.
- Fresh water should always be available.
- Some horses may not know how to use an automatic waterer if it requires the horse to push on a lever to fill the water cup.
- Water buckets or tubs should always be provided in these cases.
- Salt may need to be provided topically on the feed or in the form of a salt lick during hot weather or for horses that have diseases that create a sodium deficiency, such as colitis.

Pigs
- Pig feeding management is similar to beef cattle management in that there are breeding-farrowing (reproductive) and growing enterprises.
- Pig diets consist primarily of concentrates, along with energy, protein, mineral, and vitamin supplements.
- The farrowing unit produces baby pigs as reproductive replacements or to enter the growing unit for feeding to slaughter weight.
- The pig industry is one of the most intensively managed agricultural enterprises.
- Current pig production units are moving to total confinement farrow-to-finish operations containing many animals.
  - Within these operations, feeding groups are segregated according to nutrient requirements, with diets for lactating and gestating sows and gilts, boars, nursery pigs, and growing pigs.
- Animals in the farrowing unit are housed and fed as individuals to better control body weight and condition.
- Within the feeding operation, starting with the nursery pigs, all animals are group-housed and fed according to age and moved between groups as an entire unit.
- As omnivores, pigs have a digestive tract that can accommodate a certain level of dietary fiber.
- Given the economics of rate of gain from forages versus grains, pig diets consist primarily of concentrates, along with energy, protein, mineral, and vitamin supplements.
- All feed ingredients are thoroughly mixed and provided as a single diet, like the TMR for cattle.
- Dietary ingredients depend on the nutritional requirements of the specific group of animals being fed.

- The classic pig diet consists of corn grain and soybean meal, with a vitamin–mineral premix.
- Learning more about the specific nutrient requirements of pigs has resulted in more sophisticated diets for them.
- Crystalline amino acids, high-quality animal by-product protein meals, fiber sources, and vitamin–mineral supplements have been incorporated into specific pig diets to improve growth efficiency.

Sheep

- Sheep are managed similarly to beef cattle in that there are reproductive and lamb-growing enterprises.
- Sheep are raised under a wide variety of conditions, ranging from large flocks on western rangelands to small flocks in confinement.
- The basis of any sheep production system is forage.
- A variety of forage types, including harvested and stored forages, can be used for feeding sheep.
- As ruminants, sheep can also use a wide variety of by-product feeds efficiently.
- For the most part, sheep diets consist of vitamin–mineral supplements added to the base forage.
  - The composition of the vitamin–mineral supplement depends on the forage.
- Grazing sheep are provided with minerals as a block (salt lick) or loose from a feeder.
- Additional energy and protein supplementation may be used for late gestation, lactation, and growing diets.
- A wide variety of feed sources may be used, with cost being of primary concern.
  - These supplements may be top-dressed on (spread on top of) the forage or fed by themselves in a feed bunk.
- Commercial concentrate pellets are also available for ewes and growing lamb diets.
- Growing lambs may be sent to slaughter directly from grazing high-quality forage or after feeding in a feedlot.
- Lamb feedlots are similar in organization and feeding practices to beef feedlots.
- Lambs are acclimated from a high-forage to high-concentrate TMR diet to increase grain and feed efficiency.

Goats

- Goats are managed similarly to dairy cattle because of their milk production.
  - However, some breeds of goats are primarily used for mohair (wool) or meat production.
- Forage is the primary component of goat-feeding programs.
- Goats raised for mohair and meat are managed with grazing or browsing rangeland or pasture and appropriate energy and protein supplementation when necessary.
- Dairy goats are managed more intensively because of their higher nutritional requirements for milk production.
- Dairy goats are usually housed in smaller areas and fed stored forages, such as dry hay.

- Pasture grazing alone cannot support milk production, so supplements are necessary.
- The energy and protein feed supplements for goats are similar to those of dairy cattle.
- Many commercial concentrate products used for horses, sheep, and dairy cattle can also be fed to goats.
- The amount and nutrient composition of the supplement depend on the nutrient requirements of the animal being fed and on forage quality.
- Lactating goats require substantial energy supplementation and should be fed the highest-quality forages.
- Supplements may be top-dressed on forage in a feedbunk or provided in the milking parlor.

LIVESTOCK CLINICAL NUTRITION

- A basic understanding of nutrition can be applied to medical management of livestock.
- The most important part of clinical nutrition is obtaining an appropriate nutritional history.
- Questions one should ask in obtaining a nutritional history are outlined in Table 10.3.
- After the history taking, assess the nutritional status of the animal through physical assessment and via blood chemistry determinations.
- Physical assessment of the animal involves obtaining an accurate body weight, height measurement, and body condition score.
- Body height at the shoulders (withers) can be used to assess frame size and growth.
- Body weight and height measurements can be compared with those in standardized growth charts to assess growth performance.
- Body condition scoring is a method of subjectively quantifying subcutaneous body fat reserves.
- Changes in body condition score represent either a positive (increased) or negative (decreased) energy balance.
- A negative energy balance suggests that the diet contains insufficient energy to meet needs and that body fat reserves are being mobilized.
- Beyond this quantitative measure, physical assessment of the animal may include observations of hair coat, hoof quality, hydration status, manure consistency, and attitude.
- Assess these factors and record them in the animal's records daily for hospitalized patients. Indirect measures of nutritional status may be evaluated through metabolite concentrations in blood.

GENERAL CARE OF HORSES (EQUINE)

Bedding

- Horses can be bedded on a variety of materials.
- It is important that the bedding be clean, as dust free as possible, and relatively deep.

TABLE 10.3 Nutritional History in Livestock (Specific Information Depends on the Species of Livestock)

General Categories of Information	Specific Information
Identify the people involved	Names and telephone numbers of the owner, herdsman, veterinarian, nutritionist, others
Owner's primary concern	Pertaining to the presenting problem
Historical information about the agribusiness	Ask questions relating to years of ownership, number of hired hands, new animal purchases, acreage, other farms, etc.
Herd information	Function, breeds, average weights, and age distribution of animals on the farm
Production information	Level of performance (milk production, weaning weights, litter size, etc.) in the herd over time; use production record systems if available
Housing facilities	Type of housing, stall surfaces, and bedding used for each group of animals; adequacy of ventilation
Feeding system	Feed storage facilities, feeding system used, feed and water availability, bunk space per animal, number of times fed per day, etc.
Dietary information	Feed ingredients and their nutrient analyses, specific feeds for each feeding group; obtain feed samples if feed analysis or feed tag information is unavailable
Herd disease information	Disease prevalence for pertinent disease problems, animal culling, and mortality rates over the past month, 6 months, and year
Reproductive information	Measures of fertility, pregnancy losses, etc.
Preventive medicine practices	Vaccinations, treatments, and dewormings administered and when; ask if routine herd health visits are made by the veterinarian

From Sirois M: Principles and practice of veterinary technology, ed 3, St Louis, 2011, Mosby.

- Pine shavings are adequate for most patients, but they tend to be very dusty.
  - This may not be acceptable for horses with open wounds or respiratory disorders.
- Pine shavings with minimal dust or shredded paper bedding are preferable for horses with severe respiratory problems.
- It is best to obtain wood shavings from a known source to prevent accidental exposure to black walnut shavings, which can cause laminitis when the horse stands in the shavings.
  - Black walnut wood is darker than pine but can be difficult to recognize if the bedding is soiled or if multiple types of wood chips have been mixed.
- Straw bedding is often used for mares with newborn foals.
- Regardless of the type of bedding used, it should be kept very clean by removing soiled bedding at least once daily.
- Bedding should always be deep unless the horse has a problem that necessitates a firmer surface for standing.
- The use of rubber stall mats has also reduced the amount of bedding that has to be used.
- Recumbent adult horses must have very deep bedding to help prevent formation of decubital ulcers (pressure sores).
  - Alternatively, large mattresses or specially designed water beds can be used.

- Critically ill foals can be kept on mattresses with waterproof covers and fleece pads to keep them clean and dry.

Fly Control

- The best method of fly control is to maintain a clean barn with frequent manure removal.
- Various topical fly sprays are available.
  - Those containing permethrins, pyrethrins, or citronella sprays are the safest for sick horses.
  - Fly repellents containing organophosphates should not be applied to debilitated horses or foals.
- Overhead fly systems that release fly repellents at regular intervals can also minimize the fly population.
- A soft cloth can be used to apply fly repellent to the horse's face, taking care to apply the repellent around the eyes without getting any into the eyes.
- Fly masks are available for the face and the ears of sensitive patients, and a fly sheet can also be used to cover most of the body, except the distal parts of the legs.

Exercise

- Adult horses and foals should have some form of exercise daily unless their medical problem requires stall rest.
- Walking on soft dirt or grass surfaces is preferable to walking on concrete or asphalt.

- Foals may be allowed to run freely alongside the mare if they do not have a condition that warrants more restricted activity and if the area is properly fenced with no hazards, such as drains or moving vehicles.
- If the foal's activity must be controlled, the foal can be walked using a halter and a rope around the foal's hindquarters in the area of the semimembranosus and semitendinosus muscles. Good judgment and caution are needed to prevent the foal from rearing and flipping over backward.
- Neonates whose exercise must be limited can be walked by placing one arm in front of the foal's chest and one arm behind the foal to cradle it while walking.
- Alternatively, an adult horse halter can be used over the foal's body like a harness, with the nose piece around the foal's neck, the buckle strapped around the ventral thorax, and the rope clip located on the caudodorsal portion of the foal's back.
- The hind end of the foal may still need to be supported.

Grooming

- Equine patients should be groomed daily, unless the horse has a condition whereby vigorous grooming would be painful or damaging (e.g., severe skin infections, cutaneous burns).
- A rubber curry comb should be used in a circular motion to remove dried sweat or mud.
- Next, a stiff-bristled brush can be used to remove dirt and loose hair.
- If stiff brushes and rubber curry combs are used on the horse's face and distal limbs, they should be used gently because overly vigorous grooming may be uncomfortable for the animal. Metal curry combs should not be used on the horse's head or distal limbs.
- A soft brush can be used to finish removing loose hair and dirt.
- If needed, a damp or dry cloth can be used to remove the remaining dust from the horse's coat.
- A stiff brush, hair brush, or metal mane comb should be used on the tail and mane.

Hoof Picking

- A horse's hooves should be picked clean daily.
- Balance the hoof on your knee, hold the hoof with your left hand and the hoof pick with your right hand.
- The hoof is then cleaned with a hoof pick by removing debris from the lateral and central sulci, starting at the heel and working toward the toe, and then from the rest of the hoof (Fig. 10.2).
- A degenerative condition called **thrush** is common in feet that are infrequently cleaned or if the horse stands for long periods in damp bedding or muddy soil.

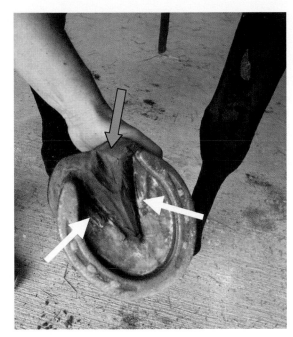

FIGURE 10.2 Central sulcus *(green arrow)* and lateral sulci *(white arrows)* of the frog. (From Sirois M: *Principles and practice of veterinary technology,* ed 3, St Louis, 2011, Mosby.)

- Thrush may occur secondary to a bacterial infection and appears as black, malodorous material in the region of the frog.
  - A 10% sodium hypochlorite (bleach) solution or 2% iodine solution can be applied to the lateral and central sulci to dry the foot and kill the bacteria.
  - Commercial formulations containing formaldehyde or copper sulfate can also be used.
- Care must always be used to avoid spilling caustic solutions on the coronary band or other parts of the horse's leg.
- Some animals with severe thrush require foot trimming to remove diseased hoof tissue and wraps to help keep the foot clean and dry during the length of the treatment program.

CARE OF CATTLE (BOVINE)

- The cattle industry can be divided into two distinctly different areas, each with its own set of production goals and management techniques.
- The beef industry uses heavily muscled breeds of cattle that are capable of efficient conversion of hay and grain into skeletal muscle mass for maximum meat production.
  - Common breeds of beef cattle include the Angus, Texas Longhorn, Brahman, and Hereford.
- The dairy industry uses other breeds of cattle that are more efficient in converting cattle food into the production of large volumes of saleable milk as the main production goal.
  - Dairy cattle breeds include Guernsey, Jersey, and Holstein.

- Labor expenses in the beef industry are mainly centered on processing and moving the cattle, with additional demands around calving time.
- The labor involved with milking cows in the dairy industry is essentially an all-day, 365-days-a-year event.
- Breeding in the beef industry still occurs by allowing bulls (intact males) to roam the pastures with cows (adult females) seeking those who are "in heat" (estrus); however, many operations are now using artificial insemination (AI) with frozen bull semen as a common method of breeding.
  - The dairy industry uses AI almost exclusively as the preferred method of breeding.
- The gestation period (pregnancy length) for cattle is about 9 months.
- The female calf is called a heifer (until she has had a calf), and the male calf is called a bull calf until he is castrated (at which time he is called a steer).
- All cattle require various vaccinations and/or blood tests before being sold or transported between states.
- Some of the vaccinations and tests must be done by an accredited veterinarian on behalf of state or federal regulatory departments that require the procedure.
  - Private practice veterinarians can become accredited by learning the required laws and rules and by passing a test to demonstrate that knowledge.
- Veterinary personnel who deliver or prescribe any medications to any food-producing animal must inform the farm manager about the proper withdrawal time for that medication.
  - The withdrawal time refers to the minimum length of time that must pass from the last administration of the medicine until the time that the animal is slaughtered for food or the milk is collected for human consumption.

CARE OF SHEEP (OVINE)

- Sheep are raised for meat and wool.
- Particular breeds are selected to do one or the other specifically.
  - All sheep have wool of some type; it just may not be very much or of as good quality as from sheep raised specifically for wool.
- Some husbandry terms related to the sheep industry include the following:
  - The ewe (adult female) gives birth to one to three lambs (lambing) that are called ram lambs (male) or ewe lambs (female).
  - The gestation for sheep is about 5 months, and breeding usually occurs in the fall of the year resulting in spring lambs.
  - The buck or ram is the name of an intact adult male, and a castrated male is called a wether.

CARE OF GOATS (CAPRINE)

- Goats are rising in popularity as an alternative farming enterprise and as pets.
  - They are also used in many teaching and research institutions as models for animal or human diseases.
- The adult female (doe) gives birth to kids (kidding) after a 5-month gestation.
- An intact adult male is called a billy or ram, and castrated males are called wethers.
- The kids are castrated at a young age with an elastrator.
- The billy goats have a strong, musky smell that is attractive to the females; however, it permeates through the entire farm as well.
- Although there is some demand for goat meat, the major use of goats today is milk production for milk or cheese.
- Goat fiber (mohair) is also marketed in the United States.

CARE OF SWINE (PORCINE)

- The present trend in swine production is the use of confinement rearing facilities.
- Confinement housing facilities allow producers to raise more pigs per farm and to market pigs in 5 to 6 months.
- The increase in pig density raises concerns in regard to prevention of disease.
- If a disease occurs, the entire herd can be affected, and the economic loss can be devastating.
- Pigs become unhealthy because of disease transmission from adjacent pigs or infections from outside sources (e.g., trucking, feed personnel, wind, other species of animals).
  - Therefore it is imperative when visiting a confinement swine unit that you follow their rules for dress and foot coverings.
- Disease is best prevented by ensuring good health status, nutrition, housing, management, and husbandry.
- The adult female (sow) gives birth to piglets (an act called farrowing) after a gestation of 3 months, 3 weeks, and 3 days (about 114 days).
- The intact adult male is a boar, and the castrated male is called a barrow. Young females are called gilts until they farrow.
- Sows enter the farrowing room a few days before expected parturition.
- The use of traditional farrowing crates limits the movement of the sows and provides an area for the piglets to avoid being laid on and stay warm and dry.
- Litter sizes range from 7 to 12, and the average birth weight is approximately 1.5 kg.
- Hypothermia is a problem in newborn piglets.
- The piglet's body temperature at birth is 102.2° F (39° C) but decreases to 98.6° F (37° C) within a few hours.
- Over the next 24 hours the piglet's body temperature returns to 102.2° F (39° C).
- An environmental temperature of 86° F to 95° F (30° to 35° C) should be maintained with heat lamps and heat mats during this time of relative hypothermia.

- Be aware that some postfarrowing sows can become very aggressive toward handlers when you are handling their newborn piglets.

CARE OF POULTRY

- Terms used to describe the anatomy of poultry as well as gender, age, and production status are in Fig. 10.3 and Box 10.1.
- The poultry industry is very diverse and can range from backyard flocks to extensive commercial operations.
- The term poultry refers to chickens, turkeys, ducks, and geese.
- There are five general segments of the poultry industry: foundation breeders, hatcheries, grow-out operations, egg production, and broiler production.
- Foundation breeders or breeding flocks are producers of parent flocks that produce eggs sold to hatcheries.
- Foundation breeders place much emphasis on fertility and rate of lay.
- Hatcheries hatch the eggs and sell the chicks as replacements for the egg production and broiler systems.
- Grow-out operations raise chicks for sale into the egg and broiler industries.
- Those producers who raise just for the egg industry are often called pullet replacement farms.
- These producers raise day-old chicks from the hatcheries until they are approximately 6 to 8 weeks old, and they are then sold into the appropriate production system.
- Some pullet farms will raise them until they are 16 to 20 weeks of age and ready to start laying eggs.
  - These facilities are equipped with brooder facilities to raise the day-old chicks which require more care.

Box 10.1 Terminology	
Hen	Female of all classes of poultry.
Pullet	Female chicken that has not yet started to lay eggs.
Layer	Hens or pullets producing eggs.
Spent Hen	A breeder or commercial-type egg hen that no longer performs at desired production levels.
Cock	A sexually mature intact male before 6 months of age.
Rooster	A male chicken usually kept for breeding.
Stag	Male chicken under 10 months of age that shows developing sex characteristics between that of a roaster and a rooster.
Broiler/ Fryer	Young chickens less than 12 weeks of age. Ready to eat at 6 lb. They are raised for meat.
Roaster	Heavy young chickens less than 12 weeks of age with live weights heavier than 7 pounds. Raised for meat.
Capon	A neutered male chicken produced for the specialty and holiday meat markets. Less than 8 months old.

From Holtgrew-Bohling KJ: Large animal clinical procedures for veterinary technicians, ed 3, St Louis, 2016, Mosby.

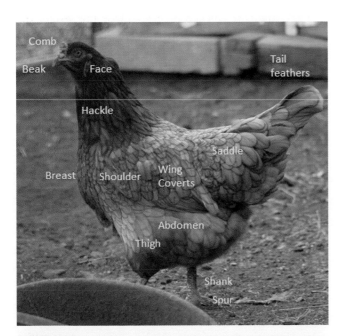

FIGURE 10.3 Anatomic locations (From Holtgrew-Bohling KJ: *Large animal clinical procedures for veterinary technicians*, ed 3, St Louis, 2016, Mosby.)

- Egg production consists of laying hens kept to produce eggs.
  - After hens have outlived their egg-laying potential, they are often marketed for meat.
  - Most laying hens are replaced after 12 to 15 months of laying.
- Broiler production systems involve the raising of poultry for meat purposes.
- The specific housing requirements for poultry vary depending on the ultimate goal of production.
- Laying housing usually consists of either an open floor system or caging system.
- Open floor systems allow the birds to wander throughout a building with several nests for egg laying.
  - If floor systems are utilized, eggs must be collected three times a day to keep the eggs at the appropriate temperature.
- Caging systems can be single, multiple, and colony-type caging.
  - Multiple caging systems often have 2 to 10 birds per cage, and colony caging systems often house 11 to 40 birds per cage.
- When cages are used, several different types of arrangements can be utilized to help maximize

light exposure, ease of egg collection, and manure removal.
- Cage laying systems often utilize automated egg collection equipment.
- Lighting is extremely important in laying houses.
  - Artificial lighting is most often utilized in windowless buildings to allow more control over the lights.
  - Dimmers are utilized to avoid abrupt changes from light to dark.
- Overheating is also a major concern in laying housing.
  - Birds are most comfortable between 45° F and 70° F (7.2° C and 21.1° C).
  - If birds get too hot, they pant because they do not have sweat glands.
  - Panting results in alkaline blood, which decreases the amount of calcium available for egg production, which results in thin-shelled eggs.
  - Systems to help keep them cool include foggers, fans, and evaporative cooling pads.

Identification

- In commercial poultry operations, the birds are often not individually identified, but identified as a group.
- In small backyard flocks or some breeding facilities, individual identification may be necessary.
- Common methods of individual identification include toe punching, wing banding, and leg banding.
- The toe punch is applied at hatching and creates a small hole in the web of the foot.
  - Caution should be used when using hole punches in ducks, as the web may grow back together.
- Wing bands are colored or plain metal and can have numbers engraved on them.
  - The band is placed by piercing the wing web of the day-old chick.
  - Caution should be taken with wing bands because occasionally they can move around the tip of the wing before the wings are fully grown, which will restrict normal growth.
- Colored, plastic, and metal leg bands are available for bird identification and are often numbered to allow for identification.
- The three types of leg bands are open, closed, and spiral.
- Closed bands are found on birds that have been banded as babies.
- Closed bands are circular and seamless; made of stainless steel, aluminum, or plastic; and come in a variety of colors and sizes.
- Application of a closed band occurs at about 2 to 3 weeks of age.
  - The band is slid over the foot to the leg portion.
  - As the bird grows, the feet become too large for the band to fall off.
- Open bands can be applied at any time. An open band is a piece of metal that has been bent into the form of a circle.

- The ends of the band do not meet and are separated by a space to enable them to be placed on a mature bird's leg.
  - After placement, the ends are then pinched together until they meet.
- Open bands are used on older birds whose feet are too large for banding with a closed band.
- Spiral leg bands work similar to a key ring.
- The bands are often larger than the chicken's leg to allow for growth and are applied just like you would put a key on a key ring.
- Caution should be taken when using leg bands—if applied when the bird is young and still growing, the band can get embedded into the leg.

Chicken Breeds

- Most commercial chicken producers have taken the standard breeds and produced hybrids specific to their operations.
- Poultry can be classified by breed, variety, type, and class.
- Breed means that they will breed true to a number of given traits that identify the breed.
- Varieties are then within breeds that can define the color of plumage and comb type.
  - They can be further defined by type as to whether they are egg producing, meat producing, or dual purpose.
- Classes generally refer to the geographic origin.
  - In general there are four classes: Mediterranean, American, English, and Asiatic.
- The American Poultry association publishes The American Standard of Perfection, which is a list describing more than 300 breeds of poultry.
- Egg-producing chicken breeds include the White Leghorn, Rhode Island Red, and Barred Plymouth Rocks.
- Meat-producing breeds include the Cornish White, New Hampshire, and White Plymouth Rock.
- Hundreds of different breeds and varieties are found in backyard flocks, such as the Brahma, Silkie, Wyandotte, Favorelle, and Ameraucana.

HORSE HANDLING AND RESTRAINT

- The size, speed, strength, and personality of horses make them potentially dangerous animals to restrain.
- Horses are suspicious creatures and are quick to detect nervousness in handlers.
- Most horses are not vicious, and most submit to properly applied restraint procedures.
- Many horses are companion animals, so it is important to always talk to them in a calm, low voice.
  - This helps keep them calm and lets them know where you are.
  - However, even cooperative horses can cause fatal injures if they are suddenly frightened or hurt.

- Because they are herd animals, horses find comfort in being with other horses and will react if other horses around them spook or get startled.
- Horses are also prey animals that have evolved a great sense of flight or fight.
  - If frightened or threatened, a horse's natural instinct is to run away.
  - If a horse cannot get away, it will fight to get away. This often causes injury to the handler or the horse.
- Horses have keen eyesight for seeing movement at great distances, but they do not see well up close, nor do they see just below their noses or directly behind themselves.
  - Never walk directly behind a horse unless you stay close and talk to the horse so that it knows you are there.
  - Never walk under a horse's neck. The horse cannot see you there and may throw its head, raise a front leg and knock you down, or rear up and come down on you.
  - Horses will run over the top of you if you are between them and freedom or if they perceive you have cornered them.
- Horses will kick as a means of protection.
  - They can kick with either back hoof directly behind themselves as well as out to the sides.
  - They can kick with both back legs at once by rocking their weight to their front legs.
  - They can strike with one front leg at a time or rock all their weight onto their back legs and rear up and strike with both front legs.
- Horses toss their heads, which can cause serious injury if you are not cautious.
- Never stand directly in front of a horse; it may strike you with its front leg or its head.
- Horses also bite; they have both upper and lower incisors that pinch, and they can lock their jaws together making it very difficult to get your body part out from between the jaws.
  - Horses use biting as a means of communication.
  - Horses use nips and outright bites to teach youngsters their place in the herd.
  - However, a horse that bites people should be disciplined quickly and without hesitation.
- Horses have elaborate body language that is learned from birth through adulthood.
- This body language can tell you if the horse is paying attention and if it is upset, angry, or in pain.
- The most expressive parts of the horse are the ears.
  - An alert horse has its ears pricked forward.
    - This shows it is aware of your approach and is curious.
  - A nervous or uncertain horse constantly flicks its ears back and forth, especially if there is activity behind it.
  - An angry or fearful horse often pins its ears back.

- Do not confuse this sign with the laid-back ears of a horse that is concentrating on a difficult task, such as calf roping or barrel racing.
- The tail also indicates a horse's attitude.
  - A wringing or circling tail indicates nervousness.
  - A tail held straight down indicates pain or sleeping.
  - A tail that is clamped tight indicates fear.
- The mouth and tongue can also indicate what the horse is thinking or how it is feeling.
- Yawning or grimacing may indicate pain.
- When asking a horse to do something new to the horse, you know the horse understands the new task when it smacks its lips or its tongue licks in and out.
  - Trainers often use this behavior as a guide to determine when the horse understands what the trainer has asked it to do.
- The horse's eyes can also tell you what it is feeling.
  - If you can see the whites all around its eyes with its head held up and its ears working furiously, the horse is probably very frightened.
  - If the horse's eyelids are droopy or half-closed, the horse may be in pain or exhausted.
- Horses can be calmed by an even tone of voice, and most cooperate if handled quietly and decisively.
- Many horses are easily bribed with lumps of sugar, horse biscuits, or grain.
- Scratching behind its ears, across its eye ridges, and along its neck also helps convince a horse that you mean it no harm and want to be friends.
- When properly restrained, you can give a horse injections, draw blood, auscultate its lungs and heart, take its temperature, administer oral medications, or perform other examinations safely and efficiently.
- If you are consistent and firm but not brutal, the horse will respond to you and try to do what you ask.

Approaching and Capturing a Horse

- Horses should be approached from the front and slightly to the near (left) side.
- The reason for approaching from the near side is that horses are accustomed to being handled from that side; they are trained to be saddled and mounted from the near side.
- The animal may become nervous if you approach or work on the far (right) side.
- You also need to stay within the horse's range of vision.
- Each eye is placed on the very edge of its head, allowing the horse to see straight forward and around to its hindquarter almost in a perfect half-circle.
- A horse does not see directly in front of it where it would have to cross or directly behind its hindquarters.
- As you approach the horse, determine the animal's behavior by looking at its body language and the positions of the ears, tail, and legs.
- Move slowly and without sudden movements because horses are easily startled.

- Once close enough to touch the animal, it is often best to scratch it behind the ears and on the side of the neck before applying a halter.
- After this introduction, slip the lead rope over the horse's neck and catch the end as it comes into your reach; tie a single overhand knot to keep the rope from slipping off.
- Most horses believe they are caught and stand peacefully, but be alert for the possibility that something may frighten the horse, causing it to bolt.
- If the horse panics and begins resisting restraint, it is better to let it go than to be injured trying to restrain it.
- Some horses quickly learn that a rope or halter slung over a human's shoulder means they must go to work, and these horses will not allow you to catch them.
  - For these horses, it is best to keep the ropes hidden from view until you are up close.
- Baling twine or a small rope works well with these horses because it is more easily concealed and need not be very strong; once the horse is caught, it usually submits quietly.
- More nervous horses must be enclosed in a smaller pen to catch them.
  - Luring them into the pen with grain is much better than chasing them in because they are then less agitated.
- The halter and lead rope are the main tools of equine restraint and should always be used when leading or working on a horse.
- Check the halter and lead rope for splits or fraying because a horse can easily break a defective lead rope or halter with a sharp jerk of its head.
- Check to make sure the halter is settled correctly on the horse's face.
  - There should be no pressure points from rings or rivets, and the straps should not be close to or over the horse's eyes.
- If you must approach a horse from the rear, as in a box stall or if the animal is tied, always let the horse know you are approaching.
  - Begin to talk quietly to the horse before you get close.
  - Remember that a horse's kicking range is 6 to 8 feet straight back, and these kicks are usually very accurate.
  - It is safest to pass behind the horse about 10 to 12 feet or more or to stay in direct physical contact by keeping your hand on the horse's rump when passing around the rear.
  - Talk to the horse before and as you approach it, so you do not surprise or startle it.

Leading a Horse

- Once you have haltered the horse, grasp the lead rope where it connects to the halter with your right hand and use your left hand to hold the loose end of the rope in neat loops, with the entire rope held in front of you.

- Never wrap the loose end of the lead rope around your hand or have the rope running behind you.
  - If the horse bolts, you will be pulled along with it and could be seriously injured.
- Always walk on the near side of the horse, close to the shoulder, and hold the lead rope with your right hand about 1 foot away from the base of the halter.
- After you stop leading a horse, stand as close to its shoulder as possible and face the same direction as the horse.
  - Be careful not to stand too far in front of the horse, as it can rear up and strike with its front foot.
  - Also, do not stand too near or the horse can accidentally step on the back of your heels as you are walking.
  - Never move under a horse's neck to get to the other side.

Tying a Horse

- If a horse is to be left unattended, it should always be tied to a sturdy object with a properly fitting halter and suitable lead rope.
- The knot used to tie the lead rope should be a quick-release knot, such as the halter tie.
  - The quick-release knot allows the horse to be released quickly if it panics, catches its foot, or falls down.
- The horse should be allowed about 2 to 3 feet of lead rope so it can adjust the angle of its neck and shift position as it desires.
  - Allowing more slack than that may cause the horse to tangle its front feet in the rope.
  - Any less slack may frustrate the horse enough for it to try to escape.
- Do not tie a horse's head too high or too low so it is at an unnatural angle.

Cross Tying

- Cross tying is another way to secure a horse's head and to keep it from rearing (Fig. 10.4).
- To cross tie, clip one lead rope to the lateral cheek rings on the left side of the horse's halter and tie the left lead, using the halter tie.
- Then walk safely around to the horse's right side and affix the second lead to the lateral cheek ring and tie the horse, again using the halter tie.

Restraint of the Head

- For almost every veterinary procedure done on a horse, the head must be restrained.
- The standard equipment for head restraint is the halter and lead rope.
- Always stand on the same side of the horse as the person who is working on the animal.
  - If the horse tries to escape, it usually will move away from you.

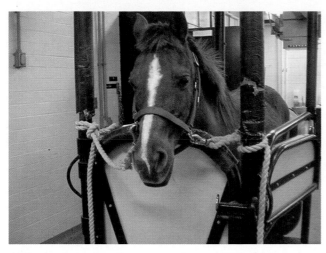

FIGURE 10.4 To cross tie, clip one lead rope to the lateral cheek rings on the left side of the horse's halter. Tie the left lead, using the halter tie. (From Sheldon CC, Topel J, Sonsthagen BS: *Animal restraint for veterinary professionals*, St Louis, 2006, Mosby.)

- If there are people on both sides of it, the animal will pick the smaller of the barriers and move over that, possibly resulting in injury to a person bending or kneeling down.
- You will also have to pay attention to the horse, as well as what is going on with the procedure.
  - Too often handlers become so wrapped up in what is going on with the procedure that they miss the signs of the horse getting restless or agitated.
- Keep the horse's head down so that its eye is looking into your eye.
  - If the horse raises its head up above your shoulders, you will not be able to keep it from moving either up or away.
  - To keep the horse's head down, place one hand over the poll, applying a gentle pressure, and pull down on the lead rope.
- Never stand directly in front of a horse; always stand to the side of the horse, and be prepared for a sudden reaction.

Distraction Techniques

Rocking an Ear
- Stand on the left side of the horse and hold the halter with your left hand over the lateral ring.
- With your right hand grasp the horse's ear at the base and gently rock it or bend it back and forth.
- Do not do this too vigorously because you can damage the cartilage and cause the horse's ear to droop.

Skin Roll
- Grasp as much skin on the shoulder as you can get with one or both hands.
- Rocking it back and forth or jiggling it provides enough distraction to allow you or another person to accomplish intravenous (IV) and intramuscular (IM) injections.

Hand Twitch
- Stand on the left side of the horse and hold its halter in your right hand so that you have good head control.
- Grasp the upper lip with your left hand and rock the lip back and forth.
- Be careful not to close off the horse's nostrils.

Blindfolds
- If a horse is afraid to enter a trailer, stock rack, or box stall or is simply obstinate, using a towel as a blindfold may help.
- The blindfolded horse usually calms down and then depends on you to guide it.
- Work slowly and talk constantly to reassure the blindfolded horse.

Leg Lift
- The last technique is quite useful when trying to take a radiograph of a leg.
- If the horse moves or is unwilling to stand still, lift and hold the leg opposite of the one being radiographed.
- This will often make the horse stand still.

Twitches
- Common types of twitches used on horses are the chain, humane (or clamp), and rope twitches.
- Twitches should be used only if you know how to apply them and often as a last resort.
- Twitches work only for a short time before the muzzle loses feeling, so the greatest effect is when it is first applied.
- To maximize the twitch's usefulness, tightening and loosening the loop around the muzzle keeps the circulation flowing and keeps the horse's attention on the twitch longer.
- Be aware that many horses try to get away or resist the twitch when it is first applied; stay with them by moving with their motions.
- If a horse continues to struggle or escalates the struggle, try another distraction technique.
- After the twitch is removed, massage the muzzle to restore circulation.
- The twitch can be applied to the lower lip of a horse as well, but this method should be used only if the horse raises strong objections to using the upper lip.
- Always curl the lip inward to protect the inner surface.
- The **chain twitch** is a flat chain loop attached to the end of a stout wooden handle to form a loop.
  - An advantage of a chain twitch is that it slips off easily when the chain is loosened.
  - The length of the handle is usually long enough for the restrainer to stand back beside the horse and hang onto the halter as well.
  - The chain can be loosened and tightened or gently wiggled for added distraction.

- If steady pressure is constantly applied, the muzzle loses circulation and becomes numb, rendering the twitch ineffective.
- A disadvantage is that sometimes the horse learns to wiggle its upper lip to dislodge the twitch.
- Another disadvantage occurs if the horse pulls the handle out of the handler's hands.
- The free handle can then become a dangerous weapon if the horse throws its head.
- The humane twitch is a metal clamplike device that pinches the upper lip between two bars.
  - The twitch usually has a length of cord with a clasp attached to it that can be wrapped around the end of the twitch and then attached to the halter.
  - Regardless of its name, this twitch is not any more humane or inhumane than the chain or rope twitch.
  - The primary disadvantage of this twitch is that it applies steady pressure that can cause the lip to lose feeling and the twitch to lose its effectiveness.
  - Also, the twitch can be dislodged and become a hazardous flying object if it is attached to the halter.
  - It is not recommended that the twitch be clipped to the halter.
  - Do not twist the muzzle while it is in the twitch because this causes more pain than is necessary.
  - Simply squeeze or jiggle the muzzle to achieve the desired effect.
  - The humane twitch will lose its effectiveness in 10 minutes because the muzzle will lose circulation and go numb.
- A rope twitch is made from small-diameter cord attached to a stout handle or ring.
  - It is applied to the horse's muzzle in the same manner as the chain twitch.
  - The advantage of a rope twitch is that it is relatively inexpensive and easily made.
  - Also, the loop tends to stay on the horse's muzzle better than a chain.
  - The disadvantage of the rope muzzle is that it tends to pinch the horse's muzzle more than the chain, often causing unnecessary pain.

Chain Shank

- The chain shank (also stud shank) is a long leather or nylon strap with about 2 feet of flat chain at its end, attached to a snap.
- It can be used as another distraction device or on horses that need more restraint than just a halter, such as many stallions.

Stocks

- Stocks are narrow enclosures with removable or semi-open sides and a gate at both ends.
- Stocks can be made of steel pipes or wooden planks, with the top bar or plank no higher than the horse's shoulder.
- The front of the stocks should have the necessary hooks for cross tying so the horse cannot jump forward or to the side if it tries to escape.
- A gate is included at both ends because horses do not like narrow, confined areas.
- The opened front gate gives the appearance of an escape route as the horse is walked into the stocks.

Tail Tying

- Much of a horse's weight can be raised or moved by its tail, which is quite strong.
- This makes the tail a handy object to use when you need to move an anesthetized horse.
- However, the tail can also be a nuisance that must be tied out of the way for certain procedures.
- Remember to always tie the tail to the animal's own body because severe injury may result if the tail is tied to an immovable object and the horse suddenly bolts.

Hobbles

- Breeding hobbles are used to prevent obstinate mares from kicking the stallion when mounting.
- These hobbles can also be used for rectal or vaginal palpation if stocks are unavailable. Start with a long rope with a bowline on a bight tied in the center.

RESTRAINT OF FOALS

- The easiest way to catch a foal is to back the mare into the corner of a large box stall and secure her in place.
- The foal naturally tries to hide behind the mare's flank.
  - When it begins to move, grasp the foal around the front of its chest with one arm and quickly around the rump, or grasp its tail with your other hand.
  - Once you have stopped the foal's forward motion, it will typically try to escape by moving backward.
  - After you have caught the foal, press it up against the wall or a sturdy partition or have another person hold the foal in the same manner on the opposite side.
  - Do not hold onto the foal's tail too tightly or press it down between the legs because this sometimes makes the foal sit down.
  - Never lift a foal off its feet; this makes foals very nervous, and they struggle fiercely to regain their feet.
  - Always talk to and comfort a foal when handling it.
  - Rough handling leads to behavior problems later in life.
- Never remove a foal from the sight of the mare.
  - Both mare and foal will fret until they are reunited, and both may injure themselves trying to get back together.

CATTLE RESTRAINT

- Dairy cattle are usually used to human handling and can be vaccinated or medicated while haltered and in a stanchion or head gate.

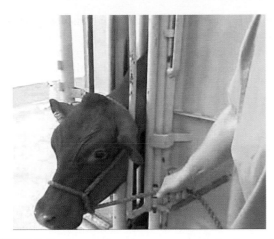

FIGURE 10.5 Cattle restrained in a squeeze chute. A rope halter has also been placed to allow further control of the head. (From Sheldon CC, Topel J, Sonsthagen BS: *Animal restraint for veterinary professionals*, St Louis, 2006, Mosby.)

- Beef cattle are not used to being handled and so should be placed in a chute and haltered for most procedures (Fig. 10.5).
- Vaccinations or medications can be given IM or subcutaneously (SQ) to cattle that are in an alley, as long as they are crowded in fairly tightly so they can't move forward or backward.
- Serious injuries can occur by being kicked.
- While working on the back end, place a bar or bale of hay behind their rear legs.
- Dairy cattle will tolerate antikicking chains being placed just above the hocks, or you can tie a foot up with a long rope.

Mechanical Devices
Squeeze Chute
- The **squeeze chute** is a restraint device used almost exclusively on beef cattle.

- A chute usually has three mechanical working parts: the head gate, tailgate, and squeeze.
- An animal is run into a chute by means of an alleyway.
- Cows will usually settle if they feel they are confined in this way.
- The head gate is closed tight enough so that the animal cannot put a foot through, but not so tight as to clamp the cow's neck to occlude the airway.
- Side panels can be opened to allow access to the cow's side or feet. The tailgate acts as a barrier between you and the cow's rear legs.
  - This allows access to the perineal area for pregnancy checking, tail bleeding, or assistance during calf delivery.
- The head gate allows you to approach the cow to place a halter or administer oral medications.
- Be aware that a cow can still stretch its neck quite a way out and can move it from side to side.
  - The danger is being butted with the head, which is usually not fatal, unless there is direct contact to your head.

Halter
- The halter used on cattle is usually a rope halter that can be adjusted to fit any sized cow or bull.
- The part of the halter that tightens when the lead is pulled goes around the nose and the lead comes off the left side of the cow's head.
- Before applying the halter, be sure the head stall is large enough to go behind the ears but not so large that you have to make major adjustments while standing close to the cow's head.
- Most people slip the nose band on first, then the headstall behind the ears (Fig. 10.6).
- Pulling the lead will cause the halter to tighten up, and the cow's head can be tied to the side of the chute.

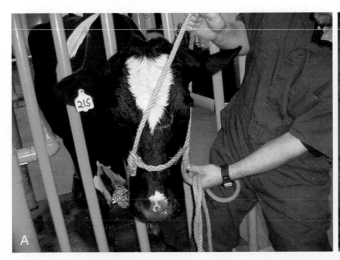
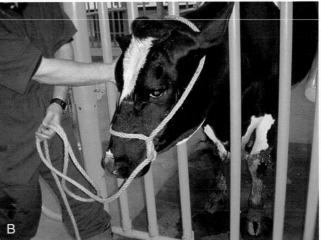

FIGURE 10.6 (A) Placing a halter on a cow. (B) Halter in position on a cow. (From Sirois M: *Principles and practice of veterinary technology*, ed 3, St Louis, 2011, Mosby.)

- Halter and tying the head to the chute allows jugular venipuncture or injections, ear tag placement, and ophthalmic procedures to be performed.

Stanchions
- A stanchion usually consists of a head gate without sidebars to restrict lateral movement.
- Dairy cattle are often placed in stanchions and are comfortable being worked on in them.
  - They are usually not substantial enough to handle beef cattle.

Hobbles
- Hobbles are usually used on dairy cattle that have a tendency to kick the milkers.
- Hobbles can be either a metal clip that is placed on each hock or a padded strap that is buckled around the lower leg.
  - With both types, it is important to keep the cow's legs squared under her.
  - If the back legs are brought in too close, she could lose her balance and fall.

Tilt Table
- Cattle, especially bulls, often need their feet trimmed.
  - This can be done in a chute, but it is easier to do on a tilt table.
- Lead the animal or use an alleyway to put the animal near the table in its vertical upright position.
  - Then sedate the animal and strap it to the table.
  - Tilt the animal so it is in lateral recumbency to allow access to all four feet at a comfortable height.

Approaching and Moving
- Cattle have the same wide-angle vision as horses.
- Cattle have a "pressure point" at the shoulders.
  - If you move past the shoulder going toward the rear of the cow, it prompts the cow to move forward.
  - If you move toward the head it will make the cow stop.
- Use this information to move cattle into a pen or down an alley without a lot of prompting with a whip or paddle.
- To move a herd or group of cattle into a pen or alley, allow them to look inside and inspect the area.
- Place one person toward the opening of the gate and one behind the group you need to move.
- The person in the back puts pressure on the group by stepping forward; the person toward the front puts pressure on the group by walking toward the rear of the group from directly behind their shoulders toward the rear.
- As the cattle start to move into the pen, the person at the front of the group continues the forward motion by stepping behind the group as he or she moves in that direction.

- Be aware that cattle will kick if frightened or pushed too hard.
- They seldom kick straight out; you can get kicked standing to the side of a cow as well as behind it.
  - Either stand right next to the rear of the cow or back at least 6 to 8 feet.
  - You can be kicked standing next to the animal, but it will not be as deadly as inside the 6-foot range.
- Sometimes it is difficult and even dangerous to separate a cow and her calf away from the herd.
  - Instinctively they try to remain with the herd for protection.
  - The best scenario is to move a small group, containing the intended cow and calf, into a pen that has a gate into another pen.
  - Remember that mothers are very protective of their calves and may chase after you if they feel threatened.
  - It is also important to lock up any dogs that may be around, even if they are trained cattle dogs.
  - Cows with young at their side will get very upset when a dog is in the pen with them and often charge the dog.

SHEEP RESTRAINT

- Sheep have a strong flocking instinct and can be moved easily as a group.
- A singled-out sheep may panic and hurt itself or the handler while trying to get back to the flock.
- Using small pens that can either crowd the sheep together or moving a single sheep out of the pen in view of the rest of the flock is a good way to handle these sensitive animals.
- Sheep have a frail skeletal system and can be injured easily if they are chased into fences.
- Never grab sheep by the wool; it is easily pulled out and the skin tears easily, causing bruising, which devalues the carcass and pelt.
- Setting a sheep up on its rump is often used for venipuncture, ID injections, and foot trimming (Fig. 10.7).
- Backing the sheep into a corner and pinning its body up against a wall with a hand under the chin will usually suffice for most procedures.
- Sheep become hyperthermic easily because of their wool and normally high body temperature (102° to 104°F [38.8° to 40°C]).
- Working in the early part of the morning with good ventilation will help keep sheep from overheating.

GOAT RESTRAINT

- Goats can often be handled like sheep; however, many milking goats are halter broken and can be led to a small stanchion or tied to a post for procedures.
- Goats can be crowded into a pen, and then an individual goat can be caught and moved out to a work area.

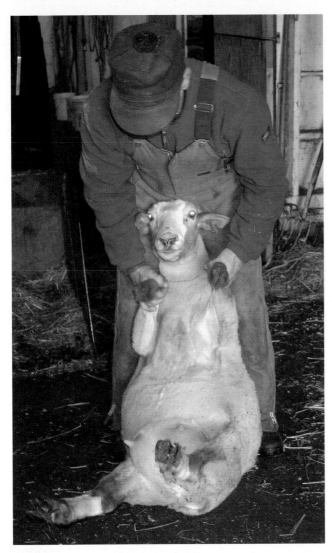

FIGURE 10.7 Setting a sheep up on its rump. (From Sheldon CC, Topel J, Sonsthagen BS: *Animal restraint for veterinary professionals*, St Louis, 2006, Mosby.)

- You can catch a goat by placing an arm around its neck and the other hand on its tail, much like a foal, and then direct its movements with forward or backward pressure.
- Goats that are handled frequently may have a collar that can be used to lead it to the work area.
- Once caught, place the goat's rear end in a corner to prevent it from backing up, and press its body against a wall to prevent lateral movement.
- Hands can be wrapped around either side of the face to lift the head for medications, IM or SQ injections, or jugular venipuncture.
- Never grab hold of a goat's horns; they resent this and will resist violently.
- They will either run at you and butt you or shake their heads vigorously. This is especially true of billy goats.

SWINE HANDLING AND RESTRAINT

- A significant animal welfare and production concern is the potential for stress from improper handling of pigs.
- Proper handling reduces stress during routine production practices, such as moving of swine, blood sampling, vaccinating, clipping tails and teeth, ear notching, detusking, castration, and administration of therapeutics.
- Pigs are not herd animals, but they tend to follow other pigs.
- When one pig becomes distressed and screams, the others may react as a group and panic, or they may come to the rescue of the "injured" pig.
- Pigs are extremely protective of their young and will come running if a piglet cries out.
- Pigs are also extremely stubborn, which can be used to advantage with various restraint procedures, particularly the hog snare.
- Pigs can become hyperthermic if chased or roughly handled, even in cool weather. Overheated pigs must be cooled immediately or they are likely to die of heat stroke.
- Pigs' main defensive weapons are their teeth.
  - They can tear flesh easily and have very strong jaws; the tusks of boars can be very dangerous.
- Sows are very dangerous when there are piglets at their side; a handler should never get into the same pen with a sow and piglets.

Driving and Catching

- Pigs can be difficult to drive in an open pen.
- Solid-paneled hurdles work well to move pigs, as well as pieces of PVC piping or a cane.
- Pigs stop when confronted with a solid barrier, such as hurdles, and pigs will move along when tapped on the rear quarters.
- Pigs should be driven into a small pen with solid walls at least as high as a pig's shoulder. They can be separated from the group again using the hurdles and pipe or cane.

Directing a Single Pig

- When moving a single pig, walk behind it with a hurdle in front of you.
- Use a cane or paddle to direct the pig by tapping it on the flank to move it forward or on the shoulder to move it right or left.
  - If it turns and moves toward you, set the edge of the hurdle on the ground and tilt it forward.
  - This prevents the pig from getting its snout under it and lifting, allowing it access to or through your legs.
  - The solid barrier will make the pig turn around.

Hog Snare

- A hog snare is used for restraining pigs for venipunctures or other injections.

- The snare is usually a metal pipe with a cable loop on one end.
- The free end of the cable runs through the hollow pipe, so the size of the loop can be controlled.
- Excessive tightening can injure the pig's snout.
- A snare should be in place for a maximum of 20 to 30 minutes.
- A rope can be used in place of the pipe and cable snare.
- If using a snare on a boar with tusks, it is important to get the snare behind the tusks.
- It is advisable to wear ear protection when using a hog snare because they scream the entire time they are held.

Restraining Piglets

- Baby pigs weighing less than 50 pounds are captured by grasping a back leg and holding the pig upside down until it can be held on your forearm close to your body or placed in a holding pen.
- If removing piglets from a sow, do it quickly and move to a different room to perform the procedure so you do not agitate the sow.
- Many farms have a cart to place the piglets in so they can be together, which makes them quiet down faster.
- Another way to quiet a piglet while holding it is to cradle its body against yours.
- Piglets can be restrained by holding both hind legs (Fig. 10.8) or placing them in a V-trough for such procedures as castration, ear notching, and cutting needle teeth.
- Piglets weighing more than 30 pounds can be held the same way, but it may take two people to hold them upside down by their hind legs.

Restraining Potbellied Pigs

- Potbellied pigs are usually kept as pets and have a docile temperament; however, some potbellied pigs may show aggression.
- Small pet pigs tend to squirm, jump, and climb on whomever is trying to restrain them.
- Ear protection is important for the handler because they can squeal as loud as a full-sized pig.

▮ COMMON PROCEDURES IN LIVESTOCK

Hoof Trimming

- Periodic trimming of the hooves is required for the comfort and humane treatment of the animals.
- Damaged or overgrown hooves can be trimmed and shaped by using various types of knives, shears, and electric grinders.
- Cattle must be properly restrained for hoof trimming by using at least a squeeze chute.
- Hydraulically operated tilt tables made specifically for trimming cattle feet make the task safe and efficient.

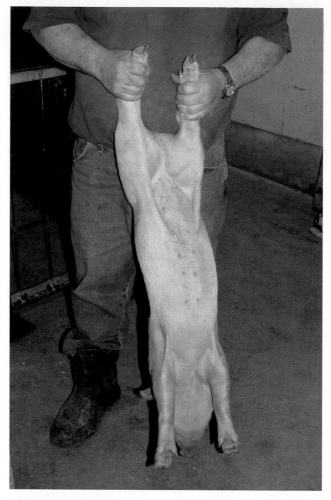

FIGURE 10.8 Holding a pig for transportation. (From Sirois M: *Principles and practice of veterinary technology*, ed 3, St Louis, 2011, Mosby.)

- The cattle are secured to the table then laid over on their side (tilted), so the operator has the legs safely restrained and the hooves at a comfortable working height.
- Sheep and goats that are not allowed to graze or that are raised in confinement tend to develop overgrown feet.
  - The sidewalls should be trimmed to keep the sole flat and the toes pointing forward.
  - Toes are normally squared off.
- Trimming is done with heavy scissors, hoof rot shears, or a sharp knife.

Crutching (or Tagging)

- Ewes close to parturition should be crutched or tagged.
  - This procedure removes the wool from around the vulva and the udder.
  - A clean vulva area facilitates passage of the lamb and allows the birthing process to proceed easily.
  - Removing the wool from around the udder assists the lambs in finding and suckling the teats.

Tail Docking and Castrating

- The tail of lambs is commonly docked to reduce the incidence of fecal material collecting on and around the anus, which can cause scalding.
  - The tail is docked or banded below the webbing on the tail using a clean tail-docking instrument, or an elastrator with an elastic band is placed around the tail, which impairs the circulation and causes the tail to fall off in about 1 week.
  - If the tail is docked too short, it can cause prolapse of the rectum.
  - Castration can also be done with the elastrator at the same time as the tail docking.
- The tail of piglets is commonly clipped to reduce the incidence of tail biting later in the grower-finisher stage.
  - The tail is docked approximately 2 cm from the base of the tail using clean, slightly dull side cutters to crush the tail.
  - Cauterizing clippers tend to reduce the amount of bleeding.
  - Cutting the tail too short may result in anal prolapse.
- After puberty male pigs may have an offensive odor or "boar taint" that is evident in pork during cooking.
- There are various techniques of castration, each determined by the age and size of the pig.
- The best time to castrate is before 3 weeks of age.
- A disadvantage to early castration is reduced detection of inguinal hernias.
- A knife blade can be used in boars of any size.
- A hooked blade (No. 12) works well with pigs weighing less than 15 kg.
- Pigs castrated between 2 weeks and 16 weeks of age can be held by the back legs, with the abdomen toward the operator and the back of the pig cradled between the restrainer's legs.
- Male calves are usually castrated at a fairly young age depending on the owner's preferences.
  - They can be castrated using an emasculator, which will surgically remove the testicle from the body.
  - Some producers will use the elastrator, an elastic band that goes around the testicle causing circulation loss, which will make the testicles fall off in about a week; however, this should not be used on calves over 1 month old; the band can fall off, and they are more prone to tetanus.
  - Dehorning is also done on young stock; the use of chemicals or a heated iron that burns the horn nub is a common technique.
  - The use of lidocaine for pain control during the burning has been found to greatly reduce the stress of this method of dehorning.

Clipping Teeth

- The newborn piglet has eight very sharp canine teeth (Fig. 10.9), referred to as wolf or **needle teeth**.

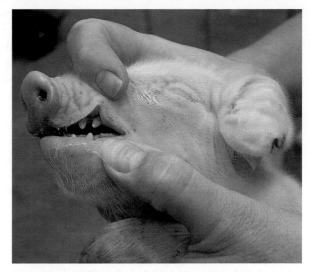

FIGURE 10.9 Needle teeth in neonatal pigs should be clipped to prevent bite injuries to the dam and littermates. (From Bassert J, Thomas J: *McCurnin's clinical textbook for veterinary technicians,* ed 8, St Louis, 2014, Saunders.)

- In large litters, if the needle teeth are left intact, the piglets scratch each other, causing infection and significant irritation to the sow's teats.
- Cutting the teeth in smaller litters may be unnecessary, but many producers clip teeth as a precaution.
- Using clean, sharp side cutters, position the side cutters parallel to the gum line and clip off the distal half of each tooth.
  - Take care not to cut the pig's gum or tongue.
  - Cutting too short may shatter the teeth, leading to gum infection.

Umbilical Cord Clipping

- The umbilical cord can act as a portal of entry for bacteria.
- If the piglet is bleeding from the umbilical cord, tie off the cord immediately using string.
- Using disinfected side cutters, cut the cord 4 to 5 cm from the abdominal wall.
- Spray with or dip the end of the cord in 2% povidone–iodine.

MONITORING HOSPITALIZED PATIENTS

- Hospitalized patients must be monitored regularly for changes in their condition.
- Horses only slightly ill can develop more severe and even life-threatening illness while receiving treatment.
  - For instance, a horse receiving antibiotic therapy for a mild respiratory infection can develop life-threatening diarrhea from changes in bowel microflora.
  - A horse receiving nonsteroidal antiinflammatory drugs for an orthopedic problem can develop gastrointestinal ulceration or renal dysfunction secondary

to the antiinflammatory medication, particularly if the animal is not eating and drinking normally.

- The heart rate, respiratory rate, rectal temperature, mucous membrane color, capillary refill time, attitude, digital pulses, urine and fecal output, gastrointestinal motility, and appetite should all be monitored at least once or twice daily.
- Critically ill neonates require more frequent monitoring, sometimes as often as every 2 hours, because their condition can deteriorate rapidly.
- Adult horses should be weighed at admission with a walk-on scale, if available, or a weight tape can be used to estimate the horse's weight.
- Neonates should be weighed at admission and then daily.

CARE OF RECUMBENT HORSES

- Nursing care for recumbent animals must be meticulous.
- Caring for a horse that is unable to rise is tedious and often unrewarding.
- Horses that remain recumbent for prolonged periods eventually develop various complications, regardless of the primary disease.
- Because of the weight of the animal, several people are needed to frequently turn the animal from one side to the other.
  - This is usually done with long ropes looped, not tied, around the pasterns so that the handlers can stand farther from the limbs of the horse, or by using a winch and harness when available.
- If the size of the horse permits, it would be preferable to flex the legs up next to the body then roll the horse's torso over the flexed legs rather than roll the horse over on its back.
  - Rolling the horse on its back may cause a twisted intestine and add another unneeded complication to an already sick or injured animal.
- When a horse is turned from one side to another, the animal often kicks, which can be very dangerous for anyone standing in the vicinity.
- The animal must be turned as frequently as possible to prevent development of decubital ulcers on the skin and edema and congestion in the dependent portion of the lung.
- Helmets can be applied to horses that tend to flail about and hit their head against the wall or ground.
- The technician and assistant should also pay particular attention to the eyes of a recumbent animal because the corneas can become ulcerated if the animal rubs its eyes on the ground.
- The primary disease must be resolved as quickly as possible so that the animal may once again stand.
- If the horse can stand but only with assistance, the hind limbs can be supported by suspending a rope attached

to the tail from a ceiling beam; the head may also need to be supported.

- Commercial slings are available that provide support for horses that have some ability to support themselves but require additional help.
- A sling cannot be used for horses with flaccid paralysis or other conditions that make them unable to support themselves at all because they can only slump down in the sling.
- Slings must be well padded to prevent development of pressure sores.
- No matter how meticulous the nursing care, decubital ulcers may develop over bony prominences, such as the tuber coxae, carpus, hock, shoulder joint, or elbow.
  - These must be cleaned with a mild antibacterial soap.
  - Topical antibacterial powders or sprays can also be used.
  - A spray that creates a "breathable" bandage may provide the best protection.
- Any bony protuberance that can be protected by wraps should be wrapped.
- Frequent cleaning can help to prevent urine scalding and reduce the severity of decubital ulcers.
- Additional bedding may also help minimize the formation of decubital sores.
- The recumbent animal may not eat or drink well.
  - Soft, highly palatable feeds should be offered.
  - Fresh, clean water should be offered to the recumbent animal every 2 hours, if possible.
  - The food and water may have to be given by nasogastric tube because the animal may aspirate feed or water into the lungs when trying to eat or drink in lateral recumbency.
  - If possible, it is preferable to feed the horse while it is in a more sternal position.
- Infusion of IV fluids may be required in more debilitated or dehydrated animals.

BANDAGING

- Materials needed to bandage the distal limbs include cotton quilts or sheet cotton (three sheets) and track wraps, brown roll gauze, or some type of conforming bandage material.
- Leg wraps can be used to protect a wound, to give additional support, or to cover a medicated area.
- The wrap should be applied with even pressure so that the tendons running along the caudal aspect of the leg (superficial and deep digital flexor tendons) are protected and pressure is evenly applied over the entire length of the tendons.

Foot Wraps

- Before applying a foot wrap, the foot is first picked clean and then washed and dried if needed.
- If the foot requires medication, this can be applied and then covered with a gauze sponge secured with a layer of rolled gauze.

- It is very important to have the ground surface of the foot wrap flat, rather than convex and bulging, so that even pressure is applied to the bottom of the foot.
- Be careful not to wrap up over the coronary band if no protective padding is in place.
  - Excessive pressure directly on the coronary band can reduce circulation to hoof tissues and cause damage or sloughing of the hoof.

Tail Bandages

- Tail wraps can consist of stall bandages, rolled brown gauze, or even commercial tail bags.
- The tail may also need to be wrapped when a mare is about to foal or for a reproductive examination.
- If the tail wrap is intended to be left on the horse for many days, it is important that the wrap not extend proximally to include the tail bones (coccygeal vertebrae) because the tail has little muscular padding, and a tight wrap can occlude blood circulation to the tail and create a tissue slough or even loss of the entire tail.
- If it is necessary to wrap more proximally on the tail, a nonconstricting wrap should be loosely applied and changed daily.
- At times it is necessary to wrap the tail of a horse with severe diarrhea to keep the tail clean. This can be done using a plastic rectal sleeve.
  - Holes can be cut in the sleeve to help keep the tail from "sweating."
  - The tail hair should first be braided and the sleeve slid over the tail and tied at the most proximal part of the braid.
  - The sleeve can also be anchored to the most proximal part of the tail with a strip of adhesive tape or duct tape placed lengthwise from the sleeve cranially along the midline of the back.

SAMPLE COLLECTION

Urine Collection

- A female generally urinates just after standing.
- Urine samples for bacteriologic, chemical, and microscopic testing can be collected directly from the bladder by inserting a catheter using aseptic technique.
- The animal should be suitably restrained and the vulva cleaned.
- For goats, a double-bladed small animal vaginal speculum is inserted into the vagina.
- Under visual control with illumination from a light, a sterile curved metal urinary catheter is inserted into the urethra.
- For cattle, a catheter is guided in with one hand in the rectum, so the feces need to be raked out and the vulva cleaned thoroughly before placing the catheter.
  - Urethral catheterization of males cannot be performed.

- The presence of a urethral diverticulum at the level of the ischial arch makes it impossible to introduce a catheter into the urinary bladder.
- Collecting urine from sheep is easier than with many other animals.
- Hold the sheep in a standing position and pinch the nostrils closed until urination occurs.
  - Generally the sheep will urinate within 30 seconds.
  - The nostrils may be held closed for up to 1 minute.
  - If the sheep does not urinate in that minute, allow the animal to rest for 1 or 2 minutes.

BLOOD COLLECTION

- Sites for venous blood sampling in horses include the jugular vein, cephalic vein, lateral thoracic vein, saphenous vein, and coccygeal vein.
- For cattle, the jugular vein is one of the most common locations for venipuncture.
- Proper restraint of the head is critical to ensure safety of personnel.
- The tail vein is another common location for blood collection in cattle because it is easily accessed if the animal has limited side-to-side mobility.
- Cattle are generally more tolerant of venipuncture in the tail than in the neck.
- The jugular vein is commonly used for blood collection in sheep and goats.
- The cephalic vein on the forearm or the femoral vein on the hindleg can also be used.
- In swine, blood collection from the tail vein is limited to adult pigs without docked tails.
- The cranial vena cava is commonly used for blood collection in swine.
  - Because the jugular vein is not as deep a structure as the cranial vena cava, it is a safer structure for access with a needle.
  - The jugular veins are not as large in diameter and may be difficult to find, especially in large or heavy animals.
- Blood samples from poultry are usually collected from either the brachial wing vein or the jugular vein.

ADMINISTRATION OF MEDICATION

Oral Administration

- Medications that are in liquid form and required in only small doses may be administered with a dose syringe or a syringe with the locking tip removed.
- The syringe is placed through the side of the mouth in the area of the diastema, or interdental space (space between the incisors and premolars) (Fig. 10.10).
- The medication is deposited on the caudal portion of the tongue if possible.

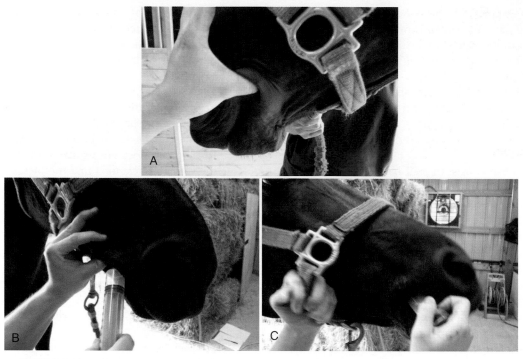

FIGURE 10.10 (A) Opening the lips before placing the oral syringe in the mouth. (B) Placement of the dose syringe near the commissure of the lips. (C) Proper positioning of the oral syringe. (From Sirois M: *Principles and practice of veterinary technology*, ed 3, St Louis, 2011, Mosby.)

- Medications in pill form can be crushed with a mortar and pestle and then mixed with something sweet, such as molasses, and given in a similar manner.
- It is best not to mix medication with the feed because horses often eat around the medication and do not consume the full dose.
- Medication that must be given in large volumes requires use of a nasogastric tube for delivery into the stomach.
- Oral administration in poultry is accomplished with tube feeding or gavage.

Balling Gun

- Boluses (large tablets), capsules, or magnets may be given per os (PO) with a balling gun. This instrument is available in various sizes for use in different species.
- Cattle require a balling gun with a large metal or flexible plastic head and a long handle.
- The plastic head produces less trauma to the pharyngeal tissue than a metal head but is easily damaged by teeth.
- Small balling guns are manufactured for use in calves, sheep/lambs, and goats/kids.
- The methods of introducing a balling gun, dose syringe, drench bottle, or Frick speculum are similar in all species.
- Commercially prepared paste syringes containing medication are inserted the same as for the balling gun. The paste is usually deposited on the tongue and not down the esophagus.
- A Frick speculum may be used to give two or more boluses to cattle.

Drenching

- Giving small volumes of liquids PO is often referred to as drenching.
- Drenching is done with a dose syringe with various-sized nozzles to fit the animal or a drench bottle
- A 60-mL catheter-tipped syringe or a bulb syringe may be used as a dose syringe in calves, lambs, and kids.
- The drench bottle should be made of strong glass and have a long, tapered neck and smooth mouth.
- The technique for drenching is similar to that described for the balling gun except you insert the bottle at the commissure of the lips in the interdental space.
- The animal's head should be held slightly elevated so that the nose is level with the animal's eye.
- The Drench-Matic dose syringe can be used to medicate a herd of animals.
- When the handles are squeezed, a set amount of medication is delivered to each animal.

Orogastric Intubation

- Orogastric administration, also called "stomach tubing," is a quick and relatively painless method to deliver large quantities of liquid medication or fluids.
- A stomach tube may be passed through the nasal cavity (nasogastric administration) in horses, but this method is not commonly used in food animals.
- In food animals, the stomach tube is usually passed through the oral cavity with the aid of a mouth speculum.

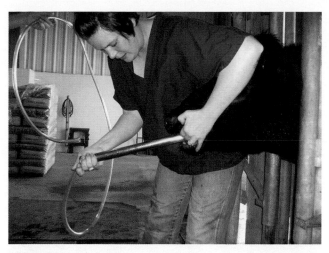

FIGURE 10.11 Placement of Frick speculum. (From Holtgrew-Bohling K: *Large animal clinical procedures for veterinary technicians*, ed 2, St Louis, 2012, Mosby.)

- An oral speculum is required to prevent damage to the soft stomach tube from the animal's teeth or be closed off by the animal biting down on the tube.
- The Frick, Drinkwater, or Bayer speculum is inserted into the mouth and held in place by an assistant or the person inserting the tube (Fig. 10.11).
- Choose an appropriately sized tube for the individual animal.
- A tube with an outside diameter of ⅝ to 1 inch is the average size used for adult cattle.
- A foal stomach tube is often used for "tubing" calves, sheep, and goats.
- A 14-Fr feeding tube will work on neonate lambs and kids.
  - A stomach pump, syringe, or funnel can be used to facilitate administration.
  - The first 3 feet of the tube should be lubricated with water or water-soluble lubricating jelly before intubation.
  - With the veterinary assistant holding an oral speculum in place, the veterinary technician inserts the tube into the speculum and advances it with gentle pressure.

Parenteral Injections

- Drugs and other liquids can be injected into a muscle (IM) or vein (IV), under the skin (SQ), or into a layer of the skin (ID).
- It is important to know which routes of administration are acceptable for each drug administered because injection by an inappropriate route can have harmful or even lethal effects on the horse.
  - For example, procaine penicillin should be given only in the muscle (IM); if given IV, the procaine component may cause excitation, seizures, and death.

- Some medications should be administered intravenously only.
- These medications can be very caustic and cause tissue sloughing if administered outside the vein (**perivascular**) or in the muscle.

Subcutaneous Injections

- SQ injections in horses usually involve items given in smaller doses, such as for allergy desensitization.
  - A 20- or 21-gauge, 1-inch needle should be used.
- Any area where the skin can easily be lifted from the underlying muscle and fascia may be used; the lateral aspect of the neck where IM injections are also given is a suitable site in horses.
- The skin is first cleaned with alcohol if necessary and then pulled laterally to form a "tent."
- SQ injections are given in the lateral aspect of the neck, over the ribs, or in front of the shoulder in cattle, sheep, and goats.
- Subcutaneous injections in pigs less than 25 kg are given primarily in the loose skin of the flank or caudal to the elbow.
  - If injecting into the flank, inject into the folds of the skin and not into the peritoneal cavity.
  - In larger pigs the preferred injection site is the loose skin caudal to the ear.
  - It is not necessary to tent the skin as in small animals if you use a short enough needle.
  - This technique is used if vaccinating numerous animals in an alley or crowd pen; otherwise, pinching the skin to make a tent works well.
- For sheep, limit the volume of medication to 5 mL per site.
  - If a large volume is to be injected, divide the dose into several portions injected at different sites.

Intramuscular Injections

- An experienced handler should always be available to properly restrain the horse when administering any IM injections in the horse.
- Various sites can be used for IM injections in horses.
- The lateral neck area can be used for administering only small volumes of medication.
  - The area to be used is a triangular portion on the side of the neck formed by the ligamentum nuchae dorsally, the spine ventrally, and the scapula caudally.
- Another common area for IM injection is in the semitendinosus and semimembranosus muscles of the hind leg.
  - This is the preferred site for IM injections in neonatal foals because they are usually the largest muscle masses available in young and minimally developed foals.
  - However, this is a very vulnerable position for the handler, and horses that are known to kick should not be injected at this site.

- Another available site would be the pectoral muscles found on the cranial chest wall between the front legs.
- A 16- or 18-gauge, 1.5-inch needle should be used for IM injections in adults.
- A 20-gauge, 1-inch needle should be used for small equines and neonates.
- The site is cleaned with alcohol if necessary, and the needle, without an attached syringe, is inserted with a quick jab.
- IM injections are not as commonly used in food animals.
- The movement to reduce injection abscesses and scarring in the muscles used for prime cuts of meat has prompted the medical community to limit IM injections to the lateral cervical muscles.
  - These muscles are cranial to the scapula, dorsal to the cervical vertebrae, and ventral to the ligamentum nuchae.
- With pigs, the area of the neck muscle caudal to the ear is used.
- Dairy cattle can be given IM injections in a stanchion or head gate; a halter is usually not necessary.
- Beef cattle should be placed in a chute and, if running a large group of cattle at one time, the injection can be given in the alleyway as they are waiting to go through the chute.
- Calves, sheep, and goats are backed into a corner and the head is restrained by placing an arm around their necks.
- Pigs will require a hog snare if they are adults; if under 40 to 50 pounds, they can be picked up by their back legs or crowded into a small pen with a marker crayon to mark each pig after an injection.

Intravenous Injections

- The jugular vein is the only appropriate vein for IV injections in horses.
  - The jugular vein runs caudally along the jugular furrow from the head and then enters the thoracic inlet on its way to the heart.
  - The carotid artery runs deep to the jugular vein in the same vicinity, but it courses deeper into the neck and is separated from the jugular vein in the more cranial portion of the neck.
- The veins most often used for IV injections in cattle, sheep, and goats are the jugular veins; in cattle, the coccygeal (tail) vein and subcutaneous abdominal (milk) veins also can be used.
  - The jugular veins are most often used for large-volume IV injections.
  - The jugular vein is always used for IV injections in calves, sheep, and goats because it is the largest accessible vessel.
- The auricular vein is used in pigs.
- The coccygeal (tail) vein is used for IV injection of small volumes (0.3 to 0.5 mL) of drugs that are noncaustic to the surrounding tissues in case it goes perivascular (Fig. 10.12).

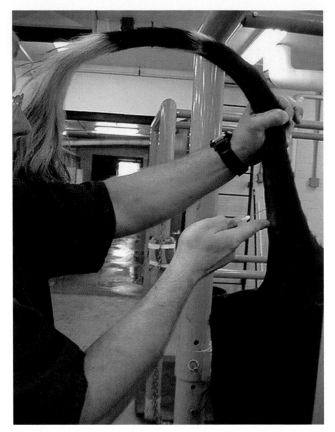

FIGURE 10.12 Coccygeal venipuncture. (From Sheldon CC, Topel J, Sonsthagen BS: *Animal restraint for veterinary professionals*, St Louis, 2006, Mosby.)

- Most dairy cattle are tolerant of tail injections; however, there is a chance of being kicked.
- This can be minimized with proper restraint, including placing a bar or bale of hay behind the back legs.
- The subcutaneous abdominal vein, also called the mammary or milk vein, is used mainly when the jugular veins are thrombosed (occluded) or cannot be located.
  - There are several disadvantages to milk vein injections.
  - The technician has an increased risk of being kicked. A second person may be required to provide additional restraint.
  - The milk vein rolls easily under the skin, making it hard to puncture the vein and thread the needle.
  - Finally, hematomas are easily formed and may result in thrombosis of the vein.
- The auricular vein in pigs is often used to deliver IV medications.
  - A winged (butterfly) infusion set can be used to access the vein and be secured with a transparent dressing that adheres well to bare skin.
  - The injection should be fairly slow because the vein will often balloon out if it is given too fast.
- Preparation for IV injection is similar for all veins.

- Cotton soaked in 70% alcohol should be applied to the injection site to remove gross contamination and increase visibility of the vein.
- IV injections should not be made through dirt or fecal material because phlebitis, septicemia, and/or contamination of medication and samples may result.
- Clipping the hair over the injection site may be necessary if it cannot be readily visualized.

Restraint
- Beef cattle are placed into a chute and their heads are haltered for the jugular vein injection. For tail injections, a bar should be placed behind their back legs to prevent kicking.
- The subcutaneous abdominal vein is rarely used on beef cattle but can be accessed by lowering the side panels on the chute.
  - Tying the back legs may be necessary because they can kick forward with their rear legs.
- Dairy cattle can be given IV injections in a stanchion.
- The veins can be easily accessed on sheep if the animal is set up on its rump.
- Goats, adult sheep, and small calves can be backed into a corner and pinned up against the wall with the restrainer's body.
- The cephalic and femoral veins may be used also, with the sheep and goats in a standing or lateral recumbency position.

- The needle selected for IV injection of large volumes of fluids varies according to personal preference, the flow rate desired, and the viscosity of the drug to be administered.
- Use the smallest needle possible because this reduces discomfort to the patient and minimizes trauma.
  - A 14-, 16-, or 18-gauge, 1.5- to 2-inch needle is best for giving large volumes to adult cattle.
  - For injections of small volumes into the jugular vein, use of a 16-, 18-, or 20-gauge, 1.5-inch needle is recommended for cows and calves.
  - Depending on the size of the sheep or goat, an 18- or 20-gauge, 1- to 1.5-inch needle and syringe can be used.
- A rubber IV line, referred to as a simplex, is used for IV infusions.
- A syringe may also be used to inject medication.
- Intravenous injections are commonly given in the auricular vein (Table 10.4) on pigs and some large cattle.
- Pigs less than 15 kg can be held, whereas larger pigs should be restrained using a snare.
- The auricular vein, near the lateral border of the ear, is prominent when held off using thumb pressure or a rubber band as a tourniquet at the base of the ear.
- A 20- to 22-gauge, ¾- to 1-inch infusion set (butterfly catheter) works very well for administration of solutions.

TABLE 10.4 Recommended Needle Sizes, Injection Volumes, and Blood Sample Volumes, Based on Pig Size

	INJECTIONS			BLOOD SAMPLING					
	IM	SC	IV	Cranial vena cava	Jugular vein	Ear vein	Medial canthus	Tail vein	Cephalic vein
Piglet Needle	18–20 gauge, 11 mm		21 gauge, 11 mm	20 gauge, 38 mm	20 gauge, 38 mm		20 gauge, 25 mm		
Quantity		1–2 mL/site			Unlimited		5–10 mL		
Weaner Needle	18–20 gauge, 18 mm		21 gauge, 25 mm	20 gauge, 38 mm	20 gauge, 38 mm		20 gauge, 25 mm		20 gauge, 38 mm
Quantity		1–2 mL/site			Unlimited		5–10 mL		5–10 mL
Grower-Finisher Needle	16 gauge, 18–25 mm		18 gauge, 25 mm	18 gauge, 65 mm	20 gauge, 38 mm	20 gauge, 25 mm	16 gauge, 38 mm		
Quantity		1–3 mL/site			Unlimited	1–2 mL	5–10 mL		
Breeding Stock Needle	14–16 gauge, 38 mm		18 gauge, 38 mm	16 gauge, 90 mm	20 gauge, 38 mm	20 gauge, 25 mm	14 gauge, 38 mm	20 gauge, 25 mm	
Quantity		1–3 mL/site			Unlimited	1–2 mL	5–10 mL	5–10 mL	

From Sirois M: Principles and practice of veterinary technology, ed 3, St Louis, 2011, Mosby.

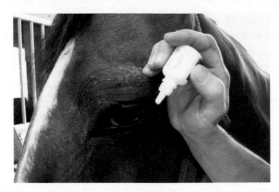

FIGURE 10.13 Proper technique for medicating the eye. Note that the hand is stabilized against the horse's head. (From Sirois M: *Principles and practice of veterinary technology*, ed 3, St Louis, 2011, Mosby.)

Eye Medication

- Topical ointments or solutions can be applied directly to the eye in horses and other livestock.
- Once the animal is adequately restrained, gently pry the eye open with clean fingers, being careful to touch only the outer lids (Fig. 10.13).
- Ointments can be applied by placing a small bead of ointment into the lower conjunctival sac.
- Ophthalmic drops can be placed in the lower conjunctival sac using the plastic dispenser vial provided or using a sterile tuberculin syringe without an attached needle if the solution is to be used on multiple horses.
- Severe corneal ulcers may require topical treatments as often as every 1 to 2 hours.
- For horses that become head shy and resentful with this frequent treatment schedule, alternative medication delivery systems can be used.
- Lavage systems can be placed in the upper eyelid (subpalpebral) or inserted into the tear duct (nasolacrimal duct), and liquid medications can then be delivered easily through either of these systems.

- Severe corneal ulcers and some other abnormalities may require extra protection for the eye.
- A protective eye cup can be used to protect the eye and keep the horse from dislodging the lavage system.
    - The black plastic cup also protects the eye from direct sunlight, which could cause pain.
    - This may be very important because many corneal ulcers require treatment with atropine to inhibit ciliary spasm.
    - This makes the horse unable to constrict the pupil when exposed to direct sunlight.
- Netted fly masks can also be used to provide some protection for the eyes.
- Horses that spend a lot of time lying down may accumulate shavings or bedding in the eyes.
- Eye cups or netted fly masks can also be used to help keep the shavings out.

RECOMMENDED READINGS

Anderson D, Rings M: *Current veterinary therapy: food animal practice*, ed 5 St Louis, 2008, Saunders.

Hanie EA: *Large animal clinical procedures for veterinary technicians*, St Louis, 2006, Mosby.

Holtgrew-Bohling, K. Large Animal Clinical Procedures for Veterinary Technicians, 3rd Edition. Mosby, 2015.

Orsini JA, Divers TJ: *Manual of equine emergencies*, ed 3, St Louis, 2009, Saunders.

Pond WG, Mersmann HJ: *Biology of the domestic pig*, Ithaca, NY, 2001, Comstock Publishing Associates.

Pugh DG: *Sheep and goat medicine*, St Louis, 2002, Mosby.

Radostits OM: *Herd health: food animal production medicine*, ed 3, St Louis, 2001, Saunders.

Reed SR, Bailey WM, Sellon DC: *Equine internal medicine*, ed 3, St Louis, 2010, Saunders.

Robinson M, Sprayberry K. *Current therapy in equine medicine*, ed 6, St Louis, 2006, Saunders.

Sirois M: *Principles and practice of veterinary technology*, ed 4, St Louis, 2016, Mosby.

Smith BP: *Large animal internal medicine*, ed 5, St Louis, 2014, Mosby.

Avian and Exotic Animal Care and Nursing

KEY TERMS

Anisodactyl
Barbering
Boar
Buck
Bumblefoot
Cavy
Cere
Choana
Cloaca
Coelom
Columella

Contour feathers
Coprodeum
Coverts
Crop
Doe
Down feathers
Flight feathers
Hobs
Jill
Keel
Lagomorphs

Malocclusion
Molting
Mouthing
Murine
Nocturnal species
Operculum
Passerines
Pneumatized
Proctodeum
Proventriculus
Psittacines

Rodents
Sow
Syrinx
Urates
Urodeum
Uropygial gland
Vent
Ventriculus

LEARNING OBJECTIVES

After reviewing this chapter, the reader will be able to:
1. State the general characteristics of mice, rats, hamsters, gerbils, guinea pigs, chinchillas, rabbits, and ferrets.
2. Discuss husbandry and principles of sanitation for small mammals.
3. Describe techniques for general nursing care of rodents, rabbits, and ferrets.
4. Describe techniques used for diagnosing and treating disease in small mammals.

5. Describe the unique features of the anatomy of birds and basic biology of common reptile species.
6. Discuss the basic behavior of birds, reptiles, and amphibians.
7. Discuss the basics of client education, husbandry, and nutrition for avian, reptile, and amphibian species.
8. Describe how to obtain a complete and thorough history of avian, reptile, and amphibian patients.

9. Explain the different capture and restraint techniques used for birds, reptiles, and amphibians.
10. Identify methods of sample collection for laboratory analysis.
11. Describe how to obtain quality diagnostic images of avian reptile and amphibian patients.

12. Discuss nursing care and supportive therapy techniques for avian, reptile, and amphibian patients.
13. Identify and discuss some common diseases of avian, reptile, and amphibian patients in the veterinary clinic.

SMALL MAMMALS

- Small mammals, also called pocket pets, include ferrets, rabbits, mice, rats, hamsters, gerbils, guinea pigs, and chinchillas.
- Although small mammals are relatively easy to care for, they require care that is different from that of dogs and cats.
- Prospective owners should be encouraged to read about a species they have never cared for before.
- Success or failure in raising an animal will depend on the knowledge that an owner has about the pet.
- Small mammals are often purchased as first pets for children.
- Children should always be supervised when handling these delicate creatures.
- Small mammals can bite, and children should be made aware of this and told that these pets are real live creatures and not stuffed animals.
- Small mammals should not be allowed free run of the house because this can prove fatal to them.
- Because the life span of most small mammals is only 2 to 4 years, children should be counseled so that an early death is not unexpected.
- Allergies to animal dander, saliva, and urinary proteins occur commonly in humans.
- Cutaneous and upper respiratory allergies to small mammals, especially rats and guinea pigs, are common.

Housing

- Caging must be escape-proof to prevent injury or fatality.
- Rodents can be housed in plastic or metal cages with slotted bars or wire mesh lids.
- Shoebox-type cages made of plastic materials are popular for housing rodents (Fig. 11.1).
- Cage flooring can be a solid bottom or wire mesh; solid flooring with bedding material is preferred.
- If mesh flooring is used, care must be taken to prevent foot injury and loss of neonates through the flooring.
- Aquariums are adequate to house pet rodents but should have a screen-type top with a locking device.
  - This type of housing unit allows easy access to the pet; however, it is heavy and can be difficult to clean.
  - Aquariums generally need more frequent cleaning to prevent ammonia buildup within the cage.

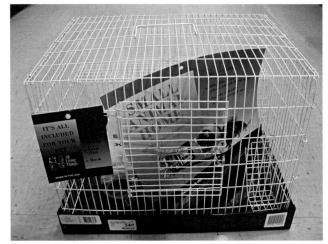

FIGURE 11.1 A typical mouse cage is made of wire and has room for a hide box and exercise wheel. (From Mitchell M, Tully TN Jr: *Manual of exotic pet practice*, St Louis, 2008, Saunders.)

- When aquariums are used for housing, care should be taken to ensure that rodents have access to food and water.
- Conventional cages such as those purchased from pet stores should have a large door to facilitate easy removal of the animal and should be easy to disassemble and clean.
- Rabbits, chinchillas, and ferrets can be housed in wire or front-opening cages with catch pans to collect urine and feces.
- Pet ferrets and rabbits can also be housed in large cat or dog carriers with a litter box.
- Rabbits and ferrets can be housed outdoors, but care must be taken to prevent heat stroke, myiasis, and dog and cat attacks.
  - Animals maintained outdoors should be provided with shelter from direct sunlight, rain, snow, and wind.
- Animals should be housed in caging that is appropriate for the animal's size and weight.
  - Some animals, such as chinchillas, are acrobatic and active and should be provided with a large cage to allow for exercise.
- Cage height should allow an animal to make normal postural adjustments.
  - For example, gerbils frequently sit upright, so the height of their caging should allow them to do so.

- The cage should be located in an area protected from climatic extremes.
- Care should be taken not to house pet rodent cages in direct sunlight because they will overheat.
- Changes in temperature and humidity and/or drafty conditions should be avoided because these can be stressful and predispose the animal to disease.
- The recommended housing temperature for mice, rats, hamsters, gerbils, and guinea pigs is 65° to 79°F (18° to 26°C); for rabbits and chinchillas it is 61° to 72°F (16° to 22°C); and for ferrets it is 39° to 64°F (4° to 18°C).
- The acceptable range of relative humidity is 30% to 70%.
- Albino rodents are susceptible to phototoxicity, so care should be taken to ensure safe illumination levels in their housing area.
- Noise should be minimized in animal housing areas because excessive sound exposure can be stressful and produce untoward effects.
- It is important to remember that many species can hear frequencies of sound that are inaudible to humans and some rodents are prone to sound-induced seizures.
- Bedding used for solid-bottom caging should be absorbent, comfortable, non-nutritive, nontoxic, and disposable.
- A variety of bedding material can be used, including paper, sawdust and soft pine, aspen, cedar, corncob, and hardwood chips.
- Cedar and soft pine shavings are frequently used for pet rodent bedding because of their pleasant aroma.
  - These are not recommended because they emit aromatic hydrocarbons that can induce liver changes and cytotoxicity.
- Burrowing rodents such as the rat and gerbil should be provided with deeper bedding to allow for this behavior.
- Cage toys can provide psychological stimulation as well as exercise for small mammals.
  - Tubes, mazes, and exercise wheels are popular.
- Timid animals such as guinea pigs and chinchillas are more comfortable if they are given a place to hide.
  - Polyvinyl chloride (PVC) plumbing pipes, especially elbows and Y and T sections, make ideal hiding places.
  - These pipes can be sanitized in the dishwasher.
- Cardboard tubes, softwood pieces, and small Nylabones can be given to rodents to gnaw on.
- Paper tissues or towels can be given to rodents who build nests, such as mice, gerbils, and hamsters.
- Metallic items such as washers can be suspended in a rabbit's cage to encourage nudging, playing, and investigative behaviors.
- Paper bags, hard plastic or metal toys, or cloth toys made for cats or babies are safe for ferrets.
- Ferrets love to run through cylindrical objects such as large mailing tubes and dryer vent tubing.
- Latex rubber toys that are intended for dogs or cats should not be given to ferrets.

Nutrition

- The rat and mouse are omnivorous, whereas the guinea pig, rabbit, chinchilla, and gerbil are herbivorous.
- The hamster is primarily granivorous.
- Ferrets are carnivorous and depend on meat proteins and fats for their dietary requirements.
- It is important to feed a balanced diet, freshly milled and formulated for that particular species.
- Pelleted foods are available commercially.
  - These diets are complete and do not require supplementation.
- Block-style pellets work well for rodents such as mice, rats, hamsters, and gerbils.
- Many types of the rodent feed found in pet stores and sold as seed mixes or treats are inadequate in protein for these species.
- Smaller pelleted foods work well for guinea pigs, chinchillas, and rabbits.
- Rabbits should be fed a high-fiber rabbit chow to prevent obesity and hairball formation.
- Rabbits, guinea pigs, and chinchillas can be fed small amounts of grass or alfalfa hay.
  - Hay not only provides them with fiber but helps reduce boredom.
- Ferrets can be fed ferret chow or commercial cat food.
  - As with dogs and cats, periodontal disease is common in ferrets.
  - Feeding dry food can help reduce tartar accumulation.
- In most cases, the food should be placed in a feeder hung in the animal's cage.
  - This prevents soiling of the food with urine and feces, keeping it dry and clean.
- If vegetables or fruit are offered to supplement the diet, they should be fresh and washed before feeding them.
  - Any uneaten vegetables or fruits should be removed daily.
- Supplements should not make up more than 10% of the animal's daily food ration.
- Animals should always have access to fresh water.

Rabbits

- The domestic rabbit, or European rabbit (*Oryctolagus cuniculus*), still exists on the European continent in three forms: wild, feral, and domestic.
- In North America, only feral and domestic rabbits exist.
- The Flemish Giant is a large breed of rabbit weighing 6 to 7 kg, the New Zealand and Californian are medium-size breeds weighing 2 to 5 kg, and the Dutch and Polish are small breeds weighing 1 to 2 kg.
  - The albino New Zealand is popularly used for meat production.
  - The smaller breeds are kept as pets.
- Rabbits make good pets; they are mild tempered, seldom bite, and can be litter box trained.

- Rabbits are **lagomorphs**, differentiated from rodents by the presence of two upper pairs of incisors that continuously grow.
  - The second set of upper incisors is smaller and is found behind the large front incisors; these are called peg teeth or wolf teeth.
- The rabbit has a life span of 5 to 6 years or longer, a body temperature of 101° to 104°F (38.5° to 40°C), heart rate of 130 to 325 beats/min, and respiratory rate of 30 to 60 breaths/min.
- Rabbits have a wide field of vision, can readily detect motion, and can see well in dim light.
- Rabbit ears are highly vascular and function in heat regulation.
- Rabbits have several unusual features in their intestinal tract, including a sacculus rotundus located at the terminal end of the ileum, a large cecum that terminates in a vermiform process or appendix, and a colon with regular sacculations called haustra.
- Rabbits are coprophagic, a term that refers to eating of feces, and pass two types of feces.
  - Soft, moist, night feces are rich in vitamins and protein and are eaten directly from the anus.
  - Firm dry pellets are passed during the daytime.
- Hairballs can be a serious, potentially fatal problem in rabbits because they cannot vomit.
  - The addition of proteolytic enzymes such as those found in unpasteurized papaya or pineapple-type products helps prevent this condition.
  - High-fiber diets are of value in trying to prevent hairballs and tend to prevent obesity, hair chewing, and enteritis.
- The color of rabbit urine varies from orange-red to brown; the pH is higher than 8 and therefore very basic.
  - A small amount of protein in the urine is normal.
  - Crystals of calcium carbonate and magnesium phosphate can be expected to be found in rabbit urine.
- Male rabbits are called **bucks** and female rabbits are called **does**.
- Determining gender can be accomplished by gently pressing the skin back from the genital opening.
  - Females have an elongated vulva, with a slit opening; males have a rounded, protruding penile sheath.
- The dewlap, a heavy fold of skin at the throat, is more prominent in females.
- Rabbits have a small skeletal mass compared with similar-sized animals and large hindquarter muscles that make them prone to back fractures.
- Back fractures are considered incurable, and the animal must be euthanized.
  - Most fractures of the spinal column result from poor handling techniques.
- When carrying a rabbit for a longer distance, its head should be tucked into the crook of the arm that is supporting the hindquarters.

- A towel wrapped around the rabbit works well for restraint, especially if the eyes are covered.
- Mechanical devices made of plastic or metal are frequently used for restraint during minor procedures, such as blood collection from an ear vein, intravenous (IV) injections, or treatments.
  - The restraining device holds the head in place and has a sliding partition that fits snugly against the rabbit's rump.
- Rabbits should never be lifted or restrained by grabbing their ears because their ears are sensitive and fragile.
- When returning a rabbit to its cage, place it in the cage rump first to prevent injury to the rabbit or handler.
  - A rabbit has a tendency to leap toward the cage if allowed to enter the cage headfirst.
- **Malocclusion** can result in overgrown incisors that may need to be trimmed every 2 to 3 weeks.
- Ear mite infections with *Psoroptes* spp. are common in pet rabbits.
  - The mites characteristically cause a dry, brown, crusty material to accumulate on the inner surface of the ears.
- Pododermatitis, a pressure necrosis of the plantar surface of the metatarsal area commonly called sore hocks or **bumblefoot**, is seen in heavy, obese rabbits.
- Rabbits are susceptible to infection with *Pasteurella multocida*.
  - Several clinical forms of the disease occur; the most common are rhinitis (snuffles) and pneumonia.
- Stressed or recently weaned rabbits are frequently infected with coccidia.

Ferrets

- The domestic ferret *(Mustela putorius furo)* belongs to the same family as weasels, mink, otter, and skunks.
- Ferrets were initially used as hunting animals for the control of rabbits and rodents and raised for their pelts.
- Ferrets have become popular pets because of their small size, ease of care, and comical and engaging personalities.
- Keeping domestic ferrets as pets is not legal in all states and/or cities.
  - It is important to be aware of legislation in your area regarding the keeping of ferrets as pets.
- The natural color of ferrets is fitch, also known as sable.
  - Fitch-colored ferrets have black guard hair with a cream-colored undercoat, black feet and tail, and a black mask on the face.
  - Two other natural colors that are seen are albino and cinnamon.
  - In addition, more than 30 color variations are recognized.
- Ferrets have long, tubular bodies with short legs and flexible spines.
  - This allows them to get into small openings and turn around easily.
- Ferrets leap and jump and can climb.

- If a ferret is allowed to run loose in the house, the house should be ferret-proofed to close up any holes or areas from which a ferret cannot be retrieved.
- Ferrets that are neutered early weigh from 0.8 to 1.2 kg when adult.
- Unneutered animals are larger, especially males.
- The ferret has a life span of 5 to 8 years, body temperature of 100° to 104°F (37.8° to 40°C), heart rate of 180 to 250 beats/min, and respiratory rate of 33 to 36 breaths/min.
- A ferret's skin is remarkably thick, especially over the neck and shoulders.
- Ferrets experience a seasonal change in body fat, losing weight in the summer and gaining it back in the winter.
  - They also molt in the spring and fall.
- Ferrets do not have sweat glands in their skin and thus are prone to heat stroke.
- Their claws are not retractable, as in cats, and need to be trimmed.
- The canine teeth are prominent, as they are in other carnivorous animals.
- Ferrets have a simple stomach and short small intestine.
  - They do not have a cecum.
- Ferrets have well-developed anal glands that produce a foul-smelling liquid when they are frightened.
- The sebaceous secretions of their skin produce the animals' odor.
- Ferrets originating from large breeding farms are routinely descented and neutered when they are 5 to 6 weeks of age before entering the pet market.
- Female ferrets are called **jills** and males are called **hobs**; young are called kits.
- A neutered female is called a sprite and a neutered male a gib.
- The preputial opening in male ferrets is located on the ventral abdomen, as in male dogs, and the os penis is readily palpable.
- The urogenital opening in female ferrets is located in the perineal region ventral to the anus.
- Most ferrets are docile and can be easily examined without undue restraint.
- Assistance is usually needed to give medications.
- Tractable ferrets can be lightly restrained on the examination table.
- An active ferret can be restrained by scruffing the loose skin on the back of the neck and suspending it off the table.
- Many animals can be distracted by feeding Nutri-Cal with a syringe or placing a small amount of it on their fur for them to lick.
- Ferrets are highly susceptible to canine distemper; they must be vaccinated against this virus because canine distemper is typically a fatal disease in ferrets.
- Ear mites are common in ferrets, and they are also susceptible to human influenza virus.
- Adrenal gland disease and insulinomas are common conditions seen in older pet ferrets.

- If female ferrets are not spayed, they frequently remain in estrus if they are not bred.
  - They can develop estrogen toxicity with bone marrow suppression and severe anemia.

Rodents

- Mice, rats, gerbils, hamsters, guinea pigs, and chinchillas are rodents.
- Rodents have four continuously erupting, chisel-like incisors and powerful jaw muscles that account for their gnawing ability.
- They are nocturnal for the most part, being more active at night rather than during the day.
- The gender of most rodents can be determined by evaluating anogenital distance; this is longer in males and shorter in females (Fig. 11.2).
- Rodents are usually prolific breeders.
- The term **murine** specifically refers to mice and rats.
- Guinea pigs and chinchillas are hystricomorph, or hedgehog-like, rodents related to porcupines.
- Although rodents do not require annual vaccinations, an annual examination is recommended to ensure good health and husbandry.

Mice

- The mouse (*Mus musculus*) is a small rodent, easily housed and handled, and relatively inexpensive to purchase and maintain as a pet.
- Mice may live up to 3 years.
- They weigh 20 to 40 g and have a rapid heart rate ($\approx$500 to 600 beats/min), rapid respiration rate, and body temperature of 97.7° to 100.4°F (36.5° to 38°C).
- Mice have a high metabolic rate and are constantly active.
- Mice spend much of their time grooming and keeping their environment organized.
- Mice can be caught and safely picked up by grasping the scruff of the neck with forceps or by grasping the base of the tail with the fingers (Fig. 11.3).
- For manipulation or examination, the animal is caught by the base of the tail and placed on a surface that it can grasp, such as the cage lid.
  - The scruff of the neck is then grasped by the thumb and forefinger, and the mouse is inverted to lie on its back with its tail positioned between the palm of your hand and little finger.
- Clear plastic restraint devices can also be used for restraint and manipulation.
- A dominant mouse sometimes chews the fur off a subordinate mouse in the facial area.
  - This harmless behavior is called **barbering**.
- Unlike female mice, male mice housed together frequently fight.
  - Bite wounds are inflicted on the back and rump.

Rats

- The common rat (*Rattus norvegicus*) found in pet stores was developed from the wild brown Norway rat.
- Rats are burrowers and communal critters.

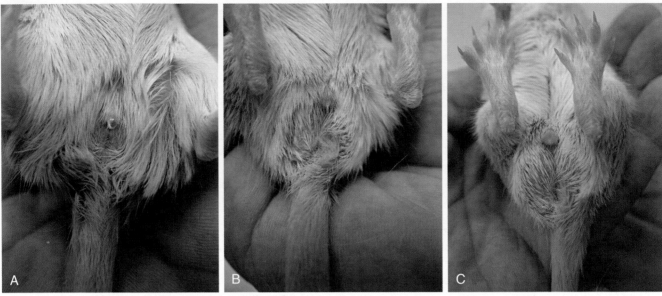

FIGURE 11.2 External genitalia of gerbils. (A) Female. (B, C) Male. Note that the anogenital distance of the female is shorter than that of the male. The adult male can also be determined by the presence of testicles in the scrotum (C), but the frightened gerbil may retract the testicles from the scrotum (B). (From Mitchell M, Tully TN Jr: *Manual of exotic pet practice*, St Louis, 2008, Saunders.)

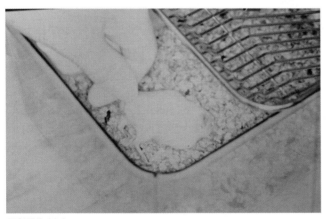

FIGURE 11.3 Proper technique for removal of a mouse from its cage. (From Sirois M: *Principles and practice of veterinary technology*, ed 3, St Louis, 2011, Mosby.)

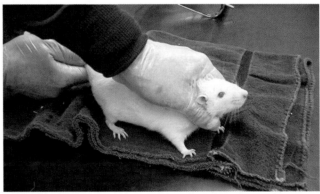

FIGURE 11.4 Restraining a rat. (Sheldon CC, Sonsthagen TF, Topel JA: *Animal restraint for veterinary professionals*, St Louis, 2006, Mosby.)

- The life span of the rat is 2.5 to 3.5 years.
- Rats weigh 250 to 500 g, with females being smaller than males.
- The body temperature of rats is 97° to 100°F (36° to 37.5°C).
- Rats have continuously erupting incisors and cheeks that close into the diastema, a space that separates the incisors from the oral cavity.
- Rats have no gallbladder.
- The Harderian gland, a lacrimal gland located caudal to the eyeball, secretes a red, porphyrin-rich secretion that lubricates the eye.
  - In times of stress or illness, red tears overflow and stain the face and nose.

- Rats can be caught and safely picked up by grasping the base of the tail to transport them a short distance, such as when changing cages.
- When rats are held upside down, they are more interested in righting themselves than in biting the handler.
- To restrain for manipulation or examination, pick up the rat by placing your hand firmly over the back and rib cage and restraining the rat's head and shoulders with your thumb and forefinger (Fig. 11.4).
  - If additional control is needed, the base of the tail may be restrained with the other hand.
- An alternative method is to pin the rat with your free hand while pulling on the base of the tail.
  - Position your index and third fingers to grasp either side of the rat's neck caudal to the mandible firmly;

the thumb and other fingers are used to restrain the chest gently.

Hamsters

- The Syrian or golden hamster *(Mesocricetus auratus)* originated in the Middle East and is the most common species of hamster in the pet trade and in research.
  - It is noted for its ease of taming, low waste production, and lack of odor.
- The golden hamster is stocky and short tailed, weighs approximately 120 g, and has a reddish–golden brown body color with a gray ventrum.
- Other color varieties, such as cinnamon, cream, white, piebald, albino, and long-haired teddy bears, are popular as pets.
- The Chinese or striped hamster *(Cricetulus griseus)* is gray-brown with a dark stripe down its back and is smaller than the golden hamster, weighing 35 g.
  - It tends to be more difficult to handle and thus is not as popular as a pet.
  - Female Chinese hamsters are belligerent and must be housed individually.
- Caging should be selected with the knowledge that hamsters are adept cage chewers and escape artists.
- Plastic tubes frequently sold as cage extensions are easily chewed through.
- Hamsters usually have a life span of 1.5 to 2 years.
- Females are usually larger than males and, unlike most mammals, tend to fight more readily and are generally more aggressive.
  - Males therefore live longer than females.
- On occasion, hamsters are cannibalistic.
- Hamsters have cheek pouches that can transport an amazing amount of food and bedding.
- A female hamster sometimes packs her whole newborn litter in her pouches to move them to another location.
- The hamster's cheek pouches are considered an immunologically privileged site; therefore they have been used in research settings for the study of transplanted tumors.
- Hamsters have extremely loose skin.
- Marking glands, called flank or hip glands, are located in the skin of both flanks and are more prominent in males.
- Hamsters are permissive hibernators, so when temperatures fall below 46°F (8°C), some hamsters become inactive for periods of 2 to 3 days.
  - During this transient state of hibernation, they have a reduced body temperature and reduced heart and respiratory rates.
  - When hamsters are group-housed, the nonhibernating hamsters will on occasion cannibalize the sleeping hamsters.
- Hamsters are sound sleepers and, on casual observation, may appear dead.
  - An important point to remember when handling a hamster is to avoid surprising it.

- Make sure that the hamster is awake and knows that the handler intends to pick it up.
- Startled or awakened hamsters often bite.
- Hamsters are most easily moved by grasping the loose skin across the shoulders or using your hands as a scoop to transfer the hamster from one cage to another.
  - They can also be picked up in a small can or cup.
- To restrain a hamster, gently grasp the loose skin across the back by curling your fingers and thumb around opposite sides of the animal to gather in as much loose skin as possible.
  - Grasp the skin, not the body, of the hamster (Fig. 11.5).
  - An alternative method is to reverse your hand so that your thumb and forefinger hold the skin at the base of the tail.

Gerbils

- The Mongolian gerbil *(Meriones unguiculatus)* is a native to desert regions of Mongolia and northeastern China.
- Gerbils are active, burrowing, social animals that tend to be more exploratory than other rodents.
- The gerbil is clean and produces little waste, is relatively odorless, is nonaggressive, and is easy to handle, making it a good pocket pet.
- The agouti or mixed-brown gerbil is the color variety most commonly seen, but black and other colors, such as piebald, white, and cinnamon, are available.
- The gerbil, or jird, as it is sometimes referred to, has an average life span of 3 years and weighs less than 100 g when mature.
- Gerbils have long hindlimbs adapted for leaping and, unlike most other rodents, they have a hair-covered tail.

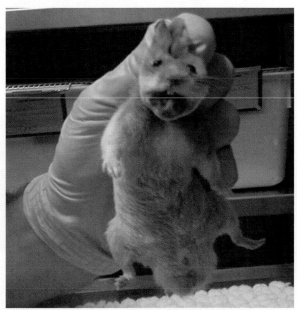

FIGURE 11.5 Holding the hamster. (Sheldon CC, Sonsthagen TF, Topel JA: *Animal restraint for veterinary professionals*, St Louis, 2006, Mosby.)

- When threatened or excited, gerbils will drum their hind legs on the cage flooring.
- Gerbils have large adrenal glands, adaptive mechanisms for temperature extremes, and a unique ability to conserve water.
- Gerbils have a high cholesterol level and lipemic serum.
- Both sexes have a distinct dark orange midventral sebaceous gland, which is used for territorial marking.

- A gerbil can be safely picked up by cupping both hands under it or by grasping the base of the tail to lift it from its cage.
- To restrain the gerbil for examination or injection, the loose skin at the nape of the neck is grasped with one hand and the base of the tail is grasped with the other hand (Fig. 11.6).
- Extreme care must be taken not to grasp the tip of the tail because the skin may tear and slip off, exposing the underlying muscle and vertebrae.

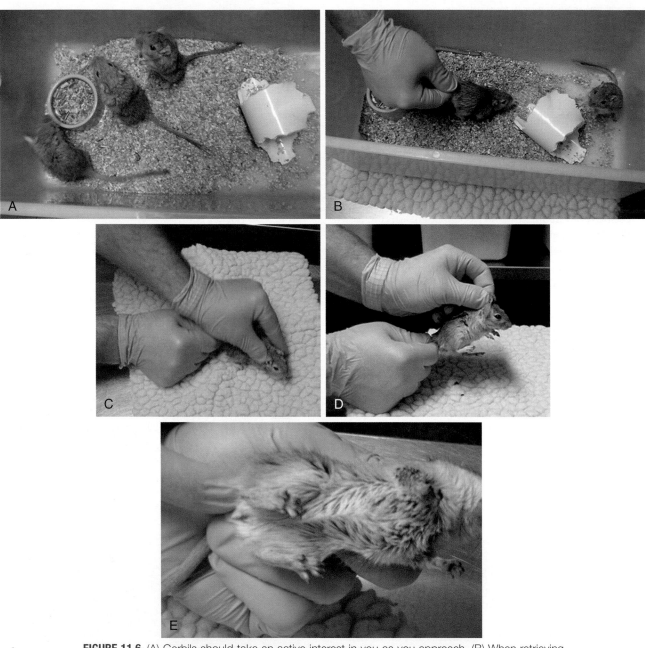

FIGURE 11.6 (A) Gerbils should take an active interest in you as you approach. (B) When retrieving the gerbil, reach into its enclosure, bringing your hand from over its head to grasp its tail firmly at the base. (C) Firmly hold the base of the animal's tail while you scruff the animal with your other hand. (D) You can then pick the animal up. (E) Once you have a good hold of the animal's scruff, you can transfer the base of its tail to your little finger on the hand with which you are scruffing so that the animal rests in the palm of your hand. (From Sheldon CC, Sonsthagen TF, Topel JA: *Animal restraint for veterinary professionals*, St Louis, 2006, Mosby.)

- Alternatively, an over-the-back grip can be used.
- Gerbils resist being placed on their back.

Guinea Pigs

- The guinea pig (*Cavia porcellus*), often referred to as a cavy, is a tailless rodent with a compact, stocky body and short legs.
- Guinea pigs originated in South America and are a hystricomorph rodent related to chinchillas and porcupines.
- The guinea pig makes a nice children's pet because it is docile and seldom bites or scratches.
- Guinea pigs have a variety of vocalizations and frequently whistle and squeak when a caregiver approaches their cage.
- Guinea pigs are messy housekeepers and commonly scatter food and bedding.
- Guinea pigs can be monocolored, bicolored, or tricolored.
- The most common pet variety is the English, American, or short-haired guinea pig.
- The Abyssinian has short, rough hair arranged in whorls or rosettes; the Peruvian or rag mop variety has long, silky hair.
- The guinea pig weighs 700 to 1200 g as an adult, has a normal body temperature of 99° to 103°F (37.2° to 39.5°C), and has a life span of 4 to 5 years.
- Guinea pigs have four digits on their front limbs and three digits on their hind limbs.
- All teeth are open rooted and erupt continuously.
- Guinea pigs have a large cecum and a long colon.
- Guinea pigs are actively coprophagic.
- Guinea pig urine is normally opaque and creamy yellow and contains crystals.
- Marking glands are located around the anus and on the rump.
- Both male and female guinea pigs have inguinal nipples.
- Sexing is difficult because, unlike other rodents, there is little difference in the anogenital distance in males and females.
  - The female has a Y-shaped anogenital opening and vaginal membrane that remains intact and closed, except during the few days of estrus and at parturition.
  - Males have scrotal pouches lateral to the anogenital line and a penis that can be protruded by manual pressure.
- The guinea pig usually responds to danger in one of two ways: either by becoming immobile for up to 20 minutes or by the scatter response, in which they run for their lives.
- Female guinea pigs are called sows, males are called boars, and the act of giving birth is called farrowing.
- The sow is polyestrous throughout the year and has an estrous cycle of 15 to 17 days.
- A sow should be bred for the first time before 6 months of age, before fusion of the pubic bones, to prevent dystocia.
- The gestation period is lengthy, averaging 68 days.
  - Larger litters have shorter gestation periods.

- Neonates are precocious and almost self-sufficient.
  - They are born fully furred, with eyes and ears open and teeth erupted.
- Young guinea pigs eat solid food within the first few days postpartum and can be weaned at 14 to 21 days.
- Guinea pigs have rigid eating habits, and any change in food or water may cause them to stop eating.
- Dietary vitamin C must be provided to guinea pigs because, like primates, they cannot synthesize their own vitamin C; lack of vitamin C causes scurvy.
- To restrain a guinea pig, lift the animal by grasping under the trunk with one hand while supporting the rear quarters with your other hand.
- It is especially important to use a two-hand support method with adult and pregnant animals.
- An alternative method is to place one hand over the shoulder area, with your thumb and forefingers just caudal to the front legs, while the other hand supports the rear quarters.
  - Use care not to compress the chest too much with this method.

Chinchillas

- The chinchilla (*Chinchilla laniger*) has a compact body, delicate limbs, large eyes, large round ears, long whiskers, and a bushy tail.
- Chinchillas have a soft, very dense hair coat that is normally bluish-gray, with yellow-white underparts.
- Chinchillas are quiet, shy animals that adapt well to humans when handled at a young age. They rarely bite and are almost odorless.
- Chinchillas are very active, agile, and like to climb and jump.
  - They require a larger cage than guinea pigs, who tend to be less active.
- The chinchilla weighs 400 to 600 g as an adult.
- Chinchillas have a normal body temperature of 99° to 100°F (37° to 38°C) and a life span of 10 years.
- Chinchillas have four toes on their front and rear feet.
- Like the guinea pig, chinchilla teeth are open rooted and ever growing.
- Chinchillas have a long gastrointestinal (GI) tract and are coprophagic.
- The female has a vaginal closure membrane that remains intact and closed except during a few days of estrus and at parturition.
- The anogenital distance is the best criterion for sexing chinchillas.
  - The female has a large urinary papilla that can be confused with a penis.
  - The penis can be protruded by manual pressure to confirm the sex.
  - Males do not have a true scrotum; the testes are contained within the open inguinal canal or abdomen.
- A tamed chinchilla will willingly come out of its cage.
- To restrain it, place one hand under the abdomen or around the scruff of the neck and hold it by the base of the tail with your other hand.

- If the chinchilla escapes from its cage, you must be fast to catch it.
  - Use care because a frightened chinchilla can lose a patch of fur where it is grasped.
  - This condition is called fur slip and is a predator avoidance mechanism.
  - It takes 6 to 8 weeks for the hairless patch to fill in.
- Access to a dust bath should be provided for 1 hour daily to prevent matted fur.
- Commercial chinchilla dust or a mixture of silver sand and Fuller earth can be used.
- One inch of dust is placed in a pan big enough for the chinchilla to roll around in and fluff its fur.
- Chinchillas are susceptible to many of the same bacterial diseases as guinea pigs.
- The bones of chinchillas are thin and fragile; it is common to see traumatic fractures.
  - The tibia is particularly fragile, being longer than the femur, and has little soft tissue covering it.
- Chinchillas are prone to heat stroke at an environmental temperature in excess of 82° to 86°F (28° to 30°C), especially when coupled with high humidity.

General Nursing Care of Small Mammals

- Because of the cost involved in hospitalization and intensive care, most pet rodents are treated on an outpatient basis, whereas rabbits and ferrets are often hospitalized.
- Pet rodents that must be hospitalized are usually critically ill.
  - These patients should be handled as little as possible.
- Fluid therapy, antibiotics, nutritional support, and proper environment are important.
- The proper ambient temperature must be maintained.
  - Incubators serve this function well; however, care must be taken not to overheat small mammals.
  - The temperature should be kept no warmer than 80°F (25°C).
  - Temperatures above this often result in death from heat stroke.
- When necessary, oxygen can be supplemented through a port on the incubator.
- Food and water should be offered, even if forced feeding is needed.
- When possible, small mammals should be isolated from other hospitalized animals, not only because of the risk of disease spread (e.g., *Bordetella* spp. passed from dogs, cats, or rabbits to guinea pigs) but also because these sick pets are extremely stressed.
- Most small mammals are prey in the wild so housing them near a natural predator such as a dog or cat may increase their stress level.

Diagnostic and Treatment Techniques

- Techniques used to diagnose disease in companion and food animals are used in small mammals.

- Some techniques such as skin scrapings can be more challenging in rodents because they are very mobile and can be difficult to restrain.
- Diagnostic testing is important because many of these pets present with vague complaints such as lethargy and lack of appetite.
- The small size of these animals makes it more difficult to obtain adequate laboratory samples.
- In the research setting, the health status of the rodent colony is often more important than the health status of an individual animal.
- Health status is frequently monitored by serologic testing of sentinel animals that are placed in the colony.

Venipuncture

- Venipuncture is a technique commonly used for ferrets and rabbits but infrequently used for pet rodents.
- Venipuncture is used for withdrawing blood for hematologic and biochemical analysis, administration of certain medications, and catheterization for administration of fluids.
- Anesthesia may be required when performing venipuncture on small mammals.
- Although each diagnostic laboratory has specific requirements for the volume of blood required for various tests, most laboratories can perform a minibattery of tests (e.g., complete blood count [CBC], chemistries, electrolytes) on 0.5 mL of blood collected in a green-topped (lithium heparin) tube.
- Special blood collection tubes (e.g., Microvette), which hold a maximum of 0.3 mL, are commercially available.
  - These are particularly useful when collecting samples from small rodents.

  Rodents
- Small blood samples can be collected from rodents by superficial venipuncture.
- The lateral saphenous vein is a good superficial vessel to use.
- Other superficial vessels that can be used include the cephalic vein, jugular vein, and tail vessels in rodents that have long tails (Fig. 11.7).
- The central vena cava of guinea pigs is easily accessible, but they must be anesthetized first.
- The orbital sinus is frequently used to collect blood from anesthetized rodents.
- Cardiac puncture can also be used in an anesthetized rodent, but is not recommended except for collection before euthanasia.

  Rabbits
- The marginal ear veins and central ear artery of the rabbit are easily visualized and can be used to collect blood (Fig. 11.8).
- Blood can be collected with a syringe and needle or by cannulating the vessel and collecting the blood in a blood tube or heparinized microhematocrit tube as it drips freely from the vessel.

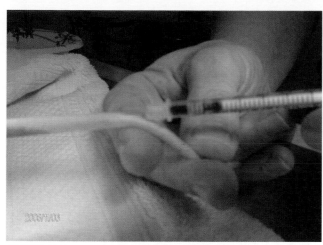

FIGURE 11.7 Blood collection from the tail vein of a rat. (From Sirois M: *Principles and practice of veterinary technology*, ed 3, St Louis, 2011, Mosby.)

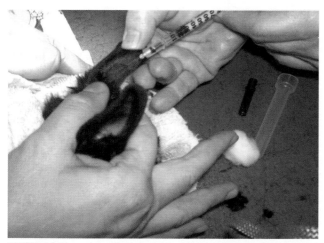

FIGURE 11.8 The marginal ear vein can be used for blood collection or small-volume IV injections in rabbits. (From Sirois M: *Principles and practice of veterinary technology*, ed 3, St Louis, 2011, Mosby.)

- Jugular venipuncture is also fairly easy and is collected in a manner similar to that used for dogs and cats.
- The veterinary assistant will restrain the rabbit in ventral recumbency.
- The cephalic vein tends to be a more difficult vessel from which to collect blood.
  Ferrets
- The cephalic vein, jugular vein, cranial vena cava, and lateral saphenous vein can be used to collect blood samples in ferrets.
- Venipuncture is most easily performed under isoflurane anesthesia maintained by face mask.
- When obtaining a jugular sample, the ferret is placed in dorsal recumbency, with the legs pulled caudally while the head and neck are extended dorsally.

- Venipuncture can be done in an awake, cooperative ferret.
- Obtaining small volumes of blood from larger ferrets is possible using the central artery of the tail.

Force Feeding

- Many small mammals present for veterinary care because of anorexia and lethargy.
  - In addition to the need for rehydration, nutritional supplementation is often required but overlooked.
- Small mammals such as rodents have high metabolic rates and thus high energy requirements.
  - Animals that are not eating are in a catabolic state.
  - Decreased food intake results in the breakdown of protein and fat for energy.
  - This can contribute to hepatic lipidosis (especially in rabbits), acidosis, azotemia, muscle wasting, impaired GI function, and decreased immunity.
  - To prevent or correct these complications, supplementation with food is important.
- Force feeding can be done in the hospital or by the owner at home if the pet will be treated on an outpatient basis.
- High-energy paste supplements such as Nutri-Cal can be given to all small mammals on a short-term basis.
- Sick rabbits often eat hay or greens, such as carrot tops and parsley, even if they refuse pellets.
  - These can be offered free choice.
  - Apples and yogurt can also be used.
- A nasogastric or gastric tube can be used to deliver a mixture of powdered pellets and water.
- Rodents' diets can be supplemented with apples and peanut butter.
  - Sweetened condensed milk is also a favorite.
  - Pedialyte or Gatorade can be fed via a small syringe for hydration, along with water.
  - Hospitalized ferrets can be force fed any of the diets suitable for cats.
- Meat-based baby foods can also be used.
- The food can be offered to the ferret to eat voluntarily or via syringe or tube.
- Warming the food slightly may increase the appetite of ferrets.

Administration of Medications

- With the exception of ferrets, small mammals are difficult to medicate with pills.
- Liquid oral medication given by eye dropper or small syringe is generally better accepted by the pet.
- Because of the small size of rodents, medications usually have to be diluted.
- For increased accuracy of dosing, it is important to have an accurate body weight and use a tuberculin syringe.
- Medication can also be administered orally by mixing the medication in the water or feed and by gavage needle.

- Rodents often do not drink medicated water because of its unpleasant taste.
- Injectable medications are usually preferred over oral medications in hospitalized small mammals.
- Extremely ill pets may have reduced intestinal function, making absorption of oral medication erratic and unpredictable.
  - Using the parenteral rather than the oral route of drug administration also decreases the possibility of GI problems in these small mammals.
- The standard routes of injection (IV, intramuscular [IM], subcutaneous [SC], intradermal [ID], intraperitoneal [IP]) are used for small mammals.
- Rodents have few readily accessible veins, making it difficult to administer drugs IV.
- Tail veins can be used in the mouse and rat.
- The marginal ear veins, located on the lateral sides of the pinna in the rabbit, are accessible and can be used for IV injections.
- Because it is difficult to carry out venous catheterization in small mammals, some doctors and technicians prefer intraosseous catheterization to administer fluids to critically ill exotic pets.
- The SC route is frequently used for fluid supplementation.
- SC fluids are given over the dorsal neck, back, and flank of small mammals.
- The small muscle mass of rodents makes it difficult to inject drugs IM.
  - For this reason, the IP route is more commonly used in rodents.
- Fluids can also be given IP in rodents, although this is least desirable because of the risk of peritonitis and laceration of internal organs.
  - When giving IP injections, it is best to use the caudal left abdominal quadrant and tilt the animal's head and forequarters ventrally.
  - This helps avoid accidental puncture of the internal organs in these animals (Fig. 11.9).

Antibiotics

- Caution must be used when administering antibiotics to rodents and rabbits.
  - These animals have a predominantly gram-positive GI flora and are sensitive to antibiotics that change the balance of the flora.
- Guinea pigs and rabbits are particularly prone to antibiotic-associated enterotoxemia.
  - Drugs such as ampicillin and penicillin will destroy susceptible gram-positive organisms and allow for the overgrowth of *Clostridium difficile* and production of its toxin.
- Safe antibacterials for use in rabbits and rodents include enrofloxacin, ciprofloxacin, trimethoprim-sulfamethoxazole, and chloramphenicol.
- If diarrhea develops, drug administration should be stopped immediately and the animal examined.
- Ferrets can be treated safely with most antibacterials used for cats.

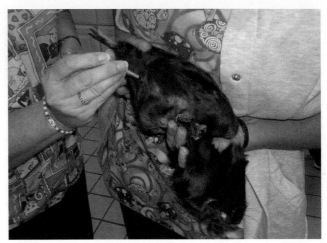

FIGURE 11.9 The guinea pig should be held with its body tilted downward when administering an IP injection. (From Sirois M: *Principles and practice of veterinary technology*, ed 3, St Louis, 2011, Mosby.)

Vaccines

- Rodents and rabbits do not currently require annual vaccines.
- Ferrets must be vaccinated against canine distemper virus with an appropriate vaccine.
  - Never use canine combination vaccines or vaccines of ferret cell origin because of the possibility of vaccine-induced disease.
  - Give ferrets a series of vaccines at 6 to 8, 10 to 12, and 14 weeks of age and then annually.
  - Vaccination against rabies is highly recommended for ferrets, especially in rabies-endemic areas.
  - An inactivated rabies vaccine approved for use in ferrets should be given SC at 3 months of age and then annually.

Fecal Analysis

- Microscopic fecal analysis is used to evaluate animals with diarrhea and any nonspecific complaint.
- A fresh fecal smear and flotation test should be performed.
- A cellophane tape test can be used on the anal region to check for the presence of pinworms in rodents.

Urinalysis

- Urine samples can be obtained by gentle manual expression of the bladder or cystocentesis.
- Rodents can be placed on a cold surface or in a cooled plastic bag until urine is voided.

BIRDS

- The common companion birds seen in a small animal veterinary hospital are typically members of the psittacine or passerine family (Box 11.1).

BOX 11.1 Common Companion Species Seen in an Avian Practice

Psittacines
- Macaw
- Cockatoo
- Amazon
- African grey
- Love bird
- Conure
- Parakeet (budgerigar)
- Cockatiel
- Caique
- Lori
- Lorikeet

Passerines
- Finches
- Canaries

From Sirois M: Principles and practice of veterinary technology, ed 3, St Louis, 2011, Mosby.

- **Psittacines**, or parrots, make up the majority of avian patients.
  - The psittacines are known as hookbills because of their curved upper beak.
  - Their feet are shaped with the second and third toes facing forward and the first and fourth toes directed backward.
  - This is referred to as zygodactyl.
- **Passerines** are usually small birds with a pointed or slightly curved beak.
  - Their feet are **anisodactyl**—three toes point forward and one toe points to the rear.
  - Many of these birds are very active and tend to hop or fly about their cage.
  - Most are not trained to sit on their owner's hand and remain inside their cages.
  - Canaries and finches are the most frequently kept passerines.

Avian Anatomy

Integument
- The body of a bird is covered by skin and its derivatives, the beak, claws, and feathers.
- The skin is delicate and has a dry, slightly wrinkled appearance.
- Underlying muscles and blood give the skin a reddish appearance in some areas.
- The skin on the legs resembles the scales of reptiles.
- The **cere**, or the area around the nostrils, the beak, and the nails, are all modified skin.
- In parakeets (budgerigars), the cere is generally blue or pink and smooth in males and brown and lumpy in females.
- Sweat glands are absent in birds.

- The one major skin gland that most birds possess is the **uropygial gland**.
  - This gland has one duct that empties into a lone papilla, found dorsally at the base of the tail.
  - It secretes a fatty sebaceous material that is spread over feathers during preening to help with waterproofing.
  - This gland is absent in the ostrich, emu, cassowaries, bustards, frogmouth, many pigeons, woodpeckers, and Amazon parrots.
- Feathers are necessary for flight; they protect the skin from trauma and exposure and assist in thermoregulation, camouflage, and communication.
- Feather follicles are located in specific tracts over the surface of the body called pterylae. These tracts are separated by nonfeathered areas of skin called apteria.
  - These tracts overlap each other to give the bird a fully feathered look.
- Birds have several types of feathers (Fig. 11.10).
  - The **contour feathers** cover the body and wings and are identified as **flight feathers** or body feathers.
  - The large, primary flight feathers (remiges) are found on the outer end of the wing.
  - The secondary flight feathers are located on the wing between the body and the primaries.
  - Body feathers, also known as **coverts**, provide surface coverage over most of the rest of the bird.
  - **Down feathers** insulate the bird and have a soft, fluffy appearance.
  - Cockatoos, cockatiels, and African greys have powder down, which breaks down to produce a white, dusty powder.
  - A healthy bird of these species will have a fine layer of this powder over most of its body, most noticeably on the beak.
- Birds spend several hours a day preening, or rearranging and conditioning their feathers.
- **Molting** occurs in all species and results in the periodic replacement of old feathers.
  - A new, growing feather has a vascular supply until it reaches full size.
  - The shafts of these so-called blood feathers appear dark and bleed profusely if broken, possibly leading to the death of the bird.

Musculoskeletal System
- The skeleton of birds is highly modified.
- Some bones are **pneumatized**, or contain air, which results in a lighter skeleton.
- The bones have thin walls, which makes them lighter but also more fragile.
- The skull bones are fused, which strengthens the beak structure.
- The vertebrae of the neck are shaped so as to create a long, flexible neck.
- The large sternum, or **keel**, supports the pectoral muscles, which are needed for flight.

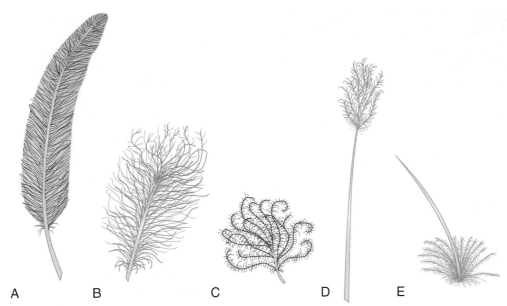

FIGURE 11.10 Types of feathers. (A) Contour. (B) Semiplume. (C) Down. (D) Filoplume. (E) Bristle. (From Colville T, Bassert JM: *Clinical anatomy and physiology for veterinary technicians*, ed 2, St Louis, 2008, Mosby.)

- A large portion of the caudal vertebrae is fused to form the synsacrum, which stabilizes the back during flight.
- The largest muscles in the body are the pectorals, which account for approximately 20% of the bird's weight.
- Because of their mass, they are used to determine the body condition of the bird and are ideal for IM injections.

Respiratory System
- Air enters the respiratory system through the nares and continues over an **operculum**, which is a cornified flap of tissue located immediately behind the nares in the nasal cavity.
- Air then travels through the many sinuses in the head and then enters the oral cavity through the slitlike opening in the roof of the mouth known as the **choana**.
- The choana is a V-shaped notch in the roof of the bird's mouth that directs air from the mouth and nasal cavities to the glottis.
  - The choana closes during swallowing.
  - This structure should be surrounded by many sharp papillae; blunted or absent papillae may indicate disease or malnutrition.
- Birds lack an epiglottis, so air travels through the glottis at the base of the tongue and down the trachea.
- The trachea is located on the left side of the cervical area, is mobile the entire length of the neck, and consists of complete cartilaginous rings that cannot expand.
- At the caudal portion of the trachea lies the **syrinx**, the voice box of birds.
  - Birds produce vocalizations by forcing air over the syrinx and vibrating membranes during the expiratory phase of respiration.

- The complexity of a bird's vocalizations depends on the species and number of muscles in the syrinx.
- The air continues into the small lungs located dorsally near the spine, where air exchange takes place.
  - There are no lobes or alveoli, so the lungs do not inflate.
- Inspiration of air occurs by extension of the intracostal joints, drawing in inspired air with a bellows-like action into the caudal air sacs.
- The **coelom** of a bird is a triangle-shaped cavity that allows for the bellows-like action during breathing.
- Both inspiration and expiration require active muscle contraction.
- Birds require the movement of their keel to achieve air exchange.
- If the keel is not allowed to expand (e.g., as with aggressive restraint), the bird cannot breathe and will go into respiratory and then cardiac arrest.
- Air flows into the air sacs, which are thin-walled hollow spaces that are lightly vascularized membranes found throughout the bird's body.
- There are a total of nine air sacs, consisting of one unpaired interclavicular air sac, located in the thoracic inlet between the clavicles, and four paired air sacs—cranial thoracic, caudal thoracic, cervical, and abdominal.
- Normal respiratory effort in the bird should not be noticeable, and the beak should remain closed.
- In some cases, there may be increased head and tail movements and increased abdominal effort after exercise; the bird should return to normal within a few minutes.

Digestive System
- The high metabolism of birds requires the ingestion of large amounts of food.

- The beak will vary with the diet and foraging strategies.
- Generally, the beak is used to grasp food and crush it with the aid of the tongue.
- Birds do not have teeth.
- The mouth consists of a hard upper palate, soft lower plate, distinctive tongue, and scattered taste buds and salivary glands.
- The mouth is relatively dry because little saliva is produced.
- When food is swallowed, it travels through the esophagus, a somewhat muscular tube that extends from the pharynx to the stomach along the right side of the neck.
- In several species, the esophagus expands into the interclavicular space to create a crop.
- The crop anatomy varies among species and can be a dilation of the esophagus, a single pouch, or a double pouch.
  - It softens food and allows continuous passage of small amounts of food to the proventriculus, or true stomach.
- The proventriculus is unique to birds; however, it is comparable to the stomach of mammals, containing digestive acid and enzymes.
- The food next passes into the ventriculus, or gizzard.
  - This is a thickly muscled organ that grinds food into smaller particles.
- Historically, it was thought that companion birds need grit, or small pieces of gravel, in the gizzard to break down hard foods; this is not true, and companion birds do not need to be given grit.
  - Grit can be problematic in some birds, and they may develop an impaction if they have access to it.
- The intestinal tract is comparable to that of mammals (Fig. 11.11).
- Birds have a pancreas, which is a relatively large gland that rests in the loop of the duodenum.
- The liver is bilobed, with the right side usually larger than the left.
- The gallbladder is absent in most parrots but is found in many other avian species.
- The duodenum or small intestine varies in length and diameter, depending on the species, and is the major organ responsible for digestion and absorption of nutrients.
- The large intestine is the segment that extends from the end of the small intestine and terminates at the cloaca.
- The cloaca is the common terminal chamber of the GI, urinary, and reproductive systems.
- The cloaca is divided into three compartments: the coprodeum, urodeum, and proctodeum.
  - The coprodeum is the cranial portion of the cloaca that receives feces from the rectum.
  - The urodeum is the middle part of the cloaca into which the ureters enter dorsolaterally on both sides; in males, the ductus deferens enters near the ureters, and in females a single oviduct enters the urodeum dorsolaterally on the left side.

- The proctodeum is the caudal part of the cloaca; if a phallus is present, it is located on the floor of the proctodeum.
- Psittacines do not have a phallus, but it is found in many other avian species.
- The external opening of the cloaca is called the vent, from which the droppings are passed.
- In most species, the vent is horizontally flattened, rather than circumferential, as in mammals.
- Normal bird droppings have three distinct components: liquid urine, semisolid white or cream urates, and feces.
  - The droppings will vary in consistency, depending on the diet.

Urinary System
- The paired kidneys of birds are closely attached to the vertebrae (see Fig. 11.11B).
- They empty into the ureters, which carry the liquid urine and semisolid urates to the cloaca.
- Urine is not concentrated in the kidneys; rather, urine moves into the coprodeum and rectum, where the resorption of water, sodium, and chloride takes place.
- Urates are the major excretion product in birds and compose the white portion of the droppings.
- Birds do not have a urinary bladder.
- A suddenly stressed bird, such as an avian patient on presentation after transport or an examination, may have an increased urine component to its droppings because the droppings pass before lower intestinal water resorption occurs; these are known as stress droppings.

Reproductive System
- In the female bird, only the left side of the reproductive tract develops fully.
  - As in mammals, an ovary, oviduct, and vagina are present.
  - Various regions of the oviduct produce the egg white and eggshell.
  - The entire process from ovulation to egg laying takes approximately 15 hours.
  - The female lays eggs even if no male is present.
- The male bird has paired testes located internally near the kidneys.
  - During periods of active breeding, they enlarge dramatically.
  - Sperm cells travel to the cloaca through the epididymis and then the ductus deferens.
  - Most birds do not have a penis or phallus, and mating takes place when the vents of the male and female birds come into contact.

Circulatory System
- The heart of birds closely resembles that of mammals, but it is proportionally about 1.5 times larger.

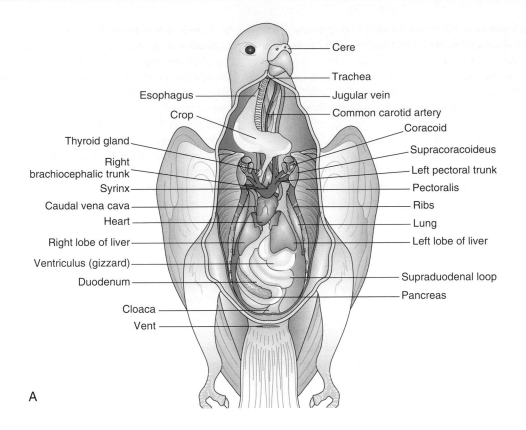

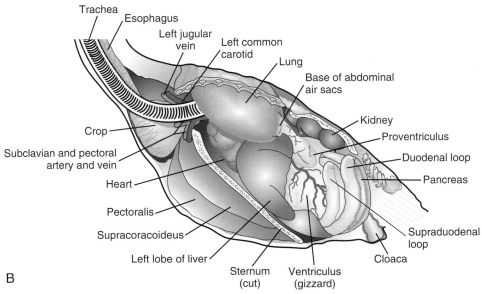

FIGURE 11.11 (A) Internal anatomy of a bird, ventrodorsal view. (B) Internal anatomy of a bird, lateral view. (From O'Malley B: *Clinical anatomy and physiology of exotic species*, Oxford, England, 2005, Saunders.)

- The heart rate ranges from 250 to 350 beats/min in large parrots and up to 1400 beats/min in the very small species.
- Blood pressure in birds is typically higher than in mammals.
- The red blood cells of birds are oval and contain a nucleus.

- Birds do not have lymph nodes and the lymphatic system is less extensive.

Special Senses

- As with mammals, birds have the traditional five senses: seeing, hearing, feeling, smelling, and tasting.

- The brain of a bird is large in proportion to its body size.
- The location and control centers within the brain that receive and process stimuli from the senses are comparable to those of mammals, with several exceptions.
- In birds, the control centers for vision and hearing are larger than those for taste, touch, and smell.
- Vision is highly developed in the avian species.
- The eyes of birds are relatively large, and a significant part of the avian skull is devoted to housing and protecting the eyes (Fig. 11.12).
- Bird eyes can be round, flat, or tubular, depending on the species.
  - Diurnal birds, birds that forage or hunt in the daytime, have round or relatively flat eyes, whereas **nocturnal species**, those that forage and hunt at night, have tubular eyes.
  - Tubular eyes have a pupil with a larger diameter than the retina, allowing more light into the eye.
- The lens and anterior chamber of the avian eye are comparable to those of mammals, with the exception of the presence of a highly vascular, ribbon-like structure called the pecten.

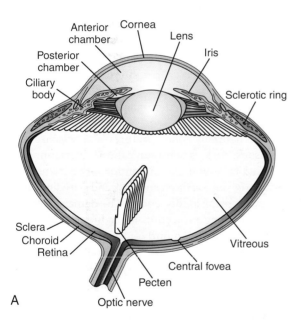

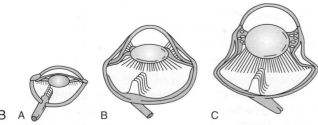

FIGURE 11.12 (A) The avian eye, transverse section. (B) Shapes of the avian eye. *A,* Flat. *B,* Round. *C,* Tubular. (From Colville T, Bassert JM: *Clinical anatomy and physiology for veterinary technicians,* ed 2, St Louis, 2008, Mosby.)

- The pecten is believed to provide nutrition to the eye.
- Bird vision is acute, and they can perceive color.
- Birds often look closely at something with one eye, tilting their head for a better view.
- In many species, the color of the iris is darker in young birds.
- The iris contains striated muscles that allow voluntary control over the size of the pupils.
  - Thus the pupillary light response is not a good diagnostic indicator in birds; however, this should always be part of a thorough physical examination.
- Blinking is done using the nictitating membrane, or third eyelid.
  - This structure is mostly transparent.
- Most birds close their eyes completely when they sleep.
- The avian ear is simpler than that of mammals but has exceptional acoustic ability.
- Located on the sides of the head and slightly below the eyes, the ears of birds are hidden from view by feathers that protect the ear during flight and yet allow sound to pass through.
- The external auditory canal funnels sound to the middle ear and tympanic membrane.
- There is a single bone in the middle ear called the **columella**, in contrast to the three bones in mammals, and it connects to the inner ear.
- The inner ear is comparable to that in mammals and consists of a membranous labyrinth that helps maintain balance and equilibrium and converts sounds into nerve impulses that are sent to the brain.
- Birds have fewer taste buds than most mammals; these are located on the roof of the mouth and scattered over the soft palate.
- The sense of smell varies greatly in birds.
  - In a few species, such as the turkey vulture, the sense of smell is highly developed for locating food, but in the average companion species it is thought that the sense of smell is poorly developed.
- The sense of touch is an important sense in many species for finding food and for defense.
- The skin of birds contains sensory nerve endings that respond to pain, heat, cold, and touch.

Basic Pet Bird Behavior

- Veterinary clinics that provide care for companion birds must also be prepared to assist clients with behavior complaints.
- Many birds are needlessly abused, ignored, abandoned at shelters or rescue societies, put up for adoption, or euthanized because the client has a lack of understanding of natural or adapted bird behaviors.
- Birds have been kept as companions for hundreds of years but are far from domestic.
  - They are genetically close to their wild ancestors and retain many of the characteristics of their wild relatives.

- Most birds have a higher-than-average intelligence, resulting in a patient that is both entertaining and challenging to alter behaviors in.

Common Behaviors

- Many of the behaviors that owners wish to modify are the result of instinctive avian reactions or related to the stresses of captivity.
- Many parrots use their agile feet to hold food while they eat or manipulate objects that they are interested in exploring.
- They tend to be good climbers, often moving around their cage using a combination of beak and feet.
- Birds will wag their tail back and forth when happy and relaxed.
- Birds grind their beak when they are comfortable and ready to fall asleep.
- Some birds will regurgitate food for those to which they are closely bonded, whether it is the owner or another bird.
- The typical behavior that indicates defecation in a calm bird is a slight wiggle of the tail, followed by a squat and an uplifted tail.
- All birds defecate frequently and more often when afraid or stressed.
- Fear is a common behavior when the bird is in the clinic; personnel should be aware of this and take appropriate measures to reduce the stress involved with the visit.
- When a bird is frightened, it may fling itself about the cage, struggle violently, flap its wings, bite, scream loudly, or take flight in response to sudden movements or unfamiliar sights or sounds.

Chewing

- Mouthing is a term used to describe a juvenile parrot that uses its tongue to explore surfaces.
- Juvenile parrots pass through an innocent beaking phase, in which they attempt to taste or chew almost anything, somewhat like puppies.
  - Contrary to puppies, birds do not grow out of this behavior.
- Clients should be counseled to supervise the parrot when out of its cage and provide the pet with safe, well-designed toys that can be destroyed.
- Toys that are safe to destroy, such as paper-based manufactured, homemade, or natural wood toys embedded with nuts, provide much-needed enrichment for these intelligent confined creatures.

Biting

- Birds bite to exhibit dominance, express fear, or exhibit jealousy or as a result of hormonal fluctuations during puberty or the breeding season.
- Biting may not be an instinctual behavior, but rather one that captive birds have developed in confinement.
- In the wild, the beak is used primarily for eating, preening, and communication.

- If a conflict arises, most birds generally fly away rather than using their beak as a weapon.
- Some protective birds may bite the owner in an effort to communicate with the person to move away from perceived danger.
- It is important for the owner to realize that the bird must not be allowed to bite as a way of controlling a situation.
- Mature parrots are more likely to bite during handling as a method of defense.
- The larger psittacines, such as macaws, can exert up to 300 pounds pressure per square inch (psi), inflicting deep bruises and lacerations.
- Birds such as cockatiels and parakeets have the potential to draw blood with their bites.
- Biting is a common behavior problem; identifying why the bird is biting is the first step to a resolution.

Dominance

- Psittacines may attempt to become dominant over their flock, and in the captive companion bird world, the flock is their human family.
- Birds should be taught consistently to step up on or down from the owner's hand when asked.
- Clipping the bird's wings to limit its flying ability can diminish dominance behaviors, such as flying down from a curtain rod to attack members of the household.
- When holding the bird, keep it at midchest level; never allowing it to sit on the head or shoulders keeps it from attaining the highest perch, a position of great power.
- Situating the cage or perches so that the bird is below eye level also discourages dominant behavior.

Vocalization

- Parrots are naturally loud creatures and vocalize for many reasons, such as communication, entertainment, exercise, and in response to discomfort or restraint.
- Birds tend to be noisy at dawn and dusk and at feeding time.
- Parrots can scream loudly enough to damage human hearing, so hearing protection is recommended when working with companion birds.
- Some of these birds have the ability to repeat what they hear; some will recite any unsavory word or derogatory phrase and bodily function sounds if these scenarios are repetitive.
- Vocalizations may become a problem in some insecure or dependent birds that call constantly to their owner.
- Some species are relatively quiet, but all birds make a certain amount of noise.
- Owners may inadvertently encourage the bird to make more noise by responding to the bird's loud calls with anger or shouting in an effort to quiet the bird.

Self-Mutilation and Feather Destructive Behavior

- Feather destructive behavior, also called feather picking or plucking, is a well-known but poorly understood condition.
- The bird uses its beak to chew on and pull out any feathers that are accessible, including any that start to grow back.

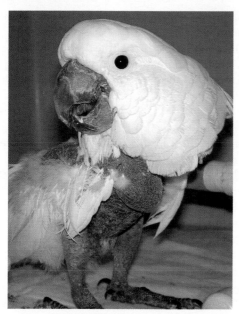

FIGURE 11.13 Some birds will remove all the feathers that they can reach, such as this cockatoo with a featherless body and fully feathered head. (From Sirois M: *Principles and practice of veterinary technology*, ed 3, St Louis, 2011, Mosby.)

- Some birds remove all but the feathers on their heads, and some may damage muscle as well as skin (Fig. 11.13).
- Some affected birds may have an underlying medical condition that initiates plucking, but some healthy birds respond to stress with self-mutilation.
- Stresses can be in the form of separation anxiety from the owner, a change in the cage location, or the addition of a new pet or family member.
  - This is a difficult problem to solve and may become a chronic condition.
  - It is most common in cockatoo species and African grey parrots.
- The most important first step in correcting this behavior is a thorough medical workup to rule out any underlying pathologic conditions.
- Once feather destructive behavior has been established, behavior modification and training may decrease the severity of the disorder but will rarely stop the habit completely.

Inappropriate Bonding
- Some owners will unintentionally allow a parrot to form a sexual bond with them by inappropriate petting.
- Petting the bird repeatedly over its back and tail sends a message to that bird that is comparable to courtship behaviors performed in the wild.
- Cuddling and feeding the bird warm foods by hand or mouth can have similar inappropriate bonding results.
- The bird may pant and masturbate; this is especially common in cockatoos.
  - Chronic masturbation can lead to medical problems that may require corrective surgery.

- Correction of behavior problems takes time, an understanding of the underlying cause, and judicious use of behavior modification.
- Prolonged physical or mental isolation of the bird, withholding food or water, and physical punishment are totally unacceptable methods of dealing with these problems.
  - All may result in permanent emotional or physical damage to the bird.

Housing and Husbandry

- Enclosures for birds come in many shapes and sizes designed to appeal to the client but that may fail to address the needs of the bird.
- The enclosure should be spacious; the minimum size would allow the bird to spread its wings without touching the sides of the cage.
- It should be easy to clean and disinfect regularly and be constructed of a durable, nontoxic material.
- Newspapers or paper towels are inexpensive, safe substrates for birds and do not promote the growth of pathogens as do other organic substrates such as wood shavings and corncob bedding.
  - Some of the latter substrates can also be ingested and create a GI foreign body with the possibility of obstruction.
- The position of the enclosure should be in a draft-free area, partially out of direct sunlight, and in an area of the house in which the family routinely congregates.
- Perches should be made from branches of clean, nontoxic hardwood trees and shrubs free of pesticides, mold, or wood rot.
- Birds need varying sizes, textures, and irregularly shaped perches to decrease the pressure placed on any one point of the foot and decrease the potential for pododermatitis.
- Food dishes, toys, mirrors and other accessories should be provided without overcrowding the bird.
- If there is insufficient room to move about, the bird may not exercise appropriately and become entrapped in parts of the accessories or toys and be injured.
- Toys should be made of nontoxic substances and of an appropriate size for the bird so as not to allow for ingestion of the pieces.
- Nutrition is an important subject and requires a handout for routine inquiries.
  - Fresh water should be provided at all times.
  - The water dish should be placed high in the bird's cage and not below any perches to decrease the possibility of fecal contamination.
  - Birds should be offered fresh food on a daily basis.
  - The optimal diet consists of a variety of pellets (70%) and fresh fruits and vegetables (30%).
  - Feeding the bird at the dinner table and from the client's mouth should be discouraged because some human foods are too high in salts and sugars and some can be toxic to the bird, such as chocolate and avocado.

- Conversion from seeds to pellets is encouraged; clients may need assistance with this task in the form of a handout and face-to-face or telephone consultations.

Beak, Wing, and Nail Trimming

Beak Trimming

- Overgrowth of the beak in psittacines is a common deformity (Fig. 11.14).
- It is important to know (or have a reference for) the normal lengths of the beaks of various species.
- In some cases, overgrowth results from malocclusion, resulting in insufficient wear on the beak; liver disease can be another cause.
- Any patient presenting for beak overgrowth should be required to have a complete workup to determine the cause.
- Reducing the length and grooming the beak can be done with a Dremel Moto-Tool (Dremel, Racine, WI).
  - Cone-shaped aluminum oxide grinding stones work well on beaks and toenails.
  - To prevent the spread of disease, it is best to have a separate grinding stone for each patient, which you can sell to the owner and the owner can bring to each visit.
- To perform this procedure, the restrainer holds the bird in an upright position.
  - The person performing the trim holds the beak closed with one hand and applies the Dremel with the other.
  - Care should be taken not to cover the nares as you hold the beak shut.

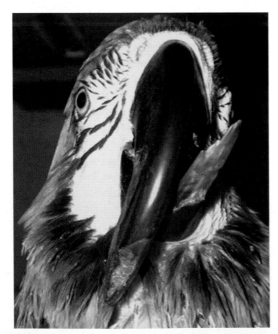

FIGURE 11.14 The need for a beak trim will be obvious in some patients. (From Sirois M: *Principles and practice of veterinary technology*, ed 3, St Louis, 2011, Mosby.)

- Monitor the patient closely for hypoxia and hyperthermia.
- Once you have achieved the desired length or shape, a small amount of mineral oil can be applied to remove the dust and make the beak aesthetically pleasing.

Wing Trimming

- Trimming a bird's wings is one method to decrease the bird's ability to fly.
  - This is done by selectively trimming some of the primary and secondary feathers.
- The flight feathers are numbered 1 through 10 from the inside out.
- There is a natural break in the direction of the feathers, with the feathers of the manus (primaries, P-1 to P-10) angled out and the feathers on the brachium and antibrachium (secondaries, S-1 to S-10) angled in.
- It is important to question the client to determine how much flight is needed and how aesthetically pleasing he or she wants the trim.
- A nice, aesthetically pleasing trim leaves the distal two primary feathers intact, trimming only four to eight feathers on each wing.
- The recommendation is to trim both wings evenly for balance.
- The general rule of wing trim is that the heavier bodied a bird is, the fewer feathers are removed.
- The trim is done up high under the coverts, so that the jagged edges of the cut feathers are not showing.
- Evaluate the feather to be trimmed and ensure that it is not a blood feather; these should be avoided.
- If one is located, the mature feather on either side should be left as support.
- Flying ability should be tested in the clinic before the bird is sent home.
- Flight distance should be limited to less than 25 feet and lift to less than 2 feet.
- Additional feathers can be trimmed after a flight test if necessary.
- Various instruments are used to perform wing trimming; these include suture scissors, cat nail trimmers, wire cutters, and sharp-sharp scissors.
- Prevent the spread of disease by sterilizing the trimmers after each use.

Nail Trimming

- A regularly requested service and important preventive care procedure is trimming of long or sharp nails.
- Excessive nail length can result in improper perching, and the nail could be traumatically avulsed.
- An overgrown nail could get caught in the grate commonly found in the bottom of most bird cages or on the carpet as the bird wanders around the house.
- Untrimmed nails can grow into the pad of the foot, causing cellulitis or abscess formation.

- The size and temperament of the bird determines the number of people required to perform the trim.
  - Towel restraint is commonly used.
- The most common tools used for nail trims include Resco trimmers (Tecla, Walled Lake, MI), the Dremel (motorized) tool, files, nail scissors, fingernail trimmers, and cautery instruments.
- The Dremel tool, typically used on large birds, uses a grinding tip to blunt the tips of the nails.
  - This handheld motorized tool is noisy and can overheat nail tissues if applied too long.
- Flat or rounded fine-toothed files are preferred by some for trimming the nails of birds of any size.
  - This method slowly blunts the nail tips, causing some birds to become impatient and struggle.
  - Clients can be trained to do this at home if the pet and owner are willing.
- Some veterinarians use electrocautery instruments to trim nails and prevent bleeding at the same time.
  - Many birds exhibit pain reactions to this procedure, presumably related to the high heat of the instrument.
  - This method of nail trimming should be done primarily on anesthetized animals.
- Any blood loss in birds should be considered serious.
- In very small birds, loss of what appears to be a minute amount of blood is potentially fatal.
- When bleeding is noticed, a hemostatic powder must be pressed immediately onto the nail.

Determination of Gender

- Pet birds often have spectacularly colorful plumage.
- It is almost impossible to determine the gender of most companion birds by appearance because males and females of each species may look identical.
  - The major exception to this rule is the eclectus parrot, in which the female is a deep reddish color, with a dark beak, and the male is bright green, with an orange beak.
- The gender of a bird can be determined by endoscopy; however, DNA sexing is a safer alternative to the surgical approach and is available through some labs around the country.
- With a very small amount of whole blood (one or two drops), the gender of a bird can be determined within a few days.
- DNA sexing uses the polymerase chain reaction (PCR) assay to analyze the DNA from the sex chromosomes of the bird.

Microchipping

- Microchipping is an identification method that uses a tiny computer chip with an identification number programmed into it that is encapsulated in a biocompatible material.
- The whole device is small enough to fit inside a hypodermic needle and can be simply injected IM, where it will stay for the life of the bird.

- The microchip provides a permanent positive identification that cannot be lost, altered, or intentionally removed.
- Before anesthetizing the bird for placement of a microchip, it is best to scan the patient to verify that there is not already a chip present.
- Scan the chip before implanting it to ensure that it works.
- The bird should be anesthetized for the procedure because the microchip is injected into the pectoral muscle via a 15-gauge needle, which can be a painful and stressful procedure.
  - The site should be aseptically prepared.
- After the chip has been inserted, scan the bird to verify that the chip is functioning correctly.

Physical Examination

History

- The first step of the physical examination is a thorough history combined with a brief visual examination.
- Husbandry-related problems are common findings with the first visit to an avian practitioner.
- Many medical conditions can be directly related to poor diet and husbandry.

Procedure Before Capture and Restraint

- The physical examination starts with observing the bird's behavior and physical appearance before capture and restraint.
- Companion birds are commonly a prey species with survival instincts and frequently alter their behavior when they are in a stressful environment, such as a clinic.
- Birds will mask their symptoms so as not to stand out in their flock, so they will not be eliminated by a predator or members of their own flock.
- The respiratory rate should be smooth and regular; a healthy bird should show no signs of increased effort.
- If the bird is exhibiting a tail bob, forward movement of the head, or open beak breathing, this could be a sign of respiratory distress and may need immediate attention.
- If the bird is trying to sleep, is droopy-eyed, is wobbling, or is barely hanging on to the perch, immediate medical attention may be necessary.
- When a bird is stressed or excited, its droppings may be mostly urine.
- Seed eaters will have drier droppings than those with a diet supplemented with fruits.
- If the bird is anorexic, the droppings will be fewer.
- Blood, parasites, or undigested seeds may be seen in the droppings.
- The feces may be green or light brown and may vary in consistency among species and according to diet.
- The urine should be clear, and the urates can appear white to a pale tan.

- In addition to the species and any disease considerations, water intake and diet influence the appearance of droppings.

Capture and Restraint

- Restraint is often required for the safety of the patient and those working with the bird.
- Capturing a bird needs to be done in a room that can be sealed and has no escape route or hiding places for the bird to access.
- Close and lock the door, close the window blinds or shades, turn off any fans, and remove any cage accessories.
- Darkening the room may help reduce the stress of capture in some cases—mainly for smaller birds that otherwise try to fly around in their cages.
- A terry cloth towel is often useful when capturing and restraining birds that range in size from cockatiels or conures to the largest parrots (Fig. 11.15).
- Paper is sometimes used when restraining parakeets, cockatiels, or conures.
- The bird should be allowed to chew on the towel if it wishes, which keeps its beak busy and makes it less likely for the holder to be bitten.
- The use of a towel to capture a bird helps keep the bird from developing a fear of hands.
- The use of gloves is discouraged because this also will create a fear of hands.
  - Gloves also reduce the handler's tactile sensation and ability to feel the patient's most subtle movements and reactions to the stress of restraint.
- Small pet birds such as finches, canaries, and parakeets are sometimes transported to the veterinarian in their own cage.
  - They must be safely and gently removed for a hands-on physical examination.

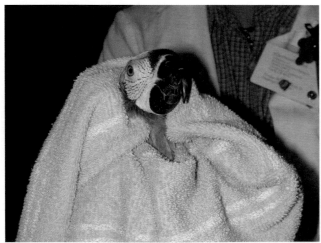

FIGURE 11.15 Small macaw captured by a terry cloth towel. (From Sirois M: *Principles and practice of veterinary technology*, ed 3, St Louis, 2011, Mosby.)

- Slow and deliberate movements minimize stress to the bird, accompanied by a quiet tone of voice for reassurance.
- Place the towel over the patient, gain control of the head, pin the wings to the body, and pick the patient up.
- Larger parrots may be caught in the cage, in the carrier, on the floor, or from a tabletop.
- Never capture a bird from the owner's shoulder; the bird might bite the owner.
- As with small birds, a slow and deliberate approach works best.
- A quiet, soothing tone of voice should be used when approaching the bird.
- Once the bird is captured, a towel can be wrapped around the bird to form a so-called birdy burrito to control the wings and the legs.
- With or without a towel, the body of the bird can be tucked under your arm once you have control of the head.
  - This will aid in restraint of the wings.
- As with all methods of restraint, you must monitor the patient carefully for stress, hypoxia, and hyperthermia.
- The restrainer is the primary person monitoring the bird's condition and stress level during the examination.
  - This allows the person performing the physical examination to proceed in a timely fashion.
- In some practices, a restraint board is used for procedures that require the awake (unanesthetized) bird to remain completely still, such as for radiographs or implantation of microchips for identification, or in other situations in which both hands may be needed to perform complicated tasks.
- Restraint boards should not be used except for radiographs, and only for heavily sedated or anesthetized companion birds.
- Proper handheld restraint allows for better observation of the bird's condition and a faster reaction time to return the bird to its cage or carrier if the patient is becoming too stressed during restraint.
- Restraint can be a stressful experience for a bird. It is not unusual for the bird to show signs of extreme distress when released.
- The bird will typically pant and exhibit open beak breathing, have hot feet, hold its wings away from its body, and fluff its feathers to allow air to cool the skin.
- Birds with featherless areas on the face, such as African greys and macaws, will blush occasionally.
- One restraint method that may be useful involves gripping the bird around the cervical region while extending its neck (Fig. 11.16).
  - This prevents the bird from dropping its head down and biting your fingers.
  - This may look like a choke hold, but it is a helpful way to restrain macaws or other birds that have

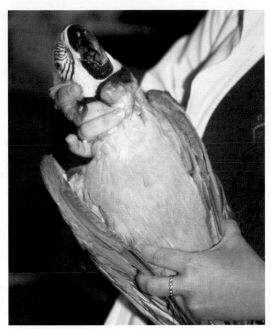

FIGURE 11.16 Choke hold restraint of a blue and gold macaw. (From Sirois M: *Principles and practice of veterinary technology*, ed 3, St Louis, 2011, Mosby.)

fragile facial skin that bruises easily with traditional restraint methods.
- With the other hand, keep the wings pinned to the sides of the body.

Performing the Physical Examination
- Table 11.1 presents physiologic data for common avian species.

- The average adult bird has a core body temperature of 100° to 109°F (38° to 42.5°C).
- A typical physical examination involves examination of the eyes, external auditory canals (or ears), nares, beak, and oral cavity.
- The crop and esophagus, neck, pectoral region, coelom and pelvic region, wings, legs, feet, and back are all palpated.
- Feather quality is evaluated, and the preen gland is checked.
- The heart, air sacs, lungs, and sinuses are auscultated.
- The cloaca is examined and the mucosa everted to examine for lesions.
- The restrainer may need to assist with opening the beak so that the oral examination can be performed.
  - The bird should be in an upright position and the oral cavity exposed by using gauze or tape strips to gently fatigue the powerful muscles controlling the beak (Fig. 11.17).
  - In smaller birds, you can use a small speculum such as a hemostat, paper clips, or small tape strips.
- When restraining the bird during examination of the wings, take care to curve the wing in the direction of the body at all times.

Weighing the Patient
- It is important to obtain an accurate weight of your patient at every visit.
- Some birds will sit on the scale nicely, but others may require that you place them in a box or small cage to weigh them.
- Weigh the patient every time it comes into the clinic, even if the bird is not sick.

TABLE 11.1 Physiologic Data for Common Avian Species

Bird	Average Weight (g)	Heart Rate (beats/min)	Respiratory Rate (breaths/min)	Sexual Maturity	Average Captive Life Span (yr)
Parakeets	30	500–600	60–70	6 mo	6
Love birds	38–56	400–600	60–80	8–12 mo	4
Cockatiels	75–125	400–500	40–50	6–12 mo	6
Conures	80–100	500–600	60–70	1–3 yr	10
Lories	100–300	300–500	35–50	2–3 yr	3
Cockatoos	300–1100	150–350	20–30	1-6 yr (species-dependent)	15
Eclectus parrots	380-450	160–300	20-30	3–6 yr	8
Amazon parrots	350–1000	160–300	20–30	4–6 yr	15
Macaws	200–1500	120–300	15–32	4–7 yr (species-dependent)	15
African greys	400–550	200–350	25–30	4–6 yr	15

Adapted from Sirois M: Principles and practice of veterinary technology, ed 3, St Louis, 2011, Mosby.

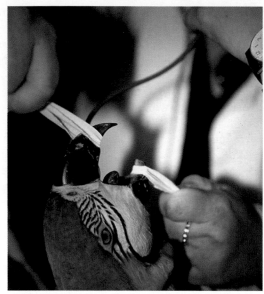

FIGURE 11.17 Oral examination method. (From Sirois M: *Principles and practice of veterinary technology*, ed 3, St Louis, 2011, Mosby.)

Diagnostic Sampling Techniques

Blood Collection

- Obtaining blood from a severely trimmed toenail is not acceptable.
  - This is painful, stressful, and can yield abnormal cell distributions and cellular artifacts.
- The medial metatarsal vein or leg vein is the vessel of choice for collecting blood in medium-to-large birds.
- You must restrain the bird securely during blood collection.
- The person taking the blood will grasp the leg and syringe in one hand while collecting the sample; this will provide more control if the patient moves.
- The jugular vein is the method of choice for small birds such as parakeets and lovebirds (Fig. 11.18) because the other vessels are usually too small.

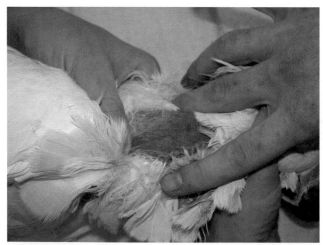

FIGURE 11.18 Jugular venipuncture. (From Sirois M: *Principles and practice of veterinary technology*, ed 3, St Louis, 2011, Mosby.)

- Birds have two jugular veins; however, the right jugular is more prominent than the left.
- The restrainer should hold the bird in left lateral recumbency.
- The phlebotomist should arch and extend the neck, part the feathers, lightly wet them with alcohol, and find the featherless track and the jugular.
- Once the sample is collected, pressure must be applied by the restrainer; this is crucial to prevent large hematomas and possible bleeding out.
- With appropriate restraint, the ulnar or basilic vein (also referred to as the wing vein) is an easily accessible vessel for venipuncture.
  - Because of the severity of the complications that can occur, it is recommended that this be attempted only on anesthetized patients.

Fecal Examinations

- The examination of feces requires a fresh sample, with little to no contaminants.
- A direct smear of the feces is the method for the detection of protozoa.
- Fecal flotation is needed to detect helminths.
- Gram staining should be included in any workup to detect yeast and bacteria.
  - Grain- and fruit-eating Psittaciformes should have a gram-positive bacterial flora, with potentially some yeast.
  - A few yeasts or gram-negative bacteria per high-power field (HPF) could be considered normal, but budding yeasts are not normal.
  - Carnivorous or insectivorous Passeriformes, raptors, Galliformes, and Anseriformes will have some gram-negative bacteria in their cloaca.
- A fecal occult blood test can also be performed.

Imaging

Radiography

- Most companion psittacine birds will require anesthesia or heavy sedation for diagnostic radiographs.
- If digital radiology is not available, high-detail rare earth cassettes with single-emulsion film provide desired results.
- Mammography film will produce even better detail but does require a higher kilovolt potential (kVP) and milliamperage (mA).
- The standard whole-body views are ventrodorsal (VD) and right lateral views.
- Plexiglas restraint boards that assist with patient positioning can be used and usually provide excellent results.
- For the VD view, place the bird on its back, legs stretched down to expose the coelomic cavity, wings stretched out symmetrically to the sides, and two pieces of masking tape or paper tape in the form of an X across each carpus.
- Palpate the keel to ensure that it is in line with the backbone.

- Positioning for the lateral view has the patient placed in right lateral recumbency, legs stretched downward, and wings pulled back together.
- Paper or masking tape is placed across the carpus to keep the wings back, and tape or gauze is used to keep the legs stretched downward.
- Once the plain films are reviewed, it may be necessary to isolate limbs for an individual shot or perform a contrast study of the GI system or an ultrasound.
- The VD and lateral views reveal the same lateral view of the wing.
- When two views are necessary, a posteroanterior (PA) view needs to be obtained.
  - The PA can be obtained by placing the bird in a dive-bombing position—head on the plate, body up in the air.
  - Extend the wing out as close to the plate as possible and collimate to the desired area (Fig. 11.19).

Standing Radiograph

- The critically ill bird or one in respiratory distress may not be able to survive the stress of restraint required for a routine diagnostic radiograph.
- The bird can be placed in a cardboard box or induction chamber or allowed to stand on a low perch to obtain a standing radiograph.

- If your machine has horizontal beam capabilities, you can obtain a lateral standing view as well.

Gastrointestinal Contrast Study

- Contrast studies are often done when abnormalities are indicated on the plain films.
- These are done with the exact positioning as mentioned earlier for plain films, with the addition of barium administered via a gavage tube into the crop.
- An immediate radiograph is taken, with subsequent views taken at 15-, 30-, 60-, and 90-minute intervals.
- To reduce the risk of aspiration of barium from the crop, the patient can be elevated on the restraint board during positioning (Fig. 11.20).
- To help prevent passive reflux of barium into the mouth during a GI contrast study, a small Vet Wrap bandage can be placed around the bird's neck, close to the mandible.
- The board can be placed level for the radiograph and then elevated again for patient repositioning.

Endoscopy

- Many veterinarians use the 2.7-mm rigid fiber-optic endoscope because it can be successfully used for birds of almost any size.

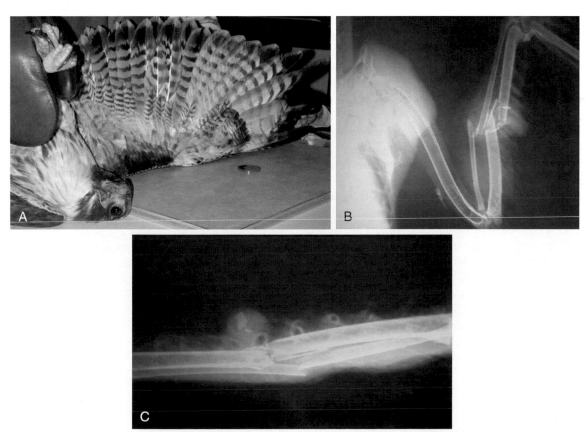

FIGURE 11.19 (A) Red-tailed hawk in posteroanterior wing position for radiographs. (B) Lateral view of the wing with a fracture. (C) Posteroanterior view of the wing with the same fracture. (From Sirois M: *Principles and practice of veterinary technology*, ed 3, St Louis, 2011, Mosby.)

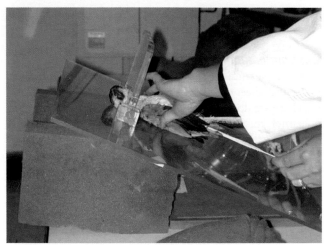

FIGURE 11.20 Elevated restraint board. (From Sirois M: *Principles and practice of veterinary technology*, ed 3, St Louis, 2011, Mosby.)

- Most endoscopic procedures are minimally invasive, and patient recovery time is more rapid than with exploratory surgery.
- Endoscopy can be used for the visual examination of any part of the body that has an orifice large enough to allow the insertion of the instrument.
- Laparoscopy, tracheoscopy, rhinoscopy, and cloacaloscopy are common diagnostic procedures.
- Using endoscopy, the veterinarian can obtain tissue biopsies and apply interlesional and topical treatments and surgical interventions, in addition to the sexing of nondimorphic species.
- The organs or system to be studied determines whether the right or left side will be the site of entry for the endoscope.
- The bird will need to be anesthetized and the endoscope insertion site aseptically prepped and draped.
- The standard approach for diagnostic evaluation of the internal organs is right lateral recumbency.
- Two approaches can be used: one with the left leg pulled caudally and the other with the left leg pulled cranially; the specific position depends on the clinician's preference.
- A small incision is made in the skin, and the muscle layer is bluntly dissected with forceps.
- The endoscope and cannula are introduced into the incision through the cranial thoracic or abdominal air sac, and the organs can be viewed. The lungs, reproductive organs, kidneys, adrenal glands, ventriculus, and other organs will typically be visualized during this examination.
- Once the endoscopy is complete, the area will need to be sutured.

Nursing Care

Hospitalization
- A separate room is needed for housing of birds.
- The room should have its own thermostat and be able to maintain a room temperature of 85° to 90°F (29° to 32°C).

- The cages and perches should be easy to disinfect, and you should have a way to isolate patients suspected of carrying infectious diseases.
- Heat lamps and water-circulating heating pads are helpful for providing extra heat to the debilitated patient, but the enclosure needs to be monitored closely so that the patient does not become overheated or destroy the pads.
- Incubator-oxygen cages can supply heat, humidity, and oxygen and are easy to disinfect.
- Avian patients are extremely intelligent and, when hospitalized, can become bored and stressed.
  - Patient enrichment is an important part of the patient's road to recovery.
  - This can be achieved by providing the patient with nontoxic, safe disposable toys and mirrors or playing a radio or television for the patient to enjoy.
  - If the patient is willing and receptive, you can spend a little time talking quietly and hand-feeding the bird in its hospital cage.

Infectious Diseases and Zoonoses
- Infectious and zoonotic diseases are critical problems for bird owners and veterinarians (Box 11.2).
- Vaccines are available to protect pet birds against some of these diseases.
- The West Nile virus is a mosquito-borne disease that primarily infects horses, humans, and birds.
  - Psittacines appear to be somewhat resistant because only a few cases have been reported from endemic areas.
  - However, keeping pet birds inside or in screened areas is suggested to prevent exposure.

BOX 11.2 Infectious and Zoonotic Diseases of Birds

- Adenoviruses
- Avian influenza
- Avian polyoma virus (APV)
- *Chlamydophila psittaci* (zoonotic)
- Eastern equine encephalitis (EEE)
- Exotic Newcastle disease virus
- Fungal infections such as *Aspergillus* spp.
- *Mycobacterium* spp. (zoonotic)
- Papillomaviruses
- Paramyxovirus-3 (PMV-3)
- Poxviruses
- Psittacid herpesviruses (PsHVs), Pacheco disease
- Psittacine beak and feather disease virus (PBFDV), circovirus
- Psittacine proventricular dilation disease (PDD)
- West Nile virus (WNV)

From Sirois M: Principles and practice of veterinary technology, ed 3, St Louis, 2011, Mosby.

- Chlamydiosis is caused by the obligate intracellular bacterium, *Chlamydophila psittaci*.
  - This is a zoonotic disease that causes psittacosis in humans and avian chlamydiosis in avian species.

Preventing the Spread of Disease in the Clinic

- Patients suspected of having infectious diseases must be isolated from other patients. Isolation areas must be out of the mainstream of the clinic, where there is minimal foot traffic.
- Ideally, the isolation room should have a ventilation system separate from that of the main clinic.
- Disposable protective shoe covers or foot baths must be used when exiting this room to prevent carrying any infectious agent out of the isolation area.
- All veterinary team members who handle animals suspected of having a zoonotic or any infectious disease must wear personal protective equipment, not only to protect themselves against infection but also to prevent transmission to others.
- Personal protective equipment includes disposable outer garments, laboratory coats or coveralls, disposable head or hair covers and gloves, safety goggles, and disposable particulate respirators approved by the National Institute for Occupational Safety and Health.
- Disposable equipment should be considered contaminated and properly disposed of after use.
- Nondisposable items such as laboratory coats and goggles should be cleaned and disinfected between uses.
- When removing contaminated protective equipment, personnel should first remove their outer garments, except for gloves, and discard them.
  - They should then remove their gloves, wash their hands with soap and water, remove their goggles and particulate respirators, and immediately wash their hands again.
- Washing your hands is the primary and best way to prevent the spread of disease, so do it between each patient, regardless of whether the patient is suspected of carrying an infectious disease.
- Using these protective measures will help prevent the spread of disease in your clinic and protect those working with the patients.
- Preparation and efficiency are essential when providing supportive care to the avian patient. Prepare each patient's medications, fluids, and food before capture.
- Make sure to treat infectious disease suspects last, wear disposable attire (or change your laboratory coat or scrub top after handling), and wash your hands well after handling all patients to prevent the spread of disease.

Oral Administration

- Medication and fluids may be administered to birds orally if the patient is alert and active.
- Primary regurgitation or vomiting, poor patient reflexes or recumbency, and oral and upper GI trauma may exclude this method.

- The oral route of administering medication is almost stress-free if the patient is tolerant.
- Medications mixed in mashed banana or fruit baby foods are often well accepted; medication of feed and water may be unreliable for some of the patients that you will see in practice.

Gavage Feeding

- Fluid therapy, nutritional support, and medication administration can be provided by gavage or tube feeding.
- Limiting factors may include patients with crop stasis, ileus, GI impactions, or other GI abnormalities that reduce motility or absorption.
- A variety of flexible and rigid feeding needles and tubes are available.
- Gavage feeding will require a number of people for larger birds, but with smaller birds a skilled person can usually do it alone (Fig. 11.21).
- In larger birds, one person holds the patient in an upright position, another opens the mouth, and another person advances the tube into place and administers the medications and food.
- Care must be taken so that the patient does not bite the tube and ingest it.
- The tube can be palpated in the crop to verify correct placement.
- If food or liquid material appears in the oral cavity while administering the medications or food, the bird should be placed back into its enclosure immediately without further handling to prevent the risk of regurgitation and potential aspiration.

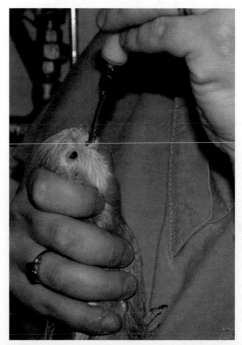

FIGURE 11.21 This experienced technician is able to gavage-feed this cockatiel alone, which is the standard accepted method. (From Sirois M: *Principles and practice of veterinary technology*, ed 3, St Louis, 2011, Mosby.)

Subcutaneous Injection Sites

- Subcutaneous sites are found in the inguinal, axillary, and dorsal regions.
- The inguinal region is the preferred site to administer SC fluids and medications (Fig. 11.22).
  - The patient is restrained in dorsal recumbency and the legs pulled straight down.
  - A small amount of alcohol is applied to the medial side of the most proximal portion of the leg, parting the feathers.
  - A small-gauge needle is inserted just under the skin.
  - Similar administration techniques are used for the axillary and dorsal regions; however, you cannot get as much fluid into these areas.

Intramuscular Injections

- For IM injections, the pectoral muscles are generally used.
- These represent the largest muscle mass on the bird and are found on both sides of the keel (Fig. 11.23).

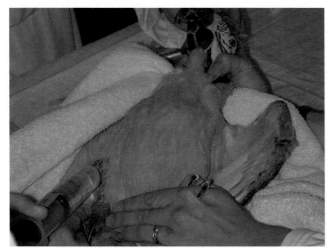

FIGURE 11.22 A blue and gold macaw is receiving a dose of SC fluids in the right inguinal region. (From Sirois M: *Principles and practice of veterinary technology*, ed 3, St Louis, 2011, Mosby.)

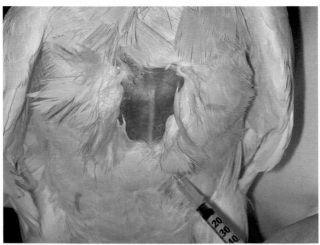

FIGURE 11.23 The pectoral muscles are the optimal site for IM injections in birds. (From Sirois M: *Principles and practice of veterinary technology*, ed 3, St Louis, 2011, Mosby.)

- A small-gauge needle is used to reduce the amount of muscle damage, and a different area of the muscle is used for any subsequent injections.
- The patient is restrained in an upright position.

Bandaging

- The figure-of-eight bandage is used when a patient presents with fractures or soft tissue injuries distal to the elbow or when you need to stabilize a wing with an intraosseous catheter.
- Soft roll gauze followed by a layer of self-adherent bandage material will provide the best results.
- Restrain the bird with the wing in a flexed position.
- The bandage is started at the carpus and the gauze wrapped around the carpus, thus creating the top of the eight in the figure eight.
- The gauze is rolled toward the elbow and wrapped around the area proximal to the elbow. This will create the lower end of the figure eight.
- A body wrap is added in addition to the figure-of-eight bandage when the patient has a humeral or pectoral girdle fracture.
- When placing a body wrap, care must be taken not to place tension on the keel, which can cause inadequate breathing.
- The body wrap is placed directly over the keel without putting pressure on the crop or coelomic cavity or interfering with the movement of the legs.
- Once the bandage is in place, the bird should be monitored for increased stress, dyspnea, and chewing or destroying the bandage.

Elizabethan Collar Placement

- Elizabethan collars (E collars) and other mechanical barriers are placed for many reasons, including prevention of self-trauma such as feather picking and self-mutilation or protection of a bandage or wound.
- Collars can be made out of old x-ray film or insulation pipe found at the hardware store, or you can purchase small versions of the ones used for canine and feline patients.
  - If you make a collar, the edges must be padded to prevent sores from forming and ensure that the bird cannot chew at the outside rim of the collar.
- Crib-type collars have an attachable disc.
  - This collar prevents the bird from dropping its head far enough to pick at the upper and lower portions of the body.
  - In some cases, the bird can still reach the area just below the lower rim of the crib collar and the tips of the wings.
  - The disc can be added to prevent any picking altogether; however, you should monitor the bird closely to ensure that it can still eat and drink.
- Commercially available bubble-style E collars can be used but may not be as effective at keeping the bird from reaching the back half of its body.
- When a collar is first placed on the bird, sedation and cage padding may be required until the collar is accepted.

- Some birds are highly stressed after the collar is placed and begin flipping in all different directions, along with flapping uncontrollably and screaming.
- Once the bird has adjusted to the collar, you can return the bird to its owner, provided that you counsel the owner about possible complications with use of the collar.
  - These include trouble eating and drinking, trouble with balance and navigating around its normal environment, and pressure sores or abrasions from the collar.

Common Diseases and Conditions

- An emergency can be defined as a sudden or unforeseen situation that requires immediate action (Box 11.3).
- Birds are primarily a species that are preyed on and tend to mask signs of illness as a means of self-preservation.
  - By hiding their illnesses, birds can be in an advanced state of debilitation by the time they are brought into the clinic.
  - In some cases, handling for examination can be contraindicated, and supportive therapy should be considered a priority.
- The bird that is having trouble perching or is fluffed may be very ill and should be considered an emergency.
- Fluffing—elevating the body feathers to trap warm air near the body—is a bird's response to loss of body heat.
- Birds often present with nonspecific signs such as being fluffed up, sitting on the cage bottom, loss of appetite, untidy appearance, lethargy or weakness, droopy eyelids, and loss of interest in their surroundings.

Respiratory Emergencies

- A bird in respiratory distress can present to your clinic for a variety of reasons, including inhaled toxins, space-occupying masses in the coelomic cavity, foreign body aspiration, tumors or other growths in the airway, or respiratory disease.

BOX 11.4 Signs of Respiratory Distress

- Tachypnea
- Labored respiration
- Open mouth respiration
- Audible respirations
- Change in vocalizations
- Tail bobbing
- Collapse

From Sirois M: Principles and practice of veterinary technology, ed 3, St Louis, 2011, Mosby.

- Upper airway emergencies can result from aspirated foreign bodies such as seeds, splinters from wooden toys, or other pieces from toys in the cage.
- Normal respiratory patterns should be slow and regular and, in the healthy bird, almost unnoticeable (Box 11.4).
- The respiratory rate can vary from 10 to 40 breaths/min, depending on the size of the bird.
- Any condition that results in tracheal obstruction can lead to an upper airway emergency (Box 11.5).
- Airborne toxins are dangerous to birds; they may die within a few minutes of exposure or develop chronic problems.
- Examples include overheated polytetrafluoroethylene (Teflon) pans, hairspray, tobacco smoke, paint fumes, strong cleaning chemicals, carbon monoxide, and dust from lead-containing paint (Box 11.6).
- Treatment for aerosol toxicity includes removing the source of the toxin and removing the bird from the toxic environment.
  - Once in the clinic, the patient should be placed in an oxygen cage.
  - These cases are best managed with minimal stress or restraint of the patient, with supportive care such as nutritional, fluid, and oxygen therapy with nebulization.
- Some respiratory emergencies may be caused by a space-occupying mass in the coelomic cavity.
- This can be the result of egg stasis, tumors, organ enlargement, or fluid buildup in the coelom.

BOX 11.3 Avian Emergencies

Dyspnea, gasping for air
Bleeding
Generalized weakness
Sudden depression
Fluffed bird
Trauma
Trouble perching
Regurgitation, vomiting, inappetence
Coelomic distention
Prolapsed cloaca

From Sirois M: Principles and practice of veterinary technology, ed 3, St Louis, 2011, Mosby.

BOX 11.5 Upper Airway Emergencies

Tracheal obstructions with:
- Tumors
- Papillomas
- Granulomas
- Transtracheal membranes

From Sirois M: Principles and practice of veterinary technology, ed 3, St Louis, 2011, Mosby.

Bleeding Emergencies

- A variety of conditions may cause bleeding emergencies (Box 11.7).
- Broken blood feathers may be the result of a traumatic fall or injury to the bird.
  - If the bird is stable, apply direct pressure, with or without styptic powder, to stop the bleeding and try to save the feather from removal.
  - If the bleeding will not stop, remove the feather using hemostats or needle-nosed pliers.

Egg Stasis or Binding

- Egg retention is defined as the failure of an egg to pass through the oviduct at a normal rate and is a commonly seen emergency in parakeets, canaries, cockatiels, finches, and lovebirds.
- These birds typically have been laying eggs for some time, thus depleting their calcium stores.
  - This causes decreased muscle activity in the oviduct, and the egg becomes trapped.
- Signs can include abdominal distention and straining, lack of droppings, depression, sitting on the cage bottom, tail wagging, and walking with widespread legs.

Prolapsed Cloaca

- Occasionally, birds will present to your clinic with a prolapsed cloaca.

- The most important immediate therapy is to keep the prolapsed tissue moist and clean.
  - If the patient is too stressed to restrain, you can place the patient in a cage lined with clean towels or gauze moistened with sterile saline.
- Many aliments can lead to a prolapsed cloaca, such as egg stasis, papillomas, chronic masturbation, and coelomic masses.

Animal Bites

- This accident normally occurs when a larger animal attacks the smaller bird, and in some cases, birds versus bird.
- Mammal bites are usually from a pet dog or cat and are true emergencies.
- Pathogenic oral bacteria from such an animal can be detrimental to the avian patient. When a wound is located, surrounding feathers are removed by plucking.
- Care must be taken when attempting to flush while cleaning the wound because of the possibility that the puncture may communicate with an air sac.

Beak Injuries and Repair

- Some birds inflict severe injuries to other birds if given the opportunity.
  - They may destroy the upper or lower beak of their victim.
  - Fractures of the mandible may occur.
- After hemorrhage is controlled, the patient is evaluated for the type of repair that will be required.

Foreign Bodies

- Foreign bodies are often ingested by a curious bird that has been roaming and chewing, a scenario similar to that found with mammals.
- Potential ingested foreign materials are toys or parts of toys, bedding, metallic items (e.g., wire, hairpins), string, fish bones, splinters, and tough plant fibers.
- A thorough physical examination and radiographs often determine the problem, but specialized studies may be required.
- Endoscopic techniques and/or surgical removal may be required to retrieve the objects.

Fractures

- Birds commonly present with a number of different scenarios resulting in a fracture.
  - These include being attacked by a larger animal, caught in its cage or cage toys, leg band entrapped in toys or other objects, flying into a window or ceiling fan, or being stepped or sat on.
- When this type of patient presents to your hospital, place the patient in a quiet, dark, well-padded environment until stable enough to restrain.
- Provide analgesics and determine the best method to stabilize the fracture.

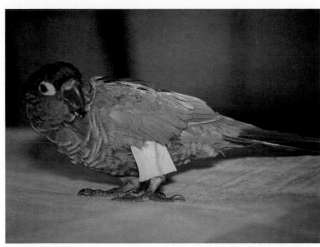

FIGURE 11.24 Tape splints are a lightweight alternative to traditional bulkier bandages for smaller birds. (From Sirois M: *Principles and practice of veterinary technology*, ed 3, St Louis, 2011, Mosby.)

- Bandages and splints are used when some support of the fracture is all that is necessary (Fig. 11.24).
- This method will make the bird more comfortable but may not allow proper healing and return to full function.
- Fractures commonly stabilized with this treatment are some wing and foot breaks.
- There are many different surgical methods and approaches to fracture repair that will be case dependent.
- In extreme cases, a traumatized leg or wing cannot be salvaged and amputation may be the only choice.
- Most psittacines do well after losing a leg because they can use their beaks to move around.
  - Most birds will perch comfortably but do run the risk of developing pododermatitis on the remaining foot.
- In pet birds, removal of a wing may cause some loss of balance, but most seem to manage rather well.

Leg and Wing Fractures
- Fractures of the wing usually are immobilized with a figure-of-eight bandage.
  - This holds the flexed wing snug against the body.
- If the humerus is fractured, a body wrap is also applied.
- An open fracture should also be cleaned and flushed, using caution because of the pneumatic bones of birds; flushing could introduce fluid into the airway.
- Appropriate supportive, antimicrobial, and analgesic therapies should be implemented as soon as possible.
- Most broken wings will need to be bandaged for 3 to 5 weeks, with routine changes.
- The bandage should be removed as soon as healing is complete.
- Complications include stiffness, muscle atrophy from disuse, and loss of flight feathers.
- Physical therapy will help the bird become limber and recover muscle mass.

- Some lower leg fractures are stabilized with a splint until healing occurs, usually in 4 to 6 weeks.
- Because of the bird's anatomy, splints will often worsen fractures of the femur and upper tibiotarsus.
  - These often require prompt surgical repair.
- Toe fractures can be treated in large birds by taping the broken toe to the neighboring intact toe.
- The Schroeder–Thomas splint can be used to treat fractures of the lower third of the tibiotarsus and the entire tarsometatarsus.
  - The bandage is changed every 1 to 3 weeks and is accompanied by passive physical therapy.
- A Robert Jones bandage can be used for simple lower leg fractures.
  - Although these are heavily padded, additional splinting materials such as tongue depressors may be needed.
  - The bandage needs to be changed at least every 2 weeks.
- A ball bandage is used for broken toes or pododermatitis.
  - A ball formed of gauze sponges is placed so that the toes curl around it.
  - The foot is covered with cotton padding and wrapped with stretchy, self-adherent bandaging. Very small birds can be difficult to splint.
- Materials such as pipe cleaners, toothpicks, paperclips, and wooden applicator sticks can be used to stabilize their fractures.
- With all splints, it is necessary to assess circulation in the foot.
  - Look for swelling of the toes, blue coloration, and coldness and change the bandage if any of these occur.
- Bandages need to be checked often for signs of chewing or moisture.
- Removal of leg bands is advised because they may cause fractures when they become caught on the cage or other objects.

Head Trauma
- Head trauma cases in which the bird flies into a window or a ceiling fan require immediate supportive therapy and evaluation.
- Place the patient in a dark, quiet, and (contrary to other situations) a cool environment to prevent vasodilation of the intracranial vessels.
- Provide supportive care as needed.

Burns
- Burns on birds commonly occur on the feet and legs.
- Birds that are left to fly freely through the house can run the risk of landing in a pot of boiling hot liquid or the burners of the stove, causing severe burns to the legs and feet.
- Burns to the oral cavity and tongue may occur if the bird bites an electrical cord.
- Treatments for burns is comparable to treating burns in other patients.

- Flush areas with copious amounts of cool water or saline and remove the surrounding feathers.
- Do not use greasy or oily medications because these can accumulate in the feathers and have an effect on thermoregulation.
- Silver sulfadiazine applied topically has antibacterial, antifungal, and analgesic effects.

Crop Burn and Crop Trauma

- Owners or breeders may bring in a baby bird that seems to have food leaking from its chest.
- A crop burn is normally caused by poorly mixed microwaved foods that are fed to neonates.
- Once the burn has occurred, normally in the right ventral portion of the crop, the crop and skin necrose, forming a fistula.
- Food will leak from this fistula, creating an alarming situation for the client and maybe an emergency.
- If the bird cannot retain enough food or water, there is a risk of dehydration and starvation.
- This will require anesthesia and a surgical closure, but recovery is usually fairly quick.

Heavy Metal Toxicosis

- Birds are naturally curious and like to investigate unfamiliar objects with their mouths.
  - When this behavior is combined with the bird being given free run of the house, the potential for ingesting foreign objects is increased.
- Some materials used for the cage or toys are made of zinc or lead.
- Because there is no quality control for toys manufactured for birds, the toys themselves can be made from toxic materials, and the client is generally unaware of this.
- Lead and zinc are the two most common heavy metal poisonings that you will encounter with avian patients.
- Typically, ingestion of curtain weights, lead clappers from bells, old-style solder, lead-based paints, plaster, foil from wine bottles, and calcium-rich dolomite or bone meal can cause lead poisoning.
- Galvanized cage wire is the usual source of ingested zinc.
- Treatment for lead and zinc toxicosis is supportive; it may include chelation therapy with calcium ethylenediaminetetraacetic acid (EDTA) and removal of the foreign body, if possible.
- Diagnosis may be based on signs and radiographic findings of heavy metal densities within the body (Box 11.8).
- Samples can be sent to an outside laboratory for heavy metal analysis.

Ingested Poisons

- As noted, birds often explore new items by mouthing them and feeling their texture with their tongues.
- Cleaning products can cause skin eruptions, GI upset (including vomiting and diarrhea), respiratory tract irritation, and esophageal damage.

BOX 11.8 Signs of Heavy Metal Toxicosis

- Lethargy
- Depression
- Anorexia
- Weakness
- Weight loss
- Anemia
- Regurgitation
- Polyuria
- Polydipsia
- Diarrhea
- Emaciation
- Ataxia
- Convulsions, paresis, paralysis
- Regenerative anemia

  Amazon parrots are the only species that will develop hematuria in acute cases. Eclectus will characteristically show biliverdinuria (greenish staining of urine). Other parrots have no urinary color changes.

From Sirois M: Principles and practice of veterinary technology, ed 3, St Louis, 2011, Mosby.

- Hydrocarbon-based compounds such as furniture polish and other petroleum products can cause central nervous system effects such as disorientation and depression, pneumonia, GI upset, kidney and liver damage, and mucous membrane and skin damage.
- Perfumes and deodorants may cause damage to the skin and mucous membranes, respiratory tract, kidneys, liver, and central nervous system.
- Shampoos lead to irritation of the eyes and diarrhea.
- Small amounts of tobacco products can result in vomiting, diarrhea, convulsions, and sudden death.
- Eating fireworks or matches can result in vomiting, diarrhea, blood in the stools, and increased respiration.

Poisonous Plants

- Many plants have been blamed for illness in birds, but plant poisoning is actually rare.
- Birds often will tear leaves without eating them, decreasing the amount ingested.
- The avian GI tract empties quickly, further reducing the chance of poisoning.
- Owners may unintentionally expose their birds to poisonous plant materials through feeding, use of poisonous plants for perches, or certain house plants (Box 11.9).
- If owners call the clinic with a bird showing unusual signs after exposure to any plant, they should be asked to bring the bird in for evaluation.
- Poisonings can be lethal without prompt intervention.
- The offending plant or a sample should be brought to the clinic. The client should try to estimate the amount ingested.

BOX 11.9 Toxic Plants

- Avocado
- Black locust*
- Clematis
- Crown vetch
- Dieffenbachia
- Foxglove
- Lily of the valley
- Lupine
- Oak*
- Oleander*
- Philodendron
- Poinsettia
- Rhododendron*
- Yew

From Sirois M: Principles and practice of veterinary technology, ed 3, St Louis, 2011, Mosby.
Should not be used for perches.

Ethical Euthanasia Techniques

- Euthanasia is sometimes necessary to alleviate patient suffering and should be done in a humane manner.
- Acceptable methods should include anesthesia to create an environment in which the patient is unaware of the injection.
- When the patient is unconscious, a commercially available euthanasia solution can be administered.
- Routes of administration are IV, intracardiac, or IP.
- The patient must be anesthetized if an intracardiac or IP route is to be used, and in all cases the patient must be monitored until its heart stops.

REPTILES AND AMPHIBIANS

- Reptiles and amphibians are a diverse group of animals that have become popular pets.
- The class Reptilia contains four orders, of which only two are commonly seen in the private clinical setting.
  - These two orders include Squamata (snakes and lizards) and Testudines (turtles and tortoises).
  - The most common lizards kept as pets in North America include iguanas, bearded dragons, geckos, chameleons, monitor lizards, and water dragons.
  - The most common snakes kept as pets in North America include boas, pythons, king snakes, rat snakes, corn snakes, and gopher snakes.
  - The most common chelonians kept as pets in North America include box turtles, red-eared sliders and other water turtles, and various tortoises.
- The class Amphibia contains three orders, which include Anura (frogs and toads), Caudata (salamanders, newts, and sirens), and Gymnophiona (caecilians).

Reptile Biology

- Reptiles are ectothermic, meaning they cannot generate their own body heat; heat is obtained from the environment.
- Reptiles are able to regulate their body heat by moving in and out of the heat or shade.
  - Each species has a specific temperature range at which it thrives.
- Reptiles have a protective layer of keratinous scales covering the skin.
- The outermost layer of the skin is shed on a regular basis.
- Species such as snakes shed their skin all at once.
- Just before the shed, the skin becomes sensitive and turns an opaque color (Fig. 11.25).
- The snake may become aggressive and anorexic just before and during the shed.
- Handling snakes should be kept to a minimum approximately 1 week before and during a shed because the skin is delicate and can be easily damaged.
- Unlike snakes, lizards and chelonians shed their skin in pieces.
- Some reptiles will have problems shedding the skin; this is called dysecdysis.
- If the patient is having problems shedding the skin, the humidity in the cage should be increased or the animal can be soaked in a warm water bath.
- Always examine the toes of lizards such as leopard geckos if they are having problems shedding their skin because the skin can become wrapped around the digits, cutting off circulation and causing necrosis.
- Like birds, reptiles lack a diaphragm to separate the thoracic and abdominal cavities. They have one visceral cavity called the coelom.
- Reptile excrement includes three components: urine, urates, and feces, similar to birds.

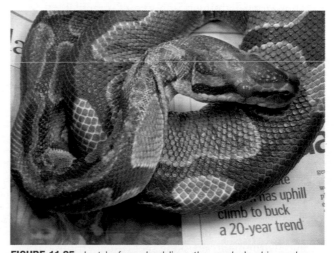

FIGURE 11.25 Just before shedding, the snake's skin and eyes turn an opaque blue color. The snake should not be handled just before and during the shed because this can damage the delicate new skin. (From Sirois M: *Principles and practice of veterinary technology*, ed 3, St Louis, 2011, Mosby.)

- The cloaca is the common opening through which the urinary, digestive, and reproductive systems empty.

Housing

- Many pet reptiles can be housed in a simple terrarium.
- The cage should be appropriately sized for the animal; in most cases, the larger the better.
- The terrarium should be easy to clean and disinfect.
- Appropriate cage furniture should also be placed in the terrarium.
- Cage furniture will vary based on the species but includes items such as logs, plants, hide boxes, and rocks.
- Cage furniture is often used by animals to help them shed.
- The terrarium setup for amphibians will vary based on the species of amphibian with which you are working and whether it is aquatic or terrestrial.
- A terrestrial amphibian cage may consist of mosses, various plants, rocks, logs, and a small amount of water in the cage.
- An aquatic cage will have a completely different set of criteria.
- If the amphibian is arboreal, you must provide height in the cage so that it can climb into a planted canopy.
- Regardless of the type of enclosure or species, the native habitat should be mimicked whenever possible.
- The substrate should be easy to remove for cleaning and replacement.
- Indoor-outdoor carpet is easy to clean and inexpensive enough to throw away when necessary.
- Other appropriate substrates include newspaper, butcher paper, hay, and commercial recycled newspaper bedding.
- Some people use wood chips and sand, but these can cause intestinal foreign bodies if eaten by the animal.
  - Shavings should not be used because they can cause irritation to the respiratory tract.
- Appropriate lighting is important for reptiles.
  - Without the proper ultraviolet (UV) lighting, many species of reptiles cannot metabolize nutrients or synthesize vitamin D adequately.
  - The light should be full spectrum, with the light source being approximately 18 to 24 inches from the animal.
  - UV bulbs need to be changed approximately every 6 months, even if they are not burnt out, because the UV portion of the light does not usually last longer than 6 months.
  - Light cycles will vary by species.
- Proper heating is critical for reptiles because they are ectothermic.
- Because reptiles thermoregulate using their surrounding environment, a basking spot (using various types of bulbs) providing increased heat should be provided, as well as a nonheated spot.
  - The reptile will move between the two spots to regulate its own body temperature.

- The basking spot should be positioned so that the animal cannot come into direct contact with the heat source.
  - Hot rocks or sizzle stones should not be used to provide heat because they often have uncontrolled hot spots that can cause thermal burns.
- Under-tank heaters can be useful in providing additional heat to the cage, but they should be used under only half of the cage so that the animal can escape the heat if necessary.
  - Under-tank heaters can cause thermal burns if not used properly.
- Humidity requirements vary among different species of reptiles.
  - Some tropical species such as the green iguana (*Iguana iguana*) require extremely high levels of humidity to stay healthy.
  - Many species of amphibians also need a temperature and humidity gradient in the cage.
- Proper sanitation of the enclosure is important.
  - The cage should be cleaned thoroughly and disinfected on a routine basis.
  - Excrement should be picked up daily.
- Owners should be aware that all reptiles have the ability to shed *Salmonella* spp. if they are positive carriers of the bacteria.
  - Owners should take precautions by wearing examination gloves during cleaning and handling of the pet.
  - Handling the animal and cleaning of the enclosure should never take place near areas where food for human consumption is prepared or stored.

Water Quality

- Water quality and care is one of the most important aspects of caring for amphibious pets.
- Amphibians are sensitive to poisoning from nitrogenous waste buildup and disinfectant residues.
- Frequent water changes and having a good filtration system on the terrarium will help keep water parameters under control.
- Several parameters should be checked on a regular basis, including temperature, pH, salinity, water hardness, alkalinity, dissolved oxygen, carbon dioxide, nonionized ammonia, nitrite, nitrate, and chlorine.

Feeding

- Improper diet and nutrition is a common cause of disease in exotic animals.
- Diets are generally species-specific and are beyond the scope of this text.
- Commercial diets are available for some reptile species but are generally not recommended.
- Reptiles must have water available at all times and the water changed daily because reptiles often defecate in the dish.
- There is no simple commercial diet available for owners to feed amphibious pets.

- Most amphibians are carnivorous or insectivorous as adults.

Snakes

- All snakes are carnivores and feed on whole prey items.
- The digestive system of snakes has evolved to digest whole prey and defecate the parts of the prey that are not digested, such as fur.
- Ingesting the entire carcass provides added nutrients such as calcium from bone.
- Further supplementation is not needed when feeding whole prey.
- Common whole prey items include rats, mice, rabbits, and guinea pigs.
- It is never appropriate to feed meat such as chicken breast, hot dogs, or raw beef because this does not provide a complete diet.
- It is suggested that prekilled or stunned food be offered to snakes so that they will not be harmed by the prey item.
  - Prekilled food can be ordered frozen from several companies.
  - If frozen mice or rats are offered, they must be thawed before being offered as food.

Lizards

- Feeding requirements vary with different species of lizards.
- Herbivores should be fed various types of dark, leafy greens and vegetables.
  - Proper leafy greens include but are not limited to kale, chard, turnip greens, and escarole.
- Most insectivores can eat worms and insects such as mealworms, silkworms, and crickets.
- Carnivorous lizards should be fed whole prey.
  - Whole prey items include mice, rats, and fish, depending on the species that you are feeding.
- Omnivores should be offered a variety of dark, leafy greens and, in most cases, insects.
- The quality and variety of food offered are important.
- Animals should not be fed the same food day after day.

Chelonians

- Most aquatic turtles are omnivorous; they generally consume food such as fish, invertebrates, algae, and leafy greens.
- Commercial diets are acceptable to feed in moderation, but it is important to make sure that they contain essential nutrients needed to maintain good health.
- Tortoises are herbivores; they eat a variety of food such as leaves, grasses, and flowers in the wild.
- In captivity, a healthy diet includes dark, leafy greens; rose petals; hay; and vegetables.
- Commercial diets can be fed in moderation and should be appropriate for herbivores.
- Do not feed dog food, tofu, monkey biscuits, or anything that has animal protein in it.

BOX 11.10 Common Diseases and Conditions of Reptiles and Amphibians

- Cutaneous bacterial infection (red leg)
- Egg binding
- Foreign body obstruction
- Gout
- Hypocalcemia
- Hypovitaminosis A*
- Metabolic bone disease
- Mycobacteriosis
- Parasitic infestations
- Poor husbandry and diet
- Reproductive organ prolapse
- Respiratory disease
- Shell rot
- Stomatitis
- Thermal burns
- Toxin exposure
- Trauma
- Ulcerative dermatitis
- Variety of bacterial, viral, and fungal infections
- Various bacterial and fungal infections

From Sirois M: Principles and practice of veterinary technology, ed 3, St Louis, 2011, Mosby.
*Chelonians only.

Taking a History

- A thorough history should be taken from the owner before the physical examination is performed.
- The owner should be asked to bring in pictures of the patient's regular enclosure.
- This will give the veterinary staff a good idea of which type of husbandry practices are being used.
- Common diseases and presentations are summarized in Box 11.10.

Capture, Restraint, and Handling

Snakes

- Most snakes can be easily captured directly out of the carrier or cage that they are in.
- When dealing with nonaggressive snakes, the restrainer can simply pick the animal up and pull it out of the cage.
- If the snake is aggressive, it may be necessary to use a towel along with leather gloves to capture it safely.
- In these cases, it is easiest to toss the towel over the snake gently and find the head.
- Once the head has been isolated and restrained, the snake can be safely taken out of the enclosure.
- If the snake is extremely aggressive or if it is a venomous snake, a snake hook should be used to pin down the head of the snake long enough to grasp its head and body safely.
- Improper use of the snake hook can cause trauma to the patient, so extreme caution should be taken.

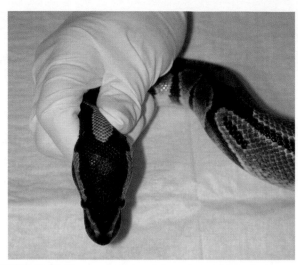

FIGURE 11.26 The snake's head is restrained by placing your hand behind the base of the skull. This will keep the snake from turning around and biting you. (From Sirois M: *Principles and practice of veterinary technology*, ed 3, St Louis, 2011, Mosby.)

- Snakes are commonly brought into the clinic in a pillowcase.
  - To remove the snake from the pillowcase safely, first find the snake's head and gently grasp it from the outside of the pillowcase.
  - Once the snake is restrained, the restrainer should put his or her free hand into the pillowcase and transfer the head to the free hand.
  - After this is accomplished, it should now be safe to take the entire snake out of the pillowcase.
- It is important to hold the snake gently, directly behind the head, with one hand (so it cannot turn around and bite) and support the body with the other hand (Fig. 11.26).
- If the snake is large, more than one person may be needed to restrain it.
  - A general rule is one person per 3 feet of snake.

Chelonians

- Although chelonians are usually the easiest to capture, they are the hardest to restrain.
- Unless working with extremely large tortoises, most chelonians can just be picked up with both hands and placed on the examination table.
- When examining large tortoises (i.e., several kilograms), it is easiest to set up an examination area within the animal's enclosure or on the floor in the clinic's examination area.
- Because there is a great deal of variation in size and strength, restraint techniques may vary between small and large chelonians.
- Once the animal's body is under control, it is imperative that the head be properly restrained.
- Although this is relatively easy when the animal is sick, it can be difficult on strong, healthy chelonians, especially large tortoises and box turtles.

- Many turtles and tortoises are curious.
  - If they are set down on the table or the ground, they may just start walking around to check things out.
  - If this is the case, the restrainer can just walk up to them and grasp the head with one hand while restraining the body with the other hand.
- To keep control of the head, it is best to position your thumb on one side of the cranial portion of the neck and position the rest of your fingers (or just the index finger, for smaller species) on the other side of the neck, just behind the base of the skull (Fig. 11.27).
- Healthy chelonians are strong, so it may take much constant but gentle force to keep the turtle or tortoise's head out of the shell.
- If the animal is extremely active, another person may be necessary to help restrain the limbs and body.
- Another way to gain control of the head is by trying to coax the animal out of its shell.
  - Many chelonians will extend their head out of the shell if food is offered to them or if they are placed in a container of shallow warm water.
  - When the head is extended, the same techniques mentioned earlier can be used to gain and keep control of the animal's head.
- If these techniques fail, it may be possible to slip a small, blunt ear curette or spay hook under the horny portion of the upper beak, known as the rhinotheca.
  - Once the probe has been placed, it can be gently pulled back to extend the neck to a position for the restrainer to grasp.
  - It is important to note that this technique can be dangerous; the beak can be chipped or broken if the animal struggles or is in poor health.

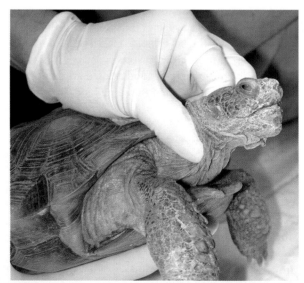

FIGURE 11.27 The tortoise is restrained by placing one hand behind the base of the skull to help keep the head and neck extended. The other hand should be used to support the body. (From Sirois M: *Principles and practice of veterinary technology*, ed 3, St Louis, 2011, Mosby.)

- If a spay hook is the tool of choice, it may be a good idea to pad the hooked portion of the instrument.
  - Padding can consist simply of tape or an elastic wrap cut to the appropriate size.
- Caution should be taken when dealing with any aquatic turtle, especially snapping turtles.
  - These species of turtles have a tendency to bite, and many of the larger turtles can cause serious bodily harm to the people working with them.
- Box turtles can be the most challenging chelonians to restrain properly.
  - Because box turtles have a hinge on their plastron, many species are able to tuck themselves completely into their shells.
  - The easiest way to extend their head is to prop open the cranial portion of the carapace (upper shell) and the plastron (lower shell) gently.
  - Extreme care must be taken when trying to prop the shell open. It is suggested that a well-padded object be used when attempting this to help avoid traumatizing or fracturing the shell.
  - Another way to extend a box turtle's head is to grasp one of the forelimbs, keeping the leg extended out of the shell until the head can be successfully pulled out and properly restrained.
  - This method works well because once the leg is extended, the turtle will usually not close its shell down on its own leg.
  - It is important to remember that any of these capture and restraint techniques can potentially cause some stress to the turtle or tortoise.
- If initial attempts at capture and restraint are not successful, chemical restraint may be necessary for any reptile, especially large tortoises and box turtles.

Lizards

- Smaller lizards are generally easy to capture but can be difficult to restrain because they tend to wriggle and squirm while they are being held.
- Most lizards can simply be picked up with both hands and taken out of the enclosure.
  - Some of the larger lizards can be difficult to capture and restrain, especially if they are aggressive.
- If the lizard is aggressive, a towel or blanket, along with leather restraint gloves, should be used.
- It is important to remember that lizards can scratch and bite when they are scared or nervous.
  - It is a good idea to wear long sleeves when possible and always keep track of where the head is.
- Long-necked lizards such as monitors can easily turn around and bite if their head is not properly restrained during capture.
- Keeping one hand on the neck, just behind the base of skull, will help prevent getting bitten.
- Never capture any species of lizard by the tail; many species of lizards have a natural predatory response to

drop or autotomize their tail voluntarily in an attempt to escape predation.
- Generally, lizards can be restrained by placing one hand around the neck and pectoral girdle region while the other hand can be used to support the body near the pelvis.
- Although it is sometimes difficult, try to avoid pressing down and damaging the dorsal spines of lizards such as iguanas when they are being restrained.
- Some lizards, such as geckos, have extremely delicate skin that can easily be damaged by capture and restraint.
  - Ensure that only soft towels are used on geckos.

Amphibians

- Amphibians can be challenging animals to capture and restrain.
- It is important to keep stress to a minimum; therefore the patient should be handled only when necessary.
- Always wear nonpowdered gloves when handling an amphibian and keep the patient moist to avoid dehydration.
- Some amphibians can release toxins from their skin that cause irritation or illness in humans; also, amphibians can absorb substances through their skin, so anything on your hands can be potentially harmful to the patient.
- Generally, amphibians can be restrained by placing one hand around the neck and pectoral girdle region while the other hand can be used to support the body near the pelvis.
- In some cases, the patient may need to be anesthetized to perform a physical examination.

Normal Physiologic Values

- Generally, normal physiologic values in reptiles have an extremely large range.
- Many reptiles can have a heart rate that ranges from approximately 10 to 80 or more beats/min.
- Heart rates and respiratory rates can vary depending on ambient temperature, age, species, and health status.
- The respiratory rate may range from 2 or 3 breaths/min to 20 breaths/min or more, depending on the factors mentioned earlier.
- The body weight of the patient will also vary depending on age, nutritional status, species, and sometimes gender.
- Patients' weight can range from as little as a few grams to several kilograms.
- A scale that weighs to the nearest gram should always be used to obtain an accurate weight on the patient.
- Body condition scoring is also performed on reptiles and follows the same guidelines used in mammalian medicine.
- The scale ranges from 1 to 9, with 1 being emaciated and 9 being grossly obese.

Determining Gender

- It is relatively easy to determine gender in many species of reptiles.

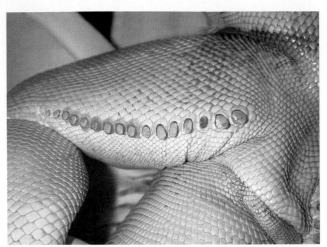

FIGURE 11.28 The femoral pores are commonly used to sex lizards such as iguanas and bearded dragons. The males (pictured) have large femoral pores, whereas females have tiny femoral pores. (From Sirois M: *Principles and practice of veterinary technology,* ed 3, St Louis, 2011, Mosby.)

- For example, male iguanas and bearded dragons have very large femoral pores compared with females (Fig. 11.28).
- Many species of male tortoises have a concave plastron, making it easier to mount the female.
- Several male water turtles have elongated nails, which are used to dangle in front of the female to impress her.
- Some species of male box turtles have brilliant red eyes.
- To determine gender in snakes, a well-lubricated metal or plastic probe is inserted into the cloaca and then directed caudolaterally.
  - In male snakes, the probe will enter the cavity in which the inverted hemipenis—one of the two reproductive organs—is located.
  - In female snakes, the probe will enter a blind diverticula.
  - Once the probe has been inserted, it is advanced slowly and gently until it will not advance any farther.
  - Your thumb should be placed on the scale where the end of the probe is located.
  - You can now pull the probe out and count the number of scales from the cloacal opening to your thumb.
  - If the number is more than 7, it is a male; if it is less than 5, it is a female.
  - If the number is in between, it is very hard to say whether the animal is a male or female.

Diagnostic Techniques
Reptile Venipuncture
- Venipuncture sites vary with different species (Table 11.2).
- Clipping toenails to obtain a blood sample is a method that some veterinary professionals may use on very small lizards or when attempts to access other venipuncture sites have failed.

TABLE 11.2 Common Venipuncture Sites in Reptiles

Species	Venipuncture Sites
Chelonians	Radiohumoral plexus sinus (brachial sinus) Dorsal venous sinus (coccygeal vein) Jugular vein Subcarapacial venous sinus Femoral vein
Lizards	Ventral and lateral aspects of the caudal tail vein
Snakes	Heart Ventral aspect of the caudal tail vein

From Sirois M: Principles and practice of veterinary technology, ed 3, St Louis, 2011, Mosby.

- Cutting toenails to the point of bleeding should not be used as a means for obtaining a blood sample; it can be painful for the animal and may introduce infection.
  - Blood from a clipped toenail also has the potential to skew blood chemistry levels (e.g., uric acid).

Snakes
- There are two common venipuncture sites in snakes, which include the caudal tail vein and heart.
- The palatine vessels are not appropriate for drawing blood samples in snakes.
- Drawing blood from the tail vein is best accomplished in large snakes; it can be difficult in small snakes because of the size of the vessel.
- The same method used to draw blood from the ventral midline in lizards is also used in snakes.
- Obtaining a blood sample from the heart (also called cardiocentesis) is generally the quickest method and will yield a large amount of blood.
- The snake should be placed in dorsal recumbency.
- The heart can then be located in the cranial third of the body.

Chelonians
- The radiohumoral plexus (brachial plexus sinus), sub-carapacial venous sinus, dorsal venous sinus (coccygeal vein), and jugular vein are the major sites from which blood can be obtained from a turtle or tortoise.
- The venipuncture site will depend on the size and species of the patient and the preference of the phlebotomist.
- If blood is drawn from the jugular vein, the turtle or tortoise should be placed in lateral recumbency.
- The head and neck should be pulled away from the shell.
- To obtain the sample, the phlebotomist will hold the head while the restrainer will keep the patient in lateral recumbency.
- The subcarapacial venous sinus is generally used when jugular venipuncture is not an option (Fig. 11.29).
- The radiohumoral plexus sinus is generally used in larger chelonians. When drawing blood from the dorsal venous sinus, the patient should be placed in sternal

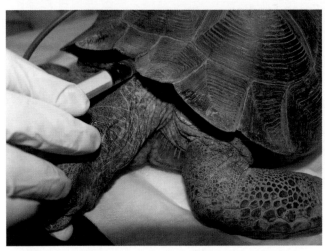

FIGURE 11.29 Blood collection from the subcarapacial venous sinus. (From Sirois M: *Principles and practice of veterinary technology*, ed 3, St Louis, 2011, Mosby.)

recumbency. The tail should be held as straight as possible, and the needle should be inserted in the midline.

Lizards

- The cephalic, jugular, and ventral abdominal vessels can be used to obtain a blood sample from various species of lizards that may be encountered in your clinic.
  - These vessels are not commonly used for several reasons.
  - The cephalic vein is usually extremely small, and the ventral abdominal vein is not generally used (especially in awake animals) because of the inability to properly restrain the animal and control hemorrhage.
  - The jugular vein is not commonly used because in many species it is a blind stick and may require a surgical cut-down to access the vessel.
  - Lymphatic fluid contamination is also common when performing venipuncture from the jugular vein.
- The most common vessel used for lizard venipuncture is the caudal tail vein, also called the ventral coccygeal vein.
- Lizards usually struggle when they are placed on their backs, making it difficult to draw blood from them.
  - It is important to keep the animal in sternal recumbency while obtaining the blood sample.
- During the blood draw, it is also important that the phlebotomist gently restrain the caudal portion of the tail with one hand and obtain the blood sample with the other.

Amphibians

- Blood collection can be challenging in amphibians.
- Alcohol should not be used to clean the venipuncture site, as it can irritate and/or desiccate the patient's skin.
  - A 1:40 diluted 2% chlorhexidine solution should be used to cleanse the site instead.
- The caudal tail vein is generally used for venipuncture in salamanders.
  - The vessel is very small and can collapse easily, so do not place a large amount of negative pressure on the syringe during collection.

- Venipuncture sites in frogs and toads include the femoral vein, ventral abdominal vein, and lingual vein, although the femoral and lingual veins are rarely used.
- The ventral abdominal vein is the easiest vessel from which to obtain a blood sample.
- The frog or toad is gently positioned on its back with the restrainer holding the pectoral girdle.
- The person drawing blood can hold the pelvic girdle with one hand and draw blood with the other hand.
- Some amphibians will need to be anesthetized for venipuncture.

Parasitology

- Reptiles and amphibians can be affected by a wide variety of parasites.
- There are several different ways to check for parasite load, including direct fecal examination, fecal flotation, and cloacal wash.
- The direct fecal examination and flotation are done in the same manner as for a dog or cat.
- The cloacal wash is done by inserting a soft rubber feeding tube attached to a syringe into the cloaca.
- Saline is then flushed into the cloaca and suctioned out, obtaining a diagnostic sample.

Radiology

- The diagnostic value of a radiograph depends on the quality of the technique and positioning of the patient.
- Digital radiology will yield the best results.
  - However, if digital radiology is not available in your hospital, high-detail rare earth cassettes with single-emulsion film provide desired results.
  - Mammography film will produce even better detail but does require a higher kVp and mA.

Amphibians

- Two views are normally taken: dorsoventral (DV) and horizontal lateral.
- A horizontal beam is essential to obtain good radiographs.
- In most cases, the patient will just sit there while the radiographs are being taken.

Snakes

- Two views are normally taken: a DV or VD and lateral views.
- Radiographs are taken in sections from head to tail and labeled with numbered lead markers to delineate each section.
- In most cases, the snake will need to be heavily sedated or anesthetized to obtain good radiographs, unless the snake is very sick.
- A plastic snake tube can be used to obtain radiographs, but often diagnostic films are not produced unless the snake cannot move within the tube and remains completely straight.

Chelonians

- Three views are normally taken: DV, horizontal lateral, and horizontal craniocaudal views.

- The craniocaudal view is taken to evaluate the left and right lung fields.
- A horizontal beam is essential to obtain good radiographs.
- Because chelonians do not have a diaphragm, placing them in lateral recumbency shifts the organs into the lung cavity, which leads to poor radiographs.
- Most chelonians do not need to be sedated for radiographs, but chemical restraint can be used if necessary.
- In most cases, the patient will just sit there or it can be placed on a plastic dish with its feet hanging in the air.

Lizards

- Two views are normally taken: DV and horizontal lateral views.
- A horizontal beam is essential to obtain good radiographs.
- Because reptiles do not have a diaphragm, placing them in lateral recumbency shifts the organs into the lung cavity, which leads to poor radiographs.
- Most lizards do not need to be sedated for radiographs, but chemical restraint can be used if necessary.
- In most cases, the patient will just sit there while the radiographs are being taken.
- You can also use vagal stimulation or the vagal response to calm the patient, if needed.
  - The vagal response in iguanas and other medium-to-large lizard species can be induced by gently applying digital pressure to both eyes for a few seconds to a few minutes.
  - The patient will usually respond with a decrease in heart rate and blood pressure.
  - The vagal response can also be induced by placing cotton balls over their eyes (Fig. 11.30).
  - The vagal response induces a short-term trancelike state, allowing time to take radiographs and, in some cases, even draw blood.

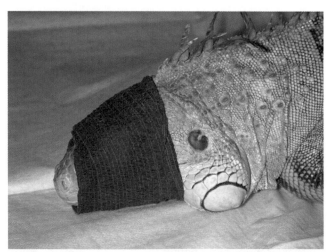

FIGURE 11.30 To induce the vagal response, place cotton balls over the eyes and lightly wrap elastic wrap around the head. This wrap takes the place of digital pressure. (From Sirois M: *Principles and practice of veterinary technology*, ed 3, St Louis, 2011, Mosby.)

Force Feeding

- Patients often present to the veterinary hospital because of anorexia or lethargy.
- Nutritional supplementation and fluid therapy are often required.
- Patients that are not eating on their own will need to be tube- or syringe-fed.
- Syringe feeding is relatively easy.
- Tube feeding is comparable to that in birds.
  - The mouth is opened with a speculum, such as a plastic spatula.
  - The tube is premeasured to estimate the location of the stomach before inserting it into the patient.
  - Unlike metal tubes that are generally used in birds, a red rubber feeding tube is typically used for most reptile and amphibian species.
- It is important to use proper syringe-feeding diets such as Carnivore Care (Oxbow Murdock, NE) for carnivores or Critical Care (Oxbow) for herbivores.
  - Other diets can be used as well, as long as they are complete and balanced.
  - Omnivorous animals can have a mixture of the two.
- Insectivores can be fed an appropriate meat-based baby food.

Administration of Fluids and Medications

- The IM and SC routes are most commonly used for the administration of medications in reptiles.
- The IV route is rarely used, but administration of fluids and some medications can be given into the caudal tail vein in reptiles or the jugular vein in chelonians (Table 11.3).
- This can be accomplished by a single injection or by placing an indwelling catheter.
- Intraosseous fluids can be given in many lizard species.

Emergency and Critical Care

- Chelonians, lizards, and snakes commonly present in emergency situations for traumatic injuries.
- Common emergencies include being hit by a car, attacked by another animal, stepped on or dropped, and thermal burns.

TABLE 11.3 Common Intravenous Catheter Sites in Reptiles

Species	Catheter Sites
Chelonians	Jugular vein
Lizards	Ventral and lateral aspects of the caudal tail vein
Snakes	Ventral aspect of the caudal tail vein

From Sirois M: Principles and practice of veterinary technology, ed 3, St Louis, 2011, Mosby.

- Wounds are treated with the same medical techniques used to treat small mammals.
- Wound care, fluid therapy, nutritional support, and pain medications should be provided as necessary.

Euthanasia

- Euthanasia can be difficult because it can sometimes be hard to access a vessel.
- For reptile patients, euthanasia barbiturate solution can be given into any vessel, the heart, or the coelomic cavity.
- If injecting into the heart, the patient must be anesthetized before the injection.
- Amphibian patients can be given ketamine for sedation or placed into a bath of tricaine methanesulfonate (MS-222, Argent Chemical Laboratories, Redmond, WA) to anesthetize the animal before injecting the euthanasia solution.
- Euthanasia solution can be given into any vessel or the coelomic cavity.
- The heart may take several minutes to several hours to stop completely, even though the patient may be clinically dead.
- Doppler ultrasound can be used to check for a heartbeat.
- The patient should be kept in the clinic for several hours or overnight to ensure that the patient has been properly euthanized before sending it home with the owner if that is the owner's preference.

RECOMMENDED READINGS

Small Mammals

Harkness JE, Turner PV, VandeWoude S, Wheler CL: *Harkness and Wagner's the biology and medicine of rabbits and rodents*, ed 5, Ames, IA, 2010, Wiley-Blackwell.

Hrapkiewicz K, Medina L, Homes D: *Clinical laboratory animal medicine: An introduction*, ed 3, Ames, IA, 2006, Wiley-Blackwell.

Quesenberry KE, Carpenter JW: *Ferrets, rabbits, rodents: Clinical medicine and surgery*, ed 3, St Louis, 2012, Saunders.

Sirois M: *Laboratory animal medicine: Principles and procedures*, St Louis, 2005, Mosby.

Companion Birds

Altman RB, Clubb SL, Dorrestein GM: *Avian medicine and surgery*, Philadelphia, 1997, WB Saunders.

Carpenter JW: *Exotic animal formulary*, ed 3, St Louis, 2005, Saunders.

Companion Parrot Online Magazine (https://companionparrotonline.com).

Harcourt-Brown C, Chitty J, editors: *BSAVA manual of psittacine birds*, Gloucester, England, 2005, British Small Animal Veterinary Association.

Harrison G, Lightfoot T: *Clinical avian medicine*, vols. 1 and 2, Palm Beach, FL, 2006, Spix.

Johnson-Delaney CA: *Exotic companion medicine handbook for veterinarians*, Lake Worth, FL, 1996, Wingers.

Mitchell M, Tully T: *Manual of exotic pet practice*, St Louis, 2009, Saunders.

O'Malley B: *Clinical anatomy and physiology of exotic species*, Oxford, England, 2005, Elsevier Saunders.

Ritchie BW: *Avian viruses*, Lake Worth, FL, 1995, Wingers.

Ritchie BW, Harrison GJ, Harrison LR: *Avian medicine: Principles and application*, Lake Worth, FL, 1994, Wingers.

Silverman S, Tell LA: *Radiology of birds: An atlas of normal anatomy and positioning*, St Louis, 2010, Saunders.

Reptiles and Amphibians

Ballard B, Cheek R: *Exotic animal medicine for the veterinary technician*, ed 2, Ames, IA, 2010, Wiley-Blackwell.

Carpenter JW: *Exotic animal formulary*, ed 3, St Louis, 2005, Saunders.

Fowler M: *Zoo and wild animal medicine*, ed 5, St Louis, 2004, Saunders.

Hatfield JW III: *Green iguana: The ultimate owner's manual*, ed 2, Ashland, OR, 2004, Dunthorpe Press.

Mader D: *Reptile medicine and surgery*, St Louis, 2006, Saunders.

Miller RA, Fowler M: *Fowler's zoo and wild animal medicine current therapy*, vol. 7, St Louis, 2011, Saunders.

Mitchell M, Tully T: *Manual of exotic pet practice*, St Louis, 2009, Saunders.

O'Malley B: *Clinical anatomy and physiology of exotic species*, Oxford, England, 2005, Elsevier Saunders.

West G, Heard D, Caulkett N: *Zoo animal and wildlife immobilization and anesthesia*, Ames, IA, 2007, Blackwell.

Wright KM, Whitaker BR: *Amphibian medicine and captive husbandry*, Malabar, FL, 2001, Krieger.

Answers available on Evolve.

CHAPTER 1 FOUNDATIONS OF VETERINARY ASSISTING

1. Which type of tissue covers the interior and exterior surfaces of the body, lines body cavities, and forms glands?
   A. Epithelial
   B. Connective
   C. Nervous
   D. Adipose

2. Which type of tissue consists of chondrocytes and various types and amounts of fibers embedded in a thick, gelatinous, intercellular substance?
   A. Muscle
   B. Nervous
   C. Cartilage
   D. Bone

3. Which vertebrae form joints with the dorsal ends of the ribs?
   A. Atlas
   B. Cervical
   C. Lumbar
   D. Thoracic

4. Which is a system consisting of glands and hormones?
   A. Integument
   B. Reproductive
   C. Endocrine
   D. Digestive

5. Which anatomic plane is perpendicular to the sagittal and transverse plane?
   A. Dorsal
   B. Midsagittal
   C. Median
   D. Cranial

6. Which term refers to a direction that is toward the nose?
   A. Cranial
   B. Proximal
   C. Dorsal
   D. Rostral

7. Which prefix refers to "insufficient" or "abnormally low"?
   A. Brady-
   B. Tachy-
   C. Hypo-
   D. Hyper-

8. What is dyspnea?
   A. Abnormal urination
   B. Difficulty breathing
   C. Dissection of the lungs
   D. Difficulty eating

9. Which description describes the term hepatopathy?
   A. Enlarged kidney
   B. Enlarged spleen
   C. Disease of the liver
   D. Study of disease

10. Which is the correct term for pus, or infection, in the uterus?
    A. Pyometra
    B. Pyrometra
    C. Pyouterus
    D. Uterinitis

CHAPTER 2 OFFICE AND HOSPITAL PROCEDURES

1. Which term refers to the specified dollar amount of a covered service that is the policyholder's responsibility once the deductible has been met?
   A. Copay
   B. Premium
   C. Per-incident limit
   D. Excluded service

2. What is the purpose of a dispensing fee added to a medication?
   A. Take additional money from the client
   B. Recover costs associated with the pill vial, label, and time to fill a script
   C. Recover costs associated with holding and ordering
   D. Recover costs associated with expired product
3. What is the recommended number of inventory turns per year?
   A. 0 to 3
   B. 4 to 5
   C. 6 to 8
   D. 8 to 12
4. Which term refers to the loss of a product without explanation?
   A. EOQ
   B. Reorder point
   C. Shrinkage
   D. Premium point
5. To what does the acronym POMR refer?
   A. Problem objective medical record
   B. Problem-oriented medical receipt
   C. Problem objective medical receipt
   D. Problem-oriented medical record
6. To what does the acronym SOAP refer?
   A. Subjective objective assessment plan
   B. Subjective-oriented assessed plan
   C. Subjective oral assessed plan
   D. Subjective objective active plan
7. What is an ideal amount of total inventory cost as a percentage of gross revenue?
   A. 0% to 10%
   B. 12% to 15%
   C. 16% to 20%
   D. 20% to 30%
8. Which document must be signed by the client indicating the consent to a medical procedure?
   A. Blanket consent form
   B. Informed consent form
   C. Client information form
   D. Patient information form
9. The receptionist should answer the phone within how many rings?
   A. One
   B. Two
   C. Three
   D. Five
10. Which law provides regulations for collection practices of overdue accounts?
    A. Fair Debt Collections Practices Act
    B. Fair Credit Reporting Act
    C. Consumer Credit Protection Act
    D. Affordable Care Act

CHAPTER 3 COMMUNICATION AND CLIENT RELATIONS

1. Which statement is the most accurate regarding communication?
   A. With the advent of the computer and email, reading and writing have become the most common forms of communication.
   B. When interacting with clients, it is possible to use so many of your senses that you overwhelm the communication.
   C. Verbal communication is the best way to get your point across.
   D. Nonverbal communication is more persuasive than verbal communication.
2. Which is a component of positive body language?
   A. Facing toward people when talking to them
   B. Looking at people's hand gestures when talking to them
   C. Watching people's body language when talking to them
   D. Keeping your hands still while talking to someone
3. Which represents the three primary categories of communication barriers?
   A. Advising, threatening, moralizing
   B. Solution sending, judging, failing to respond to others
   C. Excessive reassuring, falsely praising, diagnosing
   D. Ordering, excessive questioning, labeling (name calling)
4. Which represent active listening traits?
   A. Paraphrasing, positive head nodding, and thoughtful silence
   B. Interrupting and interjecting your comments
   C. Leaning back, crossing your arms, and keeping a straight face
   D. Watching the body language of the speaker intently, preparing to provide your input, and offering praise even if it is not warranted
5. What is the minimum safety equipment required when exposing radiographs?
   A. Lead-lined gloves and thyroid shield
   B. Lead-lined apron, gloves, and glasses
   C. Lead-lined thyroid shield, apron, and gloves
   D. Lead-lined apron and gloves
6. Which is a definition for the term ethics?
   A. General acceptance of random acts of kindness
   B. The system of moral principles that determines appropriate behavior and actions within a specific group
   C. Accepted rudeness among a specific group of professionals
   D. Political parties rationalizing each other's similarities

7. Which is a definition of the human–animal bond?
   A. Any gracious act toward a pet
   B. A nagging anticipation that a pet needs our undivided attention
   C. Feeding a pet with contempt
   D. The special, healthy relationship between people and their pets

8. What contains detailed information about every chemical found in the veterinary hospital?
   A. FLSA
   B. DSMA
   C. MSDS
   D. OSHA

9. Which activity can be performed only by a veterinarian?
   A. Administering medication
   B. Collecting diagnostic samples
   C. Administering general anesthesia
   D. Forming a diagnosis

10. Which is usually the first stage of grief?
   A. Denial
   B. Bargaining
   C. Anger
   D. Guilt

CHAPTER 4 PHARMACOLOGY AND PHARMACY

1. Which is considered a semisolid form of medication?
   A. Tablets
   B. Elixir
   C. Suspension
   D. Ointment

2. What is the total daily dose of a medication containing 100 mg/mL at a dosage of 5 mg/kg BID for a patient that weighs 50 kg?
   A. 500 mg
   B. 250 mg
   C. 50 mg
   D. 25 mg

3. What is the volume of each dose of a medication containing 100 mg/mL at a dosage of 5 mg/kg BID for a patient that weighs 50 kg?
   A. 2.5 mL
   B. 25 mL
   C. 50 mL
   D. 100 mL

4. How many 25-mg tablets must be dispensed for a medication that is prescribed for a 22-lb dog to be given at 5 mg/kg TID for 5 days?
   A. 10
   B. 20
   C. 30
   D. 50

5. Which term refers to drugs that are related to or function on the jejunum?
   A. Gastric
   B. Enteric
   C. Colonic
   D. Extrahepatic

6. Which class of medication is commonly used in the treatment of kennel cough?
   A. Antiarrhythmic medications
   B. Diuretics
   C. Antitussives
   D. Nonsteroidal antiinflammatories

7. What is the common usage for oxytocin?
   A. Modify behavior in cats
   B. Increase conditioning of feedlot cattle
   C. Increase weight
   D. Increase uterine contractions

8. Which antiinflammatory can be toxic to cats?
   A. Carprofen
   B. Meloxicam
   C. Acetaminophen
   D. Deracoxib

9. Which anticonvulsant is used for emergency treatment of seizures?
   A. Phenobarbital
   B. Diazepam
   C. Pentobarbital
   D. Phenytoin

10. Which bactericidal antimicrobial is also effective against protozoa that cause intestinal disease, such as *Giardia*?
   A. Erythromycin
   B. Chloramphenicol
   C. Metronidazole
   D. Nystatin

CHAPTER 5 EXAMINATION ROOM PROCEDURES

1. What is the most important socialization period in puppies?
   A. 2 to 7 weeks
   B. 3 to 12 weeks
   C. 3 to 6 months
   D. 6 to 12 months

2. What is the definition of the term ethology?
   A. Ethical behaviors of trainers
   B. Behavioral acts done with no obvious reason
   C. Treatment of behavior problems
   D. The study of animal behavior

3. Which term refers to the association of a particular activity with a punishment or reward?
   A. Classical conditioning
   B. Operant conditioning
   C. Instinct
   D. Imprinting

4. Which term describes the pattern of behaviors that bonds animals to their caretakers in early life?
   A. Classical conditioning
   B. Operant conditioning
   C. Instinct
   D. Imprinting

5. Which term refers to an immediate pleasant occurrence that follows a behavior?
   A. Positive reinforcement
   B. Negative reinforcement
   C. Positive punishment
   D. Negative punishment

6. What is the most common problem for which dog owners seek guidance?
   A. Aggression
   B. House soiling
   C. Separation anxiety
   D. Cognitive dysfunction

7. Which term refers to the attribution of human characteristics and emotions to animals?
   A. Imprinting
   B. Anthropomorphism
   C. Operant conditioning
   D. Habituation

8. Which term describes behaviors that animals show in situations involving social conflict?
   A. Territorial
   B. Agnostic
   C. Instinctual
   D. Investigative

9. Which term refers to the process of exposing a young animal to new experiences, people, other animals, and places with the goal of preventing fearful or anxious behavior as adults?
   A. Agnostication
   B. Reinforcement
   C. Socialization
   D. Imprinting

10. Which behavioral modification method would involve exposing a pet that is afraid of children to children using increased periods of time and decreasing distance?
    A. Extinction
    B. Avoidance therapy
    C. Desensitization
    D. Command–response–reward

CHAPTER 6 SMALL ANIMAL NURSING

1. What is the most appropriate action to take if the quick is accidentally cut during a nail trim?
   A. Apply ice packs immediately to stop the bleeding
   B. Administer pain medication
   C. Apply a cauterizing agent
   D. Notify the veterinarian immediately

2. Which is a significant concern regarding recumbent patients?
   A. Dull mentation
   B. Anorexia
   C. Decubital ulcers
   D. Petechiation

3. Which essential fatty acid is required in a cat's diet but not in a dog's?
   A. Linolenic
   B. Linoleic
   C. Threonine
   D. Arachidonic

4. Which is an essential amino acid required in the diet of dogs and cats?
   A. Linolenic
   B. Linoleic
   C. Threonine
   D. Arachidonic

5. Which is a fat-soluble vitamin?
   A. Thiamin
   B. Vitamin D
   C. Niacin
   D. Vitamin C

6. What should be the daily weight gain in a normal puppy as it relates to anticipated adult weight?
   A. 2 to 4 g/kg
   B. 8 to 10 g/kg
   C. 2 to 4 mg/kg
   D. 8 to 10 mg/kg

7. At how many weeks of age should weaning begin in small-breed puppies?
   A. 6 to 8
   B. 4 to 5
   C. 2 to 3
   D. 1 to 2

8. Which nutrient should be reduced in the diet of geriatric dogs because of its detrimental effects on the kidneys?
   A. Zinc
   B. B-complex vitamins
   C. Phosphorus
   D. Vitamin A

9. Which is a common zoonotic disease caused by a fungal organism?
   A. Psittacosis
   B. Encephalitis
   C. Newcastle disease
   D. Ringworm

10. Which common disease has signs and symptoms that include polyuria and polydipsia?
    A. Congestive heart failure
    B. Diabetes mellitus
    C. Heartworm disease
    D. Hypothyroidism

CHAPTER 7 SURGICAL PREPARATION AND ASSISTING

1. Débridement of contaminated wounds is usually completed in what part of the hospital?
   - A. Surgery room
   - B. Scrub area
   - C. Prep area
   - D. Waiting area
2. Which term refers to the destruction of all microorganisms?
   - A. Sterilization
   - B. Disinfection
   - C. Asepsis
   - D. Nosocomial
3. Which term refers to infections acquired within the hospital?
   - A. Sterilization
   - B. Disinfection
   - C. Asepsis
   - D. Nosocomial
4. Which term refers to a disinfectant that inhibits the growth of microorganisms?
   - A. Bactericidal (kills bacteria)
   - B. Bacteriostatic (inhibits growth of bacteria)
   - C. Sporicidal (kills spores)
   - D. Virucidal (kills viruses)
5. What autoclave time and temperature combination is needed to achieve complete sterilization of most items?
   - A. 9 to 15 minutes at 249.8°F (121°C)
   - B. 2 to 6 minutes at 122°F (50°C)
   - C. 6 to 8 minutes at 212°F (100°C)
   - D. 3 to 9 minutes at 167°F (75°C)
6. Which surgical tool is used to cut heavy tissue?
   - A. Metzenbaum
   - B. Mayo
   - C. Olsen–Hegar
   - D. Kelly
7. Which is an absorbable suture material?
   - A. Silk
   - B. Stainless steel
   - C. Cotton
   - D. Catgut
8. Which incision is oriented perpendicular to the long axis of the body, caudal to the last rib?
   - A. Paramedia
   - B. Ventral midline
   - C. Flank
   - D. Paracostal
9. Which procedure involves suturing the stomach to the abdominal wall to fix it in place?
   - A. Gastropexy
   - B. Enterotomy
   - C. Gastrotomy
   - D. Anastomosis
10. What size endotracheal tube would be most appropriate for a 40-pound dog?
    - A. 3 to 3.5 mm
    - B. 5 to 5.5 mm
    - C. 7 to 7.5 mm
    - D. 9 to 9.5 mm

CHAPTER 8 LABORATORY PROCEDURES

1. What is the final concentration of a 20 mg/mL solution that is diluted 1:5?
   - A. 4
   - B. 10
   - C. 12
   - D. 15
2. What is the total magnification of an item viewed under the microscope with the low-power lens?
   - A. 10
   - B. 100
   - C. 1000
   - D. 10,000
3. Which component of the microscope serves to focus the light through the object being viewed?
   - A. Rheostat
   - B. Nosepiece
   - C. Substage condenser
   - D. Aperture diaphragm
4. Which instrument is used to determine urine specific gravity?
   - A. Clinical centrifuge
   - B. Incubator
   - C. Microhematocrit centrifuge
   - D. Refractometer
5. Which type of analyzer counts and classifies cells based on their sizes?
   - A. Impedance
   - B. Laser-based
   - C. Electrochemical
   - D. Photometer
6. Which anticoagulant is preferred for routine hematologic studies because it preserves cell morphology?
   - A. Heparin
   - B. Sodium citrate
   - C. EDTA
   - D. Fluoride
7. Which can be a cause of an increased PCV?
   - A. Dehydration
   - B. Excessive plasma because of inadequate mixing of the sample
   - C. Low blood-to-anticoagulant ratio
   - D. Anemia
8. Which is the most common inherited coagulation disorder of domestic animals?
   - A. Thrombocytopenia
   - B. von Willebrand disease
   - C. Bone marrow depression
   - D. Petechia

9. Which test is used to aid in evaluation of kidney function?
   A. Glucose
   B. Bile acids
   C. Fructosamine
   D. Blood urea nitrogen
10. Which is the most common type of in-house immunologic test?
   A. Coombs
   B. Polymerase chain reaction
   C. ELISA
   D. Immunodiffusion

CHAPTER 9 DIAGNOSTIC IMAGING

1. Where are the electrons generated in the x-ray tube?
   A. Tungsten target of the anode
   B. Tungsten filament of the anode
   C. Tungsten target of the cathode
   D. Tungsten filament of the cathode
2. What causes the anode heel effect?
   A. Focal spot oriented at an angle
   B. Collimation angled at 15 degrees
   C. Unequal distribution of the x-ray beam intensity emitted from the x-ray tube
   D. The x-ray beam penetrating power being reduced
3. Which refers to the radiographic density?
   A. The difference between adjacent areas on a radiographic image
   B. The degree of blackness on a radiograph
   C. The sharpness between interfaces of tissue and organs
   D. The fuzziness between interfaces of tissue and organs
4. Which of the following refers to the radiographic contrast?
   A. The difference between adjacent areas on a radiographic image
   B. The degree of blackness on a radiograph
   C. The sharpness between interfaces of tissue and organs
   D. The fuzziness between interfaces of tissue and organs
5. If 10 mA is used for an initial film and the density of the radiograph must be doubled for subsequent films, which mA should be used?
   A. 20
   B. 12
   C. 40
   D. 25
6. Which is the equivalent to an exposure setting of 200 mA for 1/40 second?
   A. 4 mA
   B. 5 mA
   C. 8 mA
   D. 15 mA

7. Which term describes a film's inherent ability to produce shades of gray?
   A. Latitude
   B. Sensitivity
   C. Scale
   D. Contrast
8. Which term best describes an area with the same echotexture as surrounding tissues?
   A. Hyperechoic
   B. Hypoechoic
   C. Anechoic
   D. Isoechoic
9. Which is an example of a negative-contrast medium?
   A. BIPS
   B. Meglumine
   C. Barium sulfate
   D. Oxygen
10. What is the center landmark for a radiograph of the thorax?
   A. Spine of scapula
   B. Ischium
   C. Caudal border of the scapula
   D. Wings of ilium

CHAPTER 10 LARGE ANIMAL NURSING AND HUSBANDRY

1. Which term is used to describe fermented forage material?
   A. Spoilage
   B. Silage
   C. Feedstuff
   D. Concentrates
2. Which is generally low in fiber and high in energy and/or protein?
   A. Spoilage
   B. Silage
   C. Feedstuff
   D. Concentrates
3. Which body condition score would be applicable to a livestock species exhibiting minimal subcutaneous fat with individual ribs not obvious?
   A. 1.0
   B. 2.5
   C. 3.0
   D. 3.5
4. Which condition can occur in horses when the feet are infrequently cleaned or if the horse stands for long periods in damp bedding or muddy soil?
   A. Thrush
   B. Laminitis
   C. Wethers
   D. Colitis

5. Which condition can occur in horses with accidental exposure to black walnut shavings when the horse stands in the shavings?
   A. Thrush
   B. Laminitis
   C. Wethers
   D. Colitis
6. Which term describes a female chicken that has not yet started to lay eggs?
   A. Capon
   B. Hen
   C. Pullet
   D. Broiler
7. What is the approximate gestation period for cattle?
   A. 6 months
   B. 9 months
   C. 12 months
   D. 15 months
8. Which term describes a castrated male sheep?
   A. Ram
   B. Buck
   C. Wether
   D. Ewe
9. Which term describes a young female pig that has not yet farrowed?
   A. Gilt
   B. Buck
   C. Wether
   D. Sow
10. What is the vessel of choice for blood collection in swine?
   A. Jugular
   B. Cephalic
   C. Saphenous
   D. Cranial vena cava

CHAPTER 11 AVIAN AND EXOTIC ANIMAL CARE AND NURSING

1. What is the life span of most small mammals?
   A. 6 to 9 months
   B. 9 to 15 months
   C. 2 to 4 years
   D. 5 to 7 years
2. What is an acceptable humidity range for most small mammals?
   A. 10% to 25%
   B. 30% to 70%
   C. 75% to 85%
   D. 90% to 95%

3. Which is a small breed of rabbit, weighing between 2 and 6 kg?
   A. Polish
   B. New Zealand
   C. California
   D. Flemish
4. Which is a viral disease to which ferrets are susceptible and must be vaccinated against?
   A. Anemia
   B. Human influenza
   C. Insulinoma
   D. Canine distemper
5. Which can cause snuffles in rabbits?
   A. Canine distemper
   B. *Pasteurella multocida*
   C. *Psoroptes* spp.
   D. Bone marrow suppression
6. To what species does the term murine refer?
   A. Rats
   B. Guinea pigs
   C. Chinchillas
   D. Rabbits
7. Which species should be bred before six months of age before pelvic fusion can result in dystocia?
   A. Rats
   B. Ferrets
   C. Rabbits
   D. Guinea pigs
8. Which structure in avian species functions to grind food into smaller particles?
   A. Proventriculus
   B. Crop
   C. Gizzard
   D. Cloaca
9. Which shape are the eyes of nocturnal birds?
   A. Round
   B. Flat
   C. Oval
   D. Tubular
10. What is the vessel of choice for administration of fluids in chelonians?
   A. Caudal tail vein
   B. Jugular vein
   C. Ventral abdominal vein
   D. Lingual vein

Index

Note: Page numbers followed by "*b*", "*f*" and "*t*" indicate boxes, figures and tables respectively.